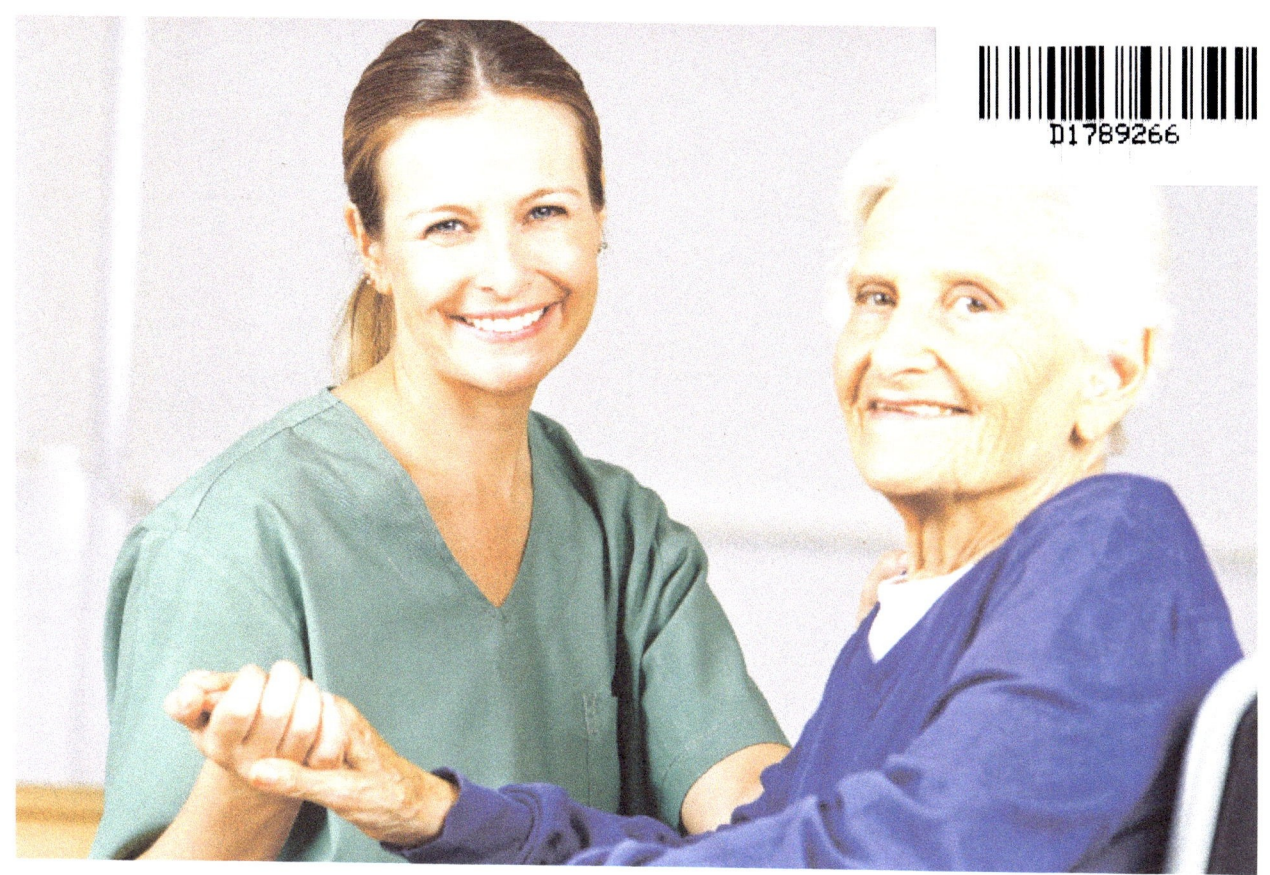

BMJ Clinical Review:

Geriatrics, Mental Health and Social Care

by
Professor Dr Babita Jyoti & Dr Ahmed Hamad

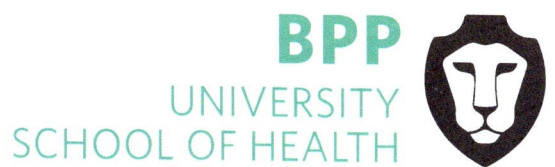

BPP
UNIVERSITY
SCHOOL OF HEALTH

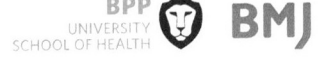

First edition April 2016

ISBN 9781 4727 4726 6
eISBN 9781 4727 4329 9
eISBN 9781 4727 4325 1

British Library Cataloguing-in-Publication Data
A catalogue record for this book is available from the British Library

Published by
BPP Learning Media Ltd
BPP House, Aldine Place
London W12 8AA

www.bpp.com/health

Printed in the United Kingdom by
CPI Antony Rowe

Bumper's Farm,
Chippenham,
Wiltshire
SN14 6LH

Your learning materials, published by BPP Learning Media Ltd, are printed on paper sourced from sustainable, managed forests.

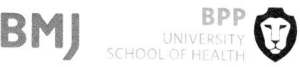

About the publisher

BPP Learning Media is dedicated to supporting aspiring professionals with top quality learning material. BPP Learning Media's commitment to success is shown by our record of quality, innovation and market leadership in paper-based and e-learning materials. BPP Learning Media's study materials are written by professionally-qualified specialists who know from personal experience the importance of top quality materials for success.

About The BMJ

The BMJ (formerly the British Medical Journal) in print has a long history and has been published without interruption since 1840. The BMJ's vision is to be the world's most influential and widely read medical journal. Our mission is to lead the debate on health and to engage, inform, and stimulate doctors, researchers, and other health professionals in ways that will improve outcomes for patients. We aim to help doctors to make better decisions. BMJ, the company, advances healthcare worldwide by sharing knowledge and expertise to improve experiences, outcomes and value.

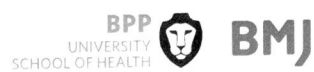

Contents

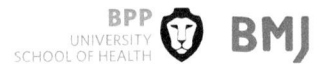

About the editors

Dr Babita Jyoti is a Radiation Oncologist with a special interest in Paediatric Proton Therapy. She graduated in Medicine in India followed by training in UK and obtained MRCP (UK) & FRCR (UK). She trained as a Clinical Oncologist at Clatterbridge Cancer Centre. She is currently working at the University of Florida Health Proton Therapy Institute in Paediatric Proton Therapy. She has been a PBL tutor and an OSCE examiner at Manchester Medical School.

Dr Ahmed Hamad is a Registrar in General Surgery with special interest in Breast Surgery at Mid Cheshire Hospitals NHS Trust. He graduated in 1992 from Cairo University School of Medicine in Egypt. Initially trained in Surgical Oncology, he received a Masters Degree in Surgery in 1997 from Cairo University. After completing his training in General Surgery, he worked as a Specialist in Surgery in different hospitals in Egypt, Saudi Arabia and Kuwait. He has become a Member of the Royal College of Surgeons of England in 2009 and in 2010, he joined the NHS, initially in General Surgery and is currently developing more experience in Breast Surgery.

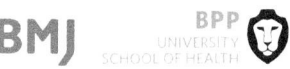

Introduction to Geriatrics, Mental Health and Social Care

Ten million people in the UK are over 65 years old. This number will have nearly doubled to approximately 19 million by 2050. Within this grand total, the number of very old people (>80 years of age) will grow even faster. There are currently three million people aged 80 years or more and this is projected to almost double by 2030 and reach eight million by 2050. While one-in-six of the UK population is currently aged 65 and over, by 2050 one in-four will be. *

Dementia is one of the main causes of disability in later life, ahead of some cancers, cardiovascular disease and stroke. Depression affects 22% of men and 28% of women aged 65 or over. This equates to just over two million people aged 65+ in England. The Royal College of Psychiatrists estimates that 85% of older people with depression receive no help at all from the NHS.

Another study estimates that depression affects 40% of older people in care homes. Poor general health can be associated with depression amongst older adults together with not living close to friends and family, poor satisfaction with accommodation and poor satisfaction with finances.

Previous figures highlight the increasing challenges facing healthcare providers dealing with an aging population as well as issues in mental health and social services which are not only a concern to elderly care physicians and psychiatrists, but also to almost all healthcare providers in the 21st century.

In this book you will find a carefully selected series of clinical reviews from The BMJ that we believe can help refresh and update knowledge on topics relevant to elderly patient care, mental health and social care.

Although systematic reviews and meta-analyses provide more comprehensive details, evidence and statistical analysis of certain topics, clinical reviews are of no less importance as they tend to be more applicable to the local situation than a systematic review, because they may take into account local shortages of equipment or personnel. **

In addition to relevance to day-to-day practice, we believe the fascinating diversity in this book is an advantage. From all areas in the United Kingdom to Canada to Australia, healthcare professionals from a broad range of specialities and at various grades in their careers including registrars, general practitioners, consultants and university professors, have participated to author these clinical reviews in their respective fields.

All articles are provided in a simple format and, at the same time, summarise tips and advice which can be of great value especially with the increasing work load and pressure experienced by healthcare professionals.

*Richard Cracknell, Key Issues for the New Parliament 2010, House of Commons Library Research

**Dr Norman Vetter, University of Wales College of Medicine, Cardiff, Wales, UK

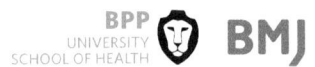

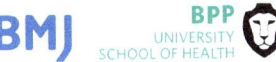

Fall assessment in older people

Jacqueline C T Close, consultant geriatrician[1][2][3], Stephen R Lord, senior principal research fellow[3]

[1]Falls and Injury Prevention Group, Neuroscience Research Australia, University of New South Wales, Randwick, Sydney, NSW 2031, Australia

[2]Prince of Wales Clinical School, University of New South Wales

[3]Falls and Balance Research Group, Neuroscience Research Australia, University of New South Wales

Correspondence to: J C T Close
j.close@neura.edu.au

Cite this as: BMJ 2011;343:d5153

DOI: 10.1136/bmj.d5153

http://www.bmj.com/content/343/bmj.d5153

Falls are common in older people and are the leading cause of injury related admissions to hospital in people of 65 years and over, accounting for about 14% of emergency admissions and 4% of all hospital admissions in this age group.[1] A fall may result from acute disease (for example, chest infection), chronic underlying pathology (for example, Parkinson's disease), or the interaction of a person with their surroundings (for example, tripping on a pavement). Evidence indicates that many falls could be prevented through appropriate assessment and intervention.[2][3][4] The terms "fall risk screening" and "fall risk assessment" are sometimes used interchangeably. Screening is a process that primarily aims to identify people at increased risk of falls, whereas assessment aims to identify factors that increase the risk of a fall that can be dealt with by subsequent intervention. In the community setting, a fall risk screen can be used at a population level to identify older people who need a more detailed fall risk assessment and intervention or onward referral (see box 1).

How best to assess risk of falling?

Many tools for screening and assessing fall risk have been developed for use in older people in community, hospital, and nursing and residential care settings. However, only some have been evaluated for reliability and predictive validity in prospective studies and have reasonable sensitivity and specificity—that is, they have acceptably high accuracy in predicting those who will or will not fall.

Screening and assessment of older people in the community

UK national and international guidelines recommend that the general practitioner or other community based health professional asks all older people (or their carers) about any falls and undertakes a brief mobility screen on an annual basis.[5][6] The "timed up and go test" is one of the more commonly used screening tests and gives a global indication of postural stability. Although results from studies vary, a time of 12 or more seconds to complete the test (for people who live in the community) is an indicator of impaired functioning and increased risk of falls.[7][8] Other community based screening tools can be found on bmj.com.

The emergency department provides a useful opportunity to screen older people for their risk of falling and to refer for assessment. However, when using screening tools that involve physical tests in this setting, interpret the results with caution because an acute injury from a fall may affect the person's ability to perform these tests. A screening tool based on questions alone may be a useful alternative (table 1).[9]

A history of two or more falls in the previous year negates the need for screening in the community and should trigger a detailed assessment (see box 2). This is consistent with the suggested algorithm in the recently published guidelines from the American Geriatric Society and British Geriatric Society[5] and the Australian Commission on Safety and Quality of Health Care.[3]

Offer further assessment to community dwelling older people who have been identified by screening as at risk of falls and to those who report two or more falls in the past year. General practitioners or other health professionals may assess fall risk using a multifactorial assessment tool that covers a range of risk factors or functional mobility assessments that focus on the physiological and functional domains of postural stability, including vision, strength, coordination, balance, and gait. Many disease processes that increase fall risk do so by impairing postural stability; examples include impaired vision from cataracts, impaired balance and proprioception from diabetic peripheral neuropathy, and reduced proximal muscle strength and reaction time because of vitamin D deficiency.

Table 1 provides example of validated assessment tools.[10][11][12][13][14][15] Other fall risk assessments can be found in the additional tables on bmj.com.[16][17][18][19][20][21][22] Most validated risk assessment tools focus on postural stability, gait, and balance. The short physical performance battery is a widely used tool for assessing the ability to rise from a chair, standing, and gait, and it has been validated against self reported disability, need for nursing home care, and mortality.[23] Assessment tools like QuickScreen assess postural stability and include additional items that may guide intervention, such as visual assessment and documentation of drug use (see box 3). The results of the assessment may show the need for direct intervention—such as reduction in dose or discontinuation of a drug that is causing postural hypotension—or onward referral for further assessment and intervention—such as referral to an ophthalmologist for cataract extraction.

Table 2 highlights risk factors that may be identified during an assessment and links them to suggested interventions. Most of these suggested interventions reflect evidence generated through randomised controlled clinical trials.[2]

Screening and assessment in hospitals

An acute admission to hospital for an older person is often associated with a change in physical or cognitive status (or both), which when combined with exposure to an unfamiliar environment presents a concomitant increase in risk of falls. Falls are one of the most common adverse events experienced in hospitals and can lead to injury, prolonged hospital stay, and death. Valid...

SUMMARY POINTS

- Fall risk screening identifies people at increased risk of falls who need detailed fall risk assessment and intervention, which can in turn prevent falls and fall related injury

- Quick validated fall risk screening tools for older people are available for community, hospital, and nursing and residential care settings

- Screen older people living in the community for fall risk every 12 months and assess for risk factors after a fall

- Fall risk in hospital inpatients is changeable because physical and cognitive abilities may alter during a hospital stay

- Although all older people in nursing and residential care are at high risk of falls, a screening tool that includes their ability to stand unaided and risk factors such as cognitive impairment, incontinence, and drug use can provide extra information about fall risk

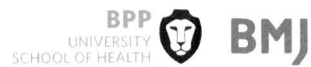

BOX 1 CASE SCENARIO

Mrs F, aged 82, has been brought to the emergency department by ambulance after tripping on a pavement while out shopping.

- **Outcome 1 (community screening and assessment):** She is assessed in the emergency department as not having a serious injury and is discharged home, advised to take simple analgesia for any pain resulting from the fall, and to consult her GP about future fall prevention.
- **Outcome 2 (hospital and residential aged care screening and assessment):** She is diagnosed with a fractured neck of femur and admitted to the hospital under the care of the orthopaedic surgeons where she undergoes surgery.

BOX 2 CASE SCENARIO (OUTCOME 1): ASSESSMENT IN THE COMMUNITY

Mrs F was discharged home from the emergency department and when she next visited her general practitioner she mentioned that she had fallen and was taken to the local emergency department by ambulance. Because this was her second fall in a year, the general practitioner undertook a more detailed fall risk assessment.

for help in getting to the toilet). In patients with delirium or cognitive impairment, changes in staff practice and environmental modifications are needed.

Screening and assessment in nursing and residential care facilities for older people

Falls are more common in older people who are in nursing and residential care facilities than in those who live in the community, and it has been argued that screening is not needed in this population because all residents are at increased risk. However, one simple validated screen looks at residents' ability to stand unaided in association with risk factors such as cognitive impairment, incontinence, and drug use and can provide additional information about fall risk in this group (table 1).[15] The screen identifies different risk factors for those who can and cannot stand unaided and draws attention to the non-linear association between fall risk and physical function—fall rates are low in those

tools are available to identify those who are most likely to fall during an inpatient stay. The two most commonly used tools are the St Thomas' risk assessment tool (STRATIFY)[19] and the modified STRATIFY (table 1).[14] Patients identified as being at increased risk of falls require further assessment to determine the nature of the increased risk so that interventions can be individually tailored. Fall risk assessment should be viewed as a dynamic process, given that a patient's physical and cognitive abilities may alter while in hospital (see box 4). It is crucial to assess cognition because strategies that require the patient's understanding and cooperation may not be feasible in people with delirium or cognitive impairment (for example, pushing the call bell

Table 1 Examples of validated tests and tools available for screening and assessment of fall risk

Test and criteria	Practical aspects
Screening in the community: timed up and go test[10-12]	
Description	This test measures the time taken for a person to rise from a chair, walk 3 m at normal pace with their usual assistive device, turn, return to the chair, and sit down
Criterion	A time of ≥12 seconds indicates increased risk of falling
Time to undertake test	1-2 minutes
Equipment	Chair and stopwatch or minute hand on watch
Assessment in the community: QuickScreen[13]	
Description	QuickScreen is a risk assessment tool designed for use by practice and rural nurses, allied health workers, and general practitioners. It allows the clinician to estimate the level of increased fall risk and determine which sensorimotor systems are impaired. The test measures previous falls, drug use, vision, peripheral sensation, lower limb strength, balance, and coordination
Criterion	A score of 4 or more indicates an increased risk of falling
Time to undertake test	10 minutes
Equipment	A low contrast eye chart, a filament for measuring touch sensation, and a small step
Screening in the emergency department: Prevention of Falls in the Elderly Trial[9]	
Description	Used in people presenting to the emergency department after a fall. Three simple questions identify people at increased risk of further falls: (1) Have you had any other falls over the past 12 months? (2) Have you fallen indoors? (3) Have you been unable to get up after a fall?
Criterion	If the patient answers yes to any of the questions further assessment and intervention are needed
Time to undertake test	1-2 minutes
Equipment	None
Screening in hospital: modified STRATIFY[14]	
Description	Six item weighted questionnaire with questions relating to falls, cognition, transfer and mobility skills, vision, and toileting practice
Criterion	A score of .9 identifies high risk fallers
Time to undertake test	1-2 minutes
Equipment	None
Screening in nursing and residential care: residential aged care falls screen[15]	
Description	Clinical algorithm based on the person's ability to stand unaided, previous falls, drug use, and continence status
Criterion	Depending on risk factors identified, outcome will be either high or low risk of falls
Time to undertake test	1-2 minutes
Equipment	Medium density 15 cm thick foam mat

STRATIFY=St Thomas' risk assessment tool.

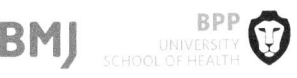

BOX 3 CASE SCENARIO (OUTCOME 1): QUICKSCREEN

Mrs F was assessed by the general practitioner using the QuickScreen assessment tool (table 1)[13] and several fall risk factors were identified—poor strength and balance because of a sedentary lifestyle, probable vitamin D deficiency from limited sunlight exposure, and the use of bifocal glasses. As a result of the assessment it was agreed that Mrs F needed to do specific exercises to improve balance and strength and to continue these exercises long term. She was started on vitamin D supplements and told that bifocal glasses pose a fall risk when worn outdoors, with the recommendation that she wear single lens glasses when away from home. Mrs F adopted the interventions, and at a follow-up fall risk assessment with her general practitioner 12 months later, she reported improved balance, increased confidence, and no further falls.

BOX 4 CASE SCENARIO (OUTCOME 2): ASSESSMENT IN HOSPITAL

On admission to the orthopaedic ward, Mrs F was assessed for risk of falls. At this point she was unable to transfer or mobilise and was not confused. The modified STRATIFY indicated that she was not at high risk of falls.[14] However, after her surgery she developed a hyperactive delirium, became impulsive and tried to get out of her bed and chair. Given the change in her clinical status, her fall risk was reassessed using the modified STRATIFY. This indicated that she was now at high risk because of her change in cognitive status and a poor performance in the mobility component. The staff moved her to an area where she could be closely observed, reviewed her pain control, and developed a plan for regular toileting. In addition, they lowered her bed to its minimum height and fitted a bed alarm to alert staff if she attempted to get up unsupervised. Finally, they asked her daughter if it would be possible for her to sit with Mrs F during the day and arrange for additional staff observation overnight until Mrs F was no longer delirious and impulsive. With these interventions in place, Mrs F did not fall during her hospital stay.

with very poor functioning (as well as those with good functioning) because of reduced exposure to risk as a result of being bed bound or wheelchair bound.[24]

As in the community setting, assessment should be linked to intervention, and several approaches have been shown to be effective in nursing and residential care facilities for older people.[3 4] Vitamin D supplementation is a simple intervention with evidence of benefit in fall prevention in older people living in nursing and residential care facilities (see box 5), particularly those with low vitamin D values (<50 nmol/L).[4] Other effective interventions deal with risk factors identified by a multifaceted assessment—factors specific to the individual (cognition, physical function, drug use, and hydration) and to the environment (such as distance to toilet or dining area and lighting at night).[4]

What are the challenges?

Despite the evidence supporting fall risk factor assessment and intervention, fall risk assessment is still not routinely undertaken, and many people who could benefit from falls and fracture interventions are not receiving guideline care.[25] This may be due, in part, to some healthcare professionals being unaware of effective approaches to intervention.

The multifactorial nature of falls and the need to assess multiple domains and involve several healthcare professionals can seem overwhelming for the patient and the clinician undertaking the initial screen or assessment. Fortunately, clearer approaches based on systematic evidence for fall prevention in different settings are now available. Time pressures are a reality in practice, and it may be necessary—as well as more appropriate for the older person—to look at one risk factor at a time and review progress in subsequent consultations. Individual perception of fall risk is also important, and many older people—as well as some healthcare professionals—describe falling as an inevitable consequence of ageing. It can be difficult to motivate older people to undertake exercise that targets balance and strength, particularly when the potential benefits are accrued over months rather than days and lost when the exercise is stopped. It is important for practitioners to prescribe exercise as an ongoing activity. Fall and fracture

Table 2 Examples of linking assessment to evidence based interventions[2]

Risk factor	Assessment	Intervention
Impaired balance and mobility	QuickScreen, short physical performance battery, physiological profile assessment, Berg balance scale, and performance oriented mobility assessment	Consider home or group based strength and balance training programme; ensure that any underlying cause for impaired balance and mobility, such as vitamin D deficiency, vitamin B-12 deficiency, use of central nervous system drugs, and pain, is dealt with if possible
Impaired vision	Snellen eye chart; Melbourne edge test; review spectacles; check for evidence of cataracts	If cataracts are impairing vision, refer for extraction; if the patient is using bifocal or multifocal glasses, recommend a separate pair of single lens glasses for use outdoors
Syncope or dizziness	Lying and standing blood pressure measurements; Holter monitoring and carotid sinus massage; Dix-Hallpike test	Review any drugs that might contribute to orthostatic hypotension; consider insertion of a pacemaker for prolonged periods of asystole; consider Epley manoeuvre if dizziness is thought to be related to benign paroxysmal positional vertigo
Feet and footwear	Foot pain and deformity	Treat pain and consider referral to podiatrist and provision of ankle strengthening and mobility exercises
Drug use	Drug review	Stop any drugs that affect the central nervous system unless there is an ongoing clinical indication; ensure calcium and vitamin D intake are sufficient and if not consider supplementation
Environment	Home assessment by an occupational therapist in people identified at high risk of falls	Modification of the home environment with provision of support and advice on safety within and outside the home
Cognition	Mini mental state examination with additional measures of cognition if indicated	Consider the effect of any cognitive deficits on the ability to engage in an intervention

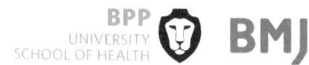

prevention may be less effective if not incorporated into the management of coexisting chronic conditions, such as diabetes, osteoporosis, and chronic obstructive pulmonary disease. This may be particularly relevant when exercise plans need to be modified to deal with a person's deficits.

Finally, evidence of the effectiveness of fall prevention initiatives is still limited in some high risk populations, including older people with dementia, Parkinson's disease, depression, and a previous stroke. Further research is needed to determine optimal interventions for these groups. In the interim, "standard" fall prevention strategies should be implemented.[3]

Conclusion

Validated fall risk screens and assessments are now available for older people in community, hospital, and nursing and residential care settings, and randomised controlled trials provide good evidence that falls can be prevented by tackling identified risk factors. A fall assessment should therefore be a key part of guideline care of older people.

SOURCES AND SELECTION CRITERIA

As well as using our personal reference collections, we used the most up to date Cochrane reviews as well as national and international guidelines, including those from the National Institute for Health and Clinical Excellence, the American and British Geriatric Society falls prevention guidelines, and the Australian national falls prevention guidelines for communities, hospitals, and residential age care facilities.

This is the third in a series of four articles about assessing older people.

Contributors: Both authors helped plan, draft, and revise the article and are guarantors.

Competing interests: Both authors have completed the ICMJE uniform disclosure form at www.icmje.org/coi_disclosure.pdf (available on request from the corresponding author) and declare: no support from any organisation for the submitted work; JCTC had no financial relationships with any organisations that might have an interest in the submitted work in the previous three years; SRL declares that the FallScreen and QuickScreen fall risk assessment tools are commercially available through Neuroscience Research Australia (NeuRA); any profits from sales of the assessments are shared between the inventors (which include SRL), the falls and balance research group at NeuRA, and the NeuRA central fund; with regard to QuickScreen, SRL's share and a matching NeuRA central fund share are transferred to the falls and balance research group for research purposes; no other relationships or activities that could appear to have influenced the submitted work.

Provenance and peer review: Commissioned; externally peer reviewed.

Patient consent not required (patient anonymised, dead, or hypothetical).

IMPROVING PRACTICE

Resources for healthcare professionals
- American Geriatric Society/British Geriatric Society. Clinical practice guidelines for falls prevention in older people. 2010. www.americangeriatrics.org/health_care_professionals/ clinical_practice/clinical_guidelines_recommendations/2010/
- Prevention of Falls Network Earth (http://profane.co/)— Interactive and up to date website combining latest evidence and practical examples of activities in falls assessment and prevention; UK focus
- Gillespie LD, Robertson MC, Gillespie WJ, Lamb SE, Gates S, Cumming RG, et al. Interventions for preventing falls in older people living in the community. *Cochrane Database Syst Rev* 2008;2:CD007146
- Cameron ID, Murray GR, Gillespie LD, Robertson MC, Hill KD, Cumming RG, et al. Interventions for preventing falls in older people in nursing care facilities and hospitals. *Cochrane Database Syst Rev* 2010;1:CD005465

BMJ Group resources
- BMJ Learning module. Discharge planning: a guide: http://learning.bmj.com/learning/search-result. html?moduleId=10017723
- Best Practice. Assessment of falls in the elderly: http:// bestpractice.bmj.com/best-practice/monograph/880.html

Resources for older people
- Aged UK. Falls awareness week. www.ageuk.org.uk/ health-wellbeing/national-falls-awareness-week/
- Aged UK. Information leaflet: Staying steady—improving your strength and balance. www.ageuk.org.uk/Global/Age-Cymru/ Information-and-Advice/AGEUKIG14%20Staying%20Steady%20 A52032pp_inf.pdf

1. Close J, Ellis M, Hooper R, Glucksman E, Jackson S, Swift C. Prevention of Falls in the Elderly Trial (PROFET): a randomised controlled trial. *Lancet* 1999;353:93-7.
2. Gillespie LD, Robertson MC, Gillespie WJ, Lamb SE, Gates S, Cumming RG, et al. Interventions for preventing falls in older people living in the community. *Cochrane Database Syst Rev* 2008;2:CD007146.
3. Australian Commission on Safety and Quality in Health Care. Falls prevention guidelines—preventing falls and harm from falls in older people: best practice guidelines for Australian hospitals, residential aged care facilities and community care. 2009. www.health.gov.au/ internet/safety/publishing.nsf/content/FallsGuidelines.
4. Cameron ID, Murray GR, Gillespie LD, Robertson MC, Hill KD, Cumming RG, et al. Interventions for preventing falls in older people in nursing care facilities and hospitals. *Cochrane Database Syst Rev* 2010;1:CD005465.
5. Panel on Prevention of Falls in Older Persons AGS, British Geriatrics S. Summary of the updated American Geriatrics Society/British Geriatrics Society clinical practice guideline for prevention of falls in older persons. *J Am Geriatr Soc* 2011;59:148-57.
6. National Institute for Health and Clinical Excellence. Falls: the assessment and prevention of falls in older people. 2004. www.nice. org.uk/CG21.
7. Shumway-Cook A, Brauer S, Woollacott M. Predicting the probability for falls in community-dwelling older adults using the Timed Up & Go Test. *Phys Ther* 2000;80:896-903.
8. Whitney JC, Lord SR, Close JCT. Streamlining assessment and intervention in a falls clinic using the timed up and go test and physiological profile assessments. *Age Ageing* 2005;34:567.
9. Close JC, Hooper R, Glucksman E, Jackson SH, Swift CG. Predictors of falls in a high risk population: results from the Prevention of Falls in the Elderly Trial (PROFET). *Emerg Med J* 2003;20:421-5.
10. Shumway-Cook A, Baldwin M, Polissar NL, Gruber W. Predicting the probability for falls in community-dwelling older adults. *Phys Ther* 1997;77:812-9.
11. Gunter K, White KN, Hayes WC, Snow C. Functional mobility discriminates non-fallers from one-time and frequent fallers. *J Gerontol A Biol Sci Med Sci* 2000;55:M672-6.
12. Rose DJ, Jones CJ, Lucchese N. Predicting the probability of falls in community-residing older adults using the 8-foot up-and-go: a new measure of functional mobility. *J Aging Phys Activ* 2002;10:466-75.
13. Tiedemann AC, Sherrington C, Lord SR. The development of a brief performance-based fall risk assessment tool (QuickScreen) for community-dwelling older people. *J Gerontol A Biol Sci Med Sci* 2010;65A:896-903.

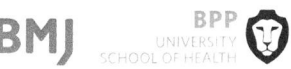

14 Papaioannou A, Parkinson W, Cook R, Ferko N, Coker E, Adachi J. Prediction of falls using a risk assessment tool in the acute care setting. *BMC Med* 2004;2:1.

15 Delbaere K, Close JCT, Menz HB, Cumming RG, Cameron ID, Sambrook PN, et al. Development and validation of fall risk screening tools for use in residential aged care facilities. *Med J Aust* 2008;189:193-6.

16 Tiedemann A, Shimada H, Sherrington C, Murray S, Lord S. The comparative ability of eight functional mobility tests for predicting falls in community-dwelling older people. *Age Ageing* 2008;37:430-5.

17 Russell MA, Hill KD, Blackberry I, Day LM, Dharmage SC. The reliability and predictive accuracy of the falls risk for older people in the community assessment (FROP-Com) tool. *Age Ageing* 2008;37:634-9.

18 Nandy S, Parsons S, Cryer C, Underwood M, Rashbrook E, Carter Y, et al. Development and preliminary examination of the predictive validity of the falls risk assessment tool (FRAT) for use in primary care. *J Public Health* 2004;26:138-43.

19 Oliver D, Britton M, Seed P, Martin FC, Happer AH. Development and evaluation of an evidence based falls risk assessment tool (STRATIFY) to predict which elderly inpatients will fall: case-control and cohort studies. *BMJ* 1997;315:1049-53.

20 Tinetti ME. Performance-oriented assessment of mobility problems in elderly patients. *J Am Geriatr Soc* 1986;34:119-26.

21 Lord SR, Menz HB, Tiedemann A. A physiological profile approach to falls risk assessment and prevention. *Phys Ther* 2003;83:237-52.

22 Sherrington C, Lord SR, Close JCT, Barraclough E, Taylor M, O'Rourke S, et al. Development of the prediction of falls in rehabilitation settings tool (Predict_FIRST): a prospective cohort study. *J Rehabil Med* 2010;42:482-8.

23 Guralnick JM, Simonsick EM, Ferruci L, Glynn RJ, Berkman LF, Blazer DG, et al. A short physical performance battery assessing lower extremity function: association with self-reported disability and prediction of mortality and nursing home admission. *J Gerontol* 1994;49:M85-94.

24 Lord SR, March LM, Cameron ID, Cumming RG, Schwarz J, Zochling J, et al. Differing risk factors for falls in nursing home and intermediate-care residents who can and cannot stand unaided. *J Am Geriatr Soc* 2003;51:1645-50.

25 Salter A, Khan K, Donaldson M, Davis J, Buchanan J, Abu-Laban R, et al. Community-dwelling seniors who present to the emergency department with a fall do not receive guideline care and their fall risk profile worsens significantly: a 6-month prospective study. *Osteoporosis Int* 2006;17:672-83.

Related links

bmj.com

- Cognitive assessment of older people (2011;343:d5042)
- Functional assessment in older people (2011;343:d4681)
- Get CME/CPD points for this article

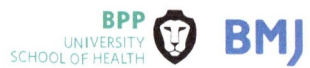

Functional assessment in older people

T J Quinn, lecturer in geriatric medicine[1], K McArthur, research fellow[1], G Ellis, consultant physician[2], D J Stott, professor of geriatric medicine[1]

[1]Institute of Cardiovascular and Medical Sciences, University of Glasgow, Glasgow, UK

[2]Department of Medicine for the Elderly, Monklands Hospital, Airdrie, UK

Correspondence to: T Quinn, Department of Academic Geriatric Medicine, Glasgow Royal Infirmary, Glasgow G4 0SF, UK terry.quinn@glasgow.ac.uk

Cite this as: BMJ 2011;343:d4681

DOI: 10.1136/bmj.d4681

http://www.bmj.com/content/343/bmj.d4681

Older people often present to healthcare services with acute and chronic problems that act together to adversely affect function. A common pathway comprises functional decline, followed by loss of independence and need for institutional care. However, this process is not necessarily inevitable or irreversible. Timely recognition of functional difficulties can lead to interventions that may prevent or arrest the decline. This article focuses on the functional assessment of older adults by generalist clinicians (see box 1 for terminology used in this broad field).

What is an assessment of functional status and why does it matter?

Decline in function itself may be a presentation of otherwise occult pathologies[4] so, not surprisingly, it is associated with increased mortality.[5] Relatively minor insults (such as changes to drugs and constipation) may precipitate substantial deterioration in function.[4] Systematic reviews have shown that intervention based on comprehensive geriatric assessment can improve physical function and reduce admission to care homes and hospital in older people.[1 6 7] The first step in this process is the recognition and description of functional problems—this task should be routine for all health professionals and not the sole preserve of the geriatrician.

It is unusual for patients themselves to identify functional decline,[8] and assessment precipitated by "crisis" remains common.[9] Because functional screening of unselected older populations has not consistently improved clinical outcomes,[10 11] opportunistic assessment is preferred and should form part of consultations for management of chronic diseases. We suggest a process of functional evaluation based on structured history and examination, which may be supplemented with standardised assessment instruments.

How is physical function best assessed?

The variable nature of presentations in older people makes it impossible to list all situations where functional assessment may be useful, but we suggest that such an assessment should always inform:

- Management of illness associated with any change in functional ability
- Consideration of transfer to a care home or integrated care setting
- The planning of major elective treatments, such as surgery.

The initial functional assessment screen does not require specialised equipment and can readily be conducted in the care home, general practice, accident and emergency department, or hospital ward or clinic. However, if the purpose is to determine how the patient would function in their own home, it is often best to perform assessments in that environment.

Throughout the assessment the focus must be on the patient: do they perceive the current level of function as problematic or do they have other difficulties that they prioritise at a higher level? For example, food preparation and outside mobility are important only if the patient still needs or wishes to engage in these tasks. The clinician should ascertain the views of the patient and carers at an early stage, including willingness to undergo investigation and expectations of treatment. Box 2 provides tips on performing a functional assessment.

History

We recommend a semi-structured approach to information gathering. The information required is not common to the usual "medical" interview, and we suggest that the descriptors used in activities of daily living (ADL) scales (box 3) guide the interview,[12] whether for initial evaluation or assessment of progress. Direct screening questions on mobility, falls, and continence are useful, given the prevalence of these problems and their potential effect on functioning.[13 14] Further assessment can be tailored to the patient's specific abilities and problems (box 4).

Patients may omit important symptoms, rationalising them as an inevitable consequence of ageing or fearing that admitting to problems may lead to placement in a care home. While exploring activities of daily living, make the distinction between what the patient wants to do, what they can do, and what they actually do—with the last descriptor being the most important.

With the patient's consent, proactively seek a history from as many perspectives as possible (family, carers, care home staff) to give a more objective description of current and previous function. Use health records, particularly to confirm extent or rate of decline. This process is easiest if information is available in a structured format such as the ADL questionnaires discussed below.

Clinical examination

A systems based physical examination may not always detect important problems that affect functional ability. Failure to appreciate the differences between functional assessment and traditional medical examination will frustrate the clinician and may deny the patient the opportunity for intervention.

SUMMARY POINTS

- In older adults functional decline is a common presentation of many disease states
- Causes and consequences are diverse, so functional assessment is not suited to a traditional medical model of system based history and examination
- Consider functional assessment "screening": where illness has caused change in function; before considering long term care; and when planning major elective procedures in older adults
- Validated scales for assessing basic and extended activities of daily living can help inform and focus history taking
- Key elements of the physical examination include subjective "end of the bed" assessment; upper and lower limbs; vision; hearing; and the patient's environment
- Functional decline is rarely related to a single problem, a problem list can guide intervention
- When functional change is evident, referral for multidisciplinary, comprehensive geriatric assessment is often needed

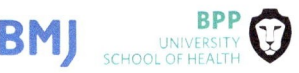

Video on bmj.com (see also http://bmj.com/video)

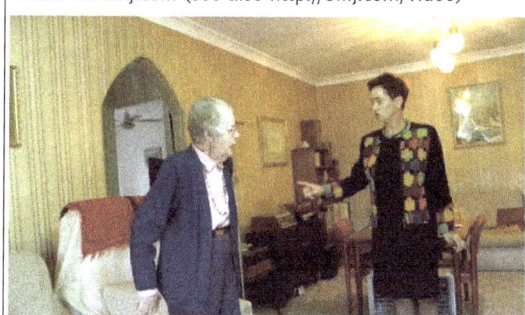

In this video, filmed in Australia, Dr Kurrle performs a functional assessment of an older adult in the home. We show some of the basic components of functional assessment that it is important for a doctor to know, some of which may be used in other settings, such as the GP surgery or on a hospital ward. In many settings an occupational therapist would provide a detailed assessment of the patient's home and their activities of daily living.

The assessment is split into stages

(1.30) – Living room: mobility, sit to stand, lighting and furniture, dexterity.

(3.00) – Kitchen: Turning on taps, cooking, holding a cup.

(4.40) – Bedroom: Dressing, transfers to and from bed.

(6.12) – Bathroom: Personal care, transfers to and from shower/bath.

(7.34) – Toilet: Transfer onto and off the toilet

(8.06) – Balcony Garden: Mobilisation out of door, hanging laundry.

(8.28) – General mobility: Walking with our without aid, climbing stairs.

(9.10) – Further assessment and interventions

BOX 1 LANGUAGE OF FUNCTIONAL ASSESSMENT

A detailed discussion on theories of function and disability is beyond the scope of this review, but an explanation of the terminology can help contextualise this complex field

- **Activities of daily living (ADL):** These are "everyday tasks," ranging from aspects of self care that are needed daily (such as toileting and eating—often described as basic or personal ADLs) through to more complex tasks (such as shopping, using a telephone—often described as instrumental or extended ADLs). When a person has difficulty with one or more basic activities, daily support (from family or carer) is needed for the person to remain safe

- **Comprehensive geriatric assessment:** The simultaneous multilevel assessment of various domains by a multidisciplinary team to ensure that problems are identified, quantified, and managed appropriately. This includes assessment of medical, psychiatric, functional, and social domains, followed by a management plan that often includes rehabilitation[1]

- **Disability:** A construct described in the World Health Organization's *International Classification of Functioning, Disability and Health* (ICF).[2] Disability (now termed activity limitation) refers to restrictions in performing usual tasks. ICF terminology recognises two other levels of function: physical impairment and handicap; all these levels of functioning are interconnected.[2] Quality of life measures seek to describe outcomes beyond participation in society and are outside the scope of WHO-ICF

- **Frailty:** A popular conceptual definition of frailty is "the propensity to deteriorate in the face of a stressor."[3] Frailty constructs range from simple measures of physical function, such as grip strength, through defined physical phenotypes, to complex multidimensional indices that are useful in research but difficult to apply in clinical practice

- **Functional ability:** Primarily refers to performance of basic and extended ADL to maintain safety. Thus functional ability is a global term and not synonymous with the more focused label "physical function." Although the focus of this review is physical function, comprehensive functional assessment should also include cognition, mood, and carer related matters

---

Where physical problems are evident from the history, explore the impact on function directly. As an example, if patients admit that they struggle to climb stairs, it is essential to observe them doing this, so ask them "could you show me?" Note patients' speed and safety in performing the task, not simply whether they complete it (box 4). Although direct observation of ADL is the most informative assessment, this is not always practical, and for certain items (toileting, bathing) may not be acceptable to the patient.

In addition we recommend a "screening" assessment, which should be useful in all older people and can direct further focused examination. As an aide memoire we suggest the mnemonic PULSE (adapted from the PULSES assessment tool[18])

P (physical condition)

A key component is the initial general inspection. Subjective "end of the bed" assessment has clinical value, and recognition of specific abnormalities (wasting of intrinsic hand muscles, abnormal posture, tremor) may direct further assessment. Problems in older people often develop in areas of the body not covered by "conventional" examination. Unless actively looked for, the clinician may miss rectifiable problems that will affect physical function. A comprehensive examination may not be possible in the initial consultation, and assessment should be directed by the history. For example, problems with mobility should prompt examination of the feet, where common problems

that affect walking, such as onychogryphosis (toenail hypertrophy and distortion) or peripheral neuropathy may be detected. Other important areas that should be actively screened, particularly in frailer patients, are pressure areas and the oral cavity; a rectal examination may be useful, particularly if constipation is suspected.

U (upper limb function)

Because this is crucial in accomplishing most activities of daily living, specific assessment is important. Tests of the ability to lift and carry objects (such as a cup) screen for proximal functional ability. Assessment of manual dexterity and fine motor ability (such as tying shoelaces or managing buttons) can serve as a screen for distal upper limb function.

L (lower limb function)

Gait and balance are fundamental components of lower limb function. Observation of walking provides useful information on strength, joint function, and balance. Begin by observing mobility around the room, with patients using their usual stick or frame.

For the non-specialist, we suggest the "get up and go test"[13] (box 5) as a lower limb assessment. This tool was developed as a screening test for falls but can be used as

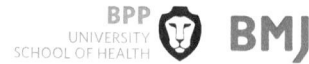

BOX 2 TIPS ON FUNCTIONAL ASSESSMENT IN OLDER PEOPLE

- **Take time:** Interviewing and examining the older patient will generally take longer than for other patients, so allow yourself and the patient enough time. Assessments may be spread over several consultations. After an initial clinic or office visit, a longer assessment in the patient's home may ultimately be more time efficient than multiple consultations in the surgery

- **Review case notes:** Patients with multiple comorbidities often attend many hospitals and other services, so taking the time to review previous correspondence before seeing the patient will make for a more efficient assessment

- **Establish effective communication:** Does the patient hear you and understand you; do you understand them?

- **Keep it simple and functional:** Assessment does not require specialist equipment. When taking a history and examining the patient, you should not simply record the pathology but include a description of the impact on physical functional ability. For example, in a stroke survivor, a report of "weakness MRC grade 4 lower limb" may be technically correct, but a functional descriptor, such as "leg weakness, leading to frequent falls and inability to climb stairs," is more useful

- **Ensure aids are used:** Aids to improve functioning are often available to the patient but may not be consistently or appropriately used. If the patient uses a hearing aid, ensure it is worn and working; ensure glasses are worn; ensure that footwear is appropriate and that mobility aids (such as a walking stick or frame) are used

- **Collate a problem list:** Often more than one problem contributes to a functional "crisis." A unifying diagnosis is less important than identifying all the modifiable contributors; multiple problems may need to be tackled in parallel (see case study, box 4)

- **Get expert help:** When physical functional problems are discovered there must be clear referral pathways to multidisciplinary rehabilitation teams that include medical assessment. Multiple agencies may be needed and are more effective when they work in unison

---

BOX 3 ACTIVITIES OF DAILY LIVING (ADL) SCALES

Barthel index of basic ADL*

This index is commonly used in UK clinical practice to describe basic ADL—these activities are considered as "core" to functional assessment.[12] Many ADL scales take the name "Barthel"[15]; the items below are adapted from the most prevalent version of the scale.[16]

- **Feeding:** Are you able to feed yourself? Can you cut up food without help?

- **Bathing:** Are you able to take a bath or shower without help? Are you confident to take a bath or shower with no one in the room or house?

- **Grooming:** Do you need help with brushing hair, shaving, or applying make-up?

- **Dressing:** Can you get dressed without help? Can you manage buttons and laces?

- **Continence:** Do you ever wet yourself if you are not able to get to the toilet in time? Do you ever soil or mess yourself with bowel motions?

- **Toileting:** Do you need help to use the toilet?

- **Transfers:** Are you able to get out of bed and on to a chair with no help?

- **Mobility:** Are you able to walk 50 yards on the flat with no help? Do you use any walking aids such as a stick or frame? Have you fallen or stumbled in the past year?

- **Stairs:** Are you able to climb a flight of stairs without help?

Extended or instrumental ADL (based on the Nottingham extended ADL scale)[17]

- **Mobility:** Are you able to walk outside on uneven surfaces? Are you able to travel on your own to local destinations? Do you feel confident to use public transport?

- **Leisure:** Are you able to continue your previous hobbies? Are you able to stay in contact with friends and family?

- **Domestic:** Are you confident in managing your finances? Are you able to go shopping for essentials? Can you manage your laundry?

- **Kitchen:** Are you able to make a hot drink or snack? Are you able to walk with a hot drink without spilling it?

This structured history includes screening questions for continence, mobility, and falls

---

a basic test of walking and transfers. Patient and observer safety is paramount when assessing mobility and transfers, and for subjects with poor mobility, assessments may have to be deferred to specialist teams with appropriate equipment and moving-handling skills.

S (sensory)

Because sensory problems are prevalent in older people and can affect function, we recommend basic assessments of vision (with a pocket Snellen chart or by asking the patient to read successively smaller print from a newspaper) and hearing (using the whispered voice test).[20] [21]

E (environment)

Environment and functional status are linked, and a comprehensive examination should ideally include some assessment of the patient's home. Patients may perform poorly in an unfamiliar ward or office, whereas the home environment may limit functional ability because of awkward stairs, clutter, and falls hazards. It can be useful if patients' usual carers are present so that you can see how they interact and help (or hinder) patients in their daily tasks.

Mood, cognition, and (if appropriate) carer stress should also be examined as part of a comprehensive assessment, but these form part of another article in the series and will not be covered further.

Standardised assessment tools

Many such tools are available for use in different settings or disease states, but no consensus exists on the optimal measure,[22] [23] [24] and detailed knowledge of scales is not essential for the general clinician.

However, awareness of some of the more prevalent instruments may help in communicating with other professionals and in interpreting older age research (box 6). Moreover, functional assessment need not involve detailed and time consuming scales. For example, the get up and go test (box 5) is as useful for predicting falls as many more complex tools.[19] If time allows, use of a longer validated assessment instrument can have added value—for example, instrumental ADL tools such as the Nottingham scale[17] (box 3) or Lawton scale (box 6)[25] give standardised quantifiable data that may avoid the ceiling effects associated with common assessments of basic activities of daily living.

Although detailed assessment of basic and extended ADL is often performed by occupational therapists, day to day observations by nursing staff or informal carers are also useful. Occupational therapy assessment may be performed

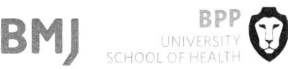

BOX 4 HYPOTHETICAL CASE STUDY IN FUNCTIONAL ASSESSMENT

Mrs A is an 84 year old woman with chronic health problems including cataract, osteoarthritis, and mild cognitive impairment. She has lived on her own since the death of her husband. She has attentive friends, but no formal support. She is brought to your general practice surgery by a concerned neighbour who feels Mrs A is "struggling to cope."

Assessment

You recognise the need for basic functional assessment. Initially Mrs A denies any problems. Using the questions in box 3 you ask specifically about basic activities of daily living, falls, continence, memory, and mood. Using these direct but non-threatening questions she admits to problems with dressing and climbing stairs. Her neighbour confirms these problems and adds that Mrs A's eyesight seems to be a problem, that she doesn't go out as much, and sometimes needs help with the shopping. You have already noticed that Mrs A used a table to steady herself when walking from the waiting area to your consulting room—"furniture walking." Focused physical examination shows general muscle wasting and no focal neurological deficits. You note that she struggles to read large print in a magazine.

You arrange for a longer home visit at the next opportunity. In the home environment you ask Mrs A to demonstrate her mobility on stairs, her ability to dress herself, and transfers on and off a chair. You note her antalgic gait, particularly on the stairs; that she uses the arms of the chair to help her get up from it, so she would need a handrail to get up from the toilet (at a similar height); and that her visual problems complicate dressing. You mention that her arthritis must make it difficult to do the shopping and cleaning, and she admits that "sometimes she relies on friends to help but that it would be nice to be able to go out more often."

Outcome

You create a problem list with important items of: visual impairment affecting reading and dressing; general deconditioning and pain from osteoarthritis impairing chair and toilet transfers and ability to go out on own, shop, and clean; lack of mobility causing some social isolation.

With Mrs A's agreement, arrangements are made for ophthalmic review; analgesia is prescribed; help with shopping, cleaning, and laundry is arranged through social services; and an occupational therapy assessment for toileting aids is requested. You recognise that a more comprehensive assessment of mobility and care needs is required and refer Mrs A for multidisciplinary assessment through the local care of the elderly team.

BOX 5 THE "GET UP AND GO TEST" AND COMMON ABNORMALITIES OF GAIT[19]

With the patient in normal footwear and using their customary walking aid, ask the patient to:

- Rise independently from an armless chair or with arms folded
- Stand still
- Then walk 3 m (10 ft)
- Turn 180 degrees
- Return to chair
- Sit down

Abnormalities that may be seen include:

- Unsteadiness
- Need for external support
- Apraxic gait (short steps, shuffling, and en-bloc turning—suggests cerebrovascular disease)
- Ataxic gait (unsteady, broad based—often seen in cerebellar dysfunction)
- Festinant gait or lack of arm swing (suggests parkinsonism)
- Hesitant gait (loss of confidence)
- Antalgic gait (may be caused by a painful hip or knee)
- Combinations of the above are common

---

practice. The assessments require some initial investment of time, but the combination of early recognition of functional decline and appropriate referral is ultimately more efficient than the multiple consultations that may result if functional problems are left to progress.

Although history taking is the cornerstone of assessment, it poses particular challenges in many older people. Barriers to communication will be more prevalent and can include cognitive impairment (delirium or dementia, or both), deafness, depression, dysphasia, and distraction caused by pain or emotional distress. General rules include the importance of speaking clearly and not too quickly while facing the patient and giving adequate time to respond. The importance of collateral history has already been emphasised.

Many older people have a complex array of medical comorbidities, functional problems, and difficult social circumstances. In these situations it is easy to feel overwhelmed, but we must avoid therapeutic nihilism. For those who perform poorly on the most basic functional assessment tasks there may still be the opportunity for meaningful improvements. A return to complete independence may not be possible for all, but small gains can greatly improve functioning and quality of life. For example, regaining the ability to move from bed to toilet independently with appropriate equipment may mean the difference between staying at home and requiring institutional care.

Busy general clinicians may feel that functional assessment is not part of their remit. With an ageing population, all clinicians are likely to encounter functional problems in their patients. Although not all clinicians have the training and infrastructural resources to offer a comprehensive assessment or rehabilitation interventions, all clinicians should screen for functional problems in older patients so that referral can be appropriately directed (box 4).[27]

TJQ drafted the manuscript and is guarantor. KM, GE, and DJS helped with the structure, content, editing, and responses to peer review.

Competing interests: All authors have completed the ICMJE uniform disclosure form at www.icmje.org/coi_disclosure.pdf (available on request from the corresponding author) and declare: no support from any organisation for the submitted work; no financial relationships

---

in wards or clinics, in purpose built environments (such as kitchens and bathrooms), or in the patient's home (through a supervised visit for inpatients).

How to use the functional assessment

When a functional assessment or screen identifies problems with physical function, this should trigger an offer of a more comprehensive multidisciplinary assessment and rehabilitation.[1 6 7] Even if no problems are identified, record details of the functional assessment because these will prove useful in monitoring progress. Because older adults are often seen by multiple healthcare professionals, robust processes are needed to allow for sharing of data and appropriate referral, while avoiding unnecessary duplication of assessments.

What are the challenges?

We recognise that functional assessment is not always straightforward. However, with the guidance offered we hope that basic assessment should be feasible in a busy

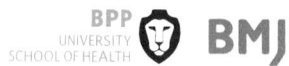

BOX 6 FUNCTIONAL ASSESSMENT TOOLS PREVALENT IN PRACTICE AND RESEARCH

These instruments are favoured by the British Rehabilitation Medicine Society and British Geriatric Society.[22 26]
Although many scales claim to be specific to a certain construct (such as impairment or disability) they often overlap, and the selection and interpretation of data from these instruments require careful consideration.

Motor function

General

- **Motor assessment scale:** Eight hierarchical scales; has proved validity and reliability but is time consuming to administer

Mobility

- **Rivermead mobility index:** Developed from a motor assessment scale; reliable and simple to administer

Upper limbs

- **Frenchay arm test:** Valid, reliable, and simple to administer; some equipment is needed, so it is not "portable"

Basic activities of daily living (ADL)

- **Barthel index:** Has proved validity, reasonable reliability, and is prevalent in practice and research. Its responsiveness to change in higher functioning subjects is limited

- **Functional assessment measure and functional independence measure:** Developed for use in brain injury. Assesses ADL but adds specific items pertinent to cognition and psychosocial issues. This test should be scored by a multidisciplinary team, which can limit its usefulness in a non-rehabilitation setting

Extended ADL

- **Nottingham extended ADL:** Describes activity in four domains; published evidence for the usefulness of this scale in non-stroke cohorts is limited

- **Lawton instrumental ADL:** Eight domain scale that can be administered via interview or as a questionnaire; there are various methods for scoring. In the original description, only five items were tested in men because it was assumed they would not participate in cooking and other duties—this highlights that ADL measures must be culture specific

SOURCES AND SELECTION CRITERIA

This review is based on the authors' clinical and research experience and is informed by a search of published literature. We searched electronic databases (Medline and Embase) from inception to December 2010 inclusive, using truncated keywords based on National Library of Medicine, medical subject headings: "aged" OR "aged, 80 or over", "rehabilitation", and "geriatric assessment". In addition, key reference works and national and international guidelines were searched for relevant papers. Particular attention was given to systematic reviews and meta-analyses. For this manuscript the intention was not to offer comprehensive systematic review, rather to give a narrative overview and critique of published literature.

IMPROVING PRACTICE

Resources for healthcare professional

- British Geriatric Society (www.bgs.org.uk/)—Comprehensive web resource with guidelines, educational materials, and original research
- American Geriatrics Society (www.geriatricsatyourfingertips.org/)—Web edition of "Geriatrics at your fingertips," available with apps for blackberry, iPhone, and android platforms (registration required)
- Barthel Index Program Training and Assessment Campus (http://barthel-english.trainingcampus.net/uas/modules/trees/windex.aspx)—Training in use of the Barthel index of activities of daily living is available through a series of online modules (registration required)

BMJ Group resources: BMJ Learning modules

- Discharge planning: a guide: http://learning.bmj.com/learning/search-result.html?moduleId=10017723
- Referring stroke patients to occupational therapy: http://learning.bmj.com/learning/search-result.html?moduleId=5001071

Resources for patients

- Age UK (www.ageuk.org.uk/)—Provides advice for older people in many areas, including health and wellbeing

3   Hogan DB, MacKnight C, Bergman H. Models, definitions and criteria of frailty. *Aging Clin Exp Res* 2003;15(suppl 3):3-29.
4   Schumacher JG. Emergency medicine and older adults: continuing challenges and opportunities. *Am J Emerg Med* 2005;23:556-60.
5   Cooper R, Kuh D, Hardy R; Mortality Review Group, FALCon and HALCyon Study Teams. Objectively measured physical capability levels and mortality: systematic review and meta-analysis. *BMJ* 2010;341:c4467.
6   Bachmann S, Finger C, Huss A, Egger M, Stuck AE, Clough-Gorr KM. Inpatient rehabilitation specifically designed for geriatric patients: systematic review and meta-analysis of randomised controlled trials. *BMJ* 2010;340:c1718.
7   Beswick AD, Rees K, Dieppe P, Ayis S, Gooberman-Hill R, Horwood J, et al. Complex interventions to improve physical function and maintain independent living in elderly people: a systematic review and meta-analysis. *Lancet* 2008;371:725-35.
8   Sinoff G, Ore L. The Barthel activities of daily living index: self-reporting versus actual performance in the old-old. *J Am Geriatr Soc* 1997;45:832-6.
9   Downing A, Wilson R. Older people's use of accident and emergency services. *Age Ageing* 2005;34:24-30.
10 Fletcher AE, Price GM, Ng ES, Stirling SL, Bulpitt CJ, Breeze E, et al. Population-based multidimensional assessment of older people in UK general practice: a cluster-randomised factorial trial. *Lancet* 2004;364:1667-77.
11 Gravelle H, Dusheiko M, Sheaff R. Impact of case management (Evercare) on frail elderly patients: controlled before and after analysis of quantitative outcome data. *BMJ* 2007;334:31-2.
12 Mahoney FI, Barthel DW. Functional evaluation: the Barthel index. *Maryland State Med J* 1965;14:61-5.
13 Ganz DA, Bao Y, Shekelle PG, Rubenstein LZ. Will my patient fall? *JAMA* 2007;297:77-86.
14 Williams EI, Wallace P. Health checks for people aged 75 and over. Occasional paper 59. Royal College of General Practitioners, 1993.
15 Quinn TJ, Langhorne P, Stott DJ. Barthel index for stroke trials: development, properties and application. *Stroke* 2011;42:1146-51.
16 Collin C, Wade DT, Davies S, Horne V. The Barthel ADL index: a reliability study. *Int Disabil Studies* 1988;10:61-3.
17 Nouri FM, Lincoln NB. An extended activities of daily living scale for stroke patients. *Clin Rehabil* 1978;1:301-5.
18 Moskowitz E. PULSES profile in retrospect. *Arch Phys Med Rehabil* 1985;66:647-8.
19 Mathias S, Nayak USL, Isaacs B. Balance in elderly patients; the "get up and go" test. *Arch Phys Med Rehabil* 1986;67:387-9.
20 Fletcher AE, Wormald RPL, Wormald RP, Ng ES, Stirling S, Smeeth L, et al. Prevalence of visual impairment in people aged 75 years and older in Britain: results from the MRC trial of assessment and management of older people in the community. *Br J Ophthalmol* 2002;86:795-800.
21 Pirozzo S, Papinczak T, Glasziou P. Whispered voice test for screening for hearing impairment. *BMJ* 2003;327:967.
22 Wade DT. Measurement in neurological rehabilitation. Oxford University Press, 1992.
23 Quinn TJ, Dawson J, Walters MR, Lees KR. Functional outcome measures in contemporary stroke trials. *Int J Stroke* 2009;4:200-5.

with any organisations that might have an interest in the submitted work in the previous three years; no other relationships or activities that could appear to have influenced the submitted work.

Provenance and peer review: Commissioned; externally peer reviewed.

1   Ellis G, Whitehead MA, Robinson D, O'Neill D, Langhorne P. Comprehensive geriatric assessment for older adults admitted to hospital. *Cochrane Database Syst Rev* 2011;7:CD006211.
2   WHO. International classification of functioning, disability and health (ICF). www.who.int/classifications/icf/en/.

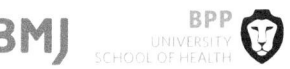

24 British Society of Rehabilitation Medicine. Basket of measures. 2000.
    www.bsrm.co.uk/ClinicalGuidance/OutcomeMeasuresB3.pdf.

25 Lawton MP, Brody EM. Assessment of older people: self maintaining
    and instrumental activities of living. *Gerontologist* 1968;9:179-86.

26 Pearson V. Assessment of function. In: Kane RL, ed. Assessing older
    persons: measures, meaning and practical applications. Oxford
    University Press, 2000:17-48.

27 Stott DJ, Langhorne P, Knight PV. Multidisciplinary care for elderly
    people in the community. *Lancet* 2008;371:699-700.

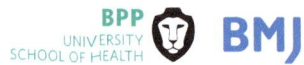

Prescribing for older people

James C Milton, specialist registrar in geriatric and general medicine[1], Ian Hill-Smith, general practitioner[2], Stephen H D Jackson, professor of clinical gerontology[1]

[1]Clinical Age Research Unit, Department of Clinical Gerontology, King's College Hospital Foundation Trust, London SE5 9PJ

[2]Stopsley Group Practice, Churchfield Medical Centre, Luton LU2 9SB

Correspondence to: J C Milton jim_milton@hotmail.com

Cite this as: BMJ 2011;343:d6838

DOI: 10.1136/bmj.39503.424653.80

http://www.bmj.com/content/336/7644/606

About a fifth of the population in the United Kingdom is 60 years or older,[1] yet people in this age group receive 59% of dispensed prescriptions and account for more than half of NHS drug costs.[2] Older people often have several coexisting medical problems and take multiple drugs. Increasing age is associated with changes in pharmacokinetics and pharmacodynamics, so prescribing in this age group can be problematic.[3]

Many randomised controlled trials involving older patients focus on managing a single disease state, such as hypertension or osteoporosis, but people in this age group often have many interacting conditions and are taking many drugs, so guidance on their treatment often has to be based on consensus and involves extrapolating data derived from healthier patients. This review highlights some of the difficulties in prescribing in older patients and offers guidance for appropriate prescribing.

Sources and selection criteria

We searched the National Library for Health, PubMed, and Embase databases using the keywords "elderly" and "prescribing", including synonyms by the MeSH or major descriptor headings. Our search was limited to studies undertaken in humans that were published in English during the past five years. We displayed abstracts of interest using Abstract Plus before obtaining the full text of articles of interest. In addition, we searched the Cochrane Library and our own personal archives of references

What physiological changes occur with ageing?

Pharmacokinetic and pharmacodynamic changes

With age the body undergoes several changes that can affect the distribution, metabolism, and excretion of drugs. These changes included a reduction in renal clearance, liver size, and lean body mass.[4] Hepatic enzyme activity and serum albumin may also be reduced in the presence of chronic disease. The most clinically important of these changes is the reduction in renal clearance, which results in reduced excretion of water soluble drugs. This is especially important for drugs with a narrow therapeutic window (ratio of desired effect to toxic effect), such as digoxin, lithium, and gentamicin.

As well as changes in pharmacokinetics, older people are also more sensitive to the effects of some drugs, especially those that act on the central nervous system, such as benzodiazepines, which are associated with an increase in postural sway and risk of falls.

Multiple pathology and polypharmacy

Polypharmacy is common in older people—around 20% of people over 70 take five or more drugs.[5] In the past decade, the average number of items prescribed to people aged 60 and over has almost doubled from 21.2 to 40.8 items for each person each year.[6] Previously, polypharmacy implied inappropriate prescribing, but this is not necessarily true, because all of the prescribed drugs may have an appropriate indication.

Polypharmacy is associated with increases in many adverse outcomes, including drug interactions, adverse drug reactions, falls, hospital admissions, length of hospital stay, readmission rate soon after discharge, and mortality rate.[5] [7] [8] However, these effects may result from polypharmacy acting as a marker of multiple pathology or frailty, as opposed to being an independent risk factor.

What is inappropriate prescribing?

Inappropriate prescribing for older patients encompasses all of the normal indicators of inappropriate prescribing for adults in general, but the problem is especially relevant to older patients because they often take a large number of drugs. Not only does this increase their chance of having an adverse event, but it means that unnecessary drugs may be obscured by the large number of necessary ones. Dose, formulation, and delivery need to be adjusted according to the age and frailty of the patient, and some drugs are best avoided altogether. This is familiar territory to general practitioners, who also see very young patients and routinely adjust drug dose according to the British National Formulary for Children—perhaps we need an equivalent publication for older patients to highlight the importance of taking age into account. Problems arise when older patients are assumed to respond to drugs in the same way that an average adult does.[9] In addition, as patients grow older, it is easy to forget to adjust drug doses appropriately. This is where a review by someone other than the usual prescriber can be particularly helpful.

Which drugs should we avoid in older patients?

Some adverse drug reactions occur at a similar prevalence regardless of age, such as cough induced by angiotensin converting enzyme inhibitors. However, a greater prevalence of adverse drug reactions may be seen as a result of the pharmacokinetic or pharmacodynamic changes seen with ageing. An American consensus guideline known as the Beers criteria—first published in 1991 and last updated in 2003—provides a list of drugs that the panel of experts thought to be particularly problematic for older patients.[10] The table gives examples from this list that are especially relevant to prescribing in the United Kingdom.

What drugs should we routinely consider in older patients?

Older people have been under-represented in clinical trials of new drugs, but there is a solid evidence base using some newer treatments in this population. Warfarin reduces strokes in patients with atrial fibrillation, with no significant

SUMMARY POINTS

- Prescribing for older people is problematic
- Older people are often prescribed unnecessary drugs, drugs that are contraindicated in their age group, or the wrong dose for their age
- Misconceptions about age may prevent them being given drugs with a specific indication and evidence base
- Inappropriate prescribing may be reduced by reviewing drugs regularly, electronic prescribing, regular auditing, and limiting the number of prescribers

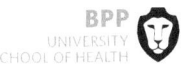

Drugs that pose a particular risk for older people[10]

Drug	Adverse drug reactions
Long term non-steroidal anti-inflammatory drugs	Gastrointestinal haemorrhage, renal impairment, hypertension
Benzodiazepines	Falls caused by impaired balance
Anticholinergic drugs	Unmasking Alzheimer's disease, urinary retention
Tricyclic antidepressants	Orthostatic hypotension, sedation
Chlorpropramide	Hypoglycaemia
Doxazosin	Orthostatic hypotension, dry mouth, urinary problems

TIPS FOR NON-SPECIALISTS

- Older people's drugs should be reviewed regularly. People taking fewer than four drugs should be reviewed at least annually. People taking four or more should be reviewed at least every six months
- Patients taking several drugs who have multiple comorbidities may benefit from a specialist review by a geriatrician. The referral should include a history of adverse events or intolerances as well as a list of drugs that are currently being taken

BOX 1 GUIDELINES FOR GOOD PRESCRIBING IN ELDERLY PATIENTS

- Carry out a regular medication review and discuss and agree all changes with the patient
- Stop any current drugs that are not indicated
- Prescribe new drugs that have a clear indication
- If possible, avoid drugs that have known deleterious effects in elderly patients, such as benzodiazepines, and recommend dosage reduction when appropriate
- Use the recommended dosages for elderly patients
- Use simple drug regimens and appropriate administration systems
- Consider using once daily or once weekly formulations and using fixed dose combinations when possible
- Consider non-pharmacological treatments if appropriate
- Limit the number of people prescribing for each patient if possible
- Where possible, avoid treating adverse drug reactions with further drugs

increase in the risk of bleeding, and it is recommended for most patients over 75 years with atrial fibrillation.[11][12]

Recent reviews also provide convincing evidence for the use of angiotensin converting enzyme inhibitors and β blockers in left ventricular systolic dysfunction, statins in hypercholesterolaemia, and bisphosphonates in osteoporosis in older patients.[13][14][15][16] These drugs were well tolerated in older people, but few studies included patients who were taking several drugs at the same time.[11][13][14][15][16] We therefore advise monitoring the introduction of new agents carefully, often starting with low doses and titrating upwards.

How can inappropriate prescribing in older people be reduced?

Good prescribing practice
Box 1 offers some guidelines to aid prescribing in older patients. Some of these guidelines, such as using as few prescribers as possible, are evidence based,[17] but because of the paucity of evidence in this area, most are consensus opinion.

Medication review
The national service framework for older people recommends regular medication reviews, with patients taking four or more drugs being reviewed every six months and those taking fewer reviewed annually.[18] General practitioners, who do most of the prescribing, can set the authorisation of repeat prescriptions for a period of time or a number of repeats, and automatically generate a recall using their clinical software. A medication review for all patients being prescribed four or more repeat medicines is part of the quality and outcomes framework of the general practitioner contract, and the National Prescribing Centre has issued detailed guidance on how it should be done.[19] However, the government has recently threatened to withdraw funding this target in favour of extended opening hours.

The medication review not only examines the indication for taking existing drugs and checks their dosage, but it also provides an opportunity to identify and treat new conditions, such as atrial fibrillation, cardiac failure, or Alzheimer's disease, which increase in prevalence with advancing age. Older people with complex medication or medical needs should be referred for a specialist review by a geriatrician.[18]

A systematic review of the effects of pharmacist led interventions in reducing polypharmacy identified only 14 trials that met the inclusion criteria, and these tended to report cost savings rather than benefits to the patients.[20] A recent randomised controlled trial found that regular telephone counselling by a hospital pharmacist increased concordance and reduced all cause mortality without altering the total number of drugs taken,[21] but it would be difficult to implement this intervention in the wider community. The 2005 contract for community pharmacists included a review of the use of drugs as the first advanced level service to be implemented,[22][23] but the aim of this review is to ensure that drugs are taken and taken properly. Without the clinical records pharmacists cannot review the indications for treatment. Community pharmacists have an important role in spotting adverse drug reactions, drug interactions, and concordance problems, even though we have no evidence that this reduces mortality or emergency admissions.[24]

Using as few prescribers as possible
In the UK, most prescribing is done by the patient's general practitioner, but it is often started or adjusted in secondary care, so good communication is crucial. Unintentional discrepancies in medication are found in half of older patients after they have left hospital, an error rate that can be halved if the community pharmacist is sent a copy of the discharge summary.[25]

A recent study in the United States found that the incidence of adverse drug reactions is directly related to the number of doctors who prescribe for a patient.[17] The effects of non-medical prescribing, by nurses and other health professionals, have not been studied. It results in a similar number of prescriptions to physician prescribing,[26] but does increase the potential number of prescribers (although independent nurse prescribers cooperate closely with the patient's general practitioner).

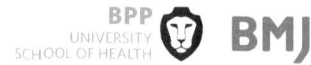

Education

A Cochrane review concluded that educational outreach visits are a promising way to modify the behaviour of health professionals, especially prescribing behaviour.[27] In a UK study of 75 randomly selected general practices, those assigned educational outreach had a small improvement in prescribing practice.[28] Interestingly, smaller practices (two or fewer full time equivalent practitioners) improved by 13.5%, whereas larger practices did not improve significantly. This may have been because a greater proportion of doctors in smaller practices attended the outreach meetings. A randomised controlled trial showed that similar interventions can also change prescribing in hospital practice.[29]

Electronic prescribing

Electronic prescribing (ePrescribing) aims to reduce prescribing and administration errors by eliminating the risk of errors when generating or reading paper prescriptions.[30] This is one step in the overall goal of integrating the entire patient record across the health service as a way to minimise errors or delays in communication between service providers. Prescribing advice software can be integrated within this structure. This promises to be of particular benefit to older patients with several morbidities who are taking multiple drugs, but setting up ePrescribing is only half the challenge—patients may need help and encouragement to use it initially.[31]

Before and after studies in a surgical ward of a London teaching hospital provide an early indication of benefit. The introduction of closed loop electronic prescribing resulted in fewer prescribing errors, fewer errors related to medication administration, and fewer prescription endorsements by a pharmacist.[32] [33]

Audit

Auditing of prescribing is integral to providing good clinical care, but the traditional audit loop of data gathering, data interpretation, and feedback produces a long delay between an action and its feedback, which reduces any effect on behaviour. Furthermore, amalgamated data distance the prescriber from specific errors and make it harder to see obvious ways to improve. Audit does not necessarily change behaviour,[34] but prescribing indicators have been developed for older patients,[35] [36] [37] which could provide immediate feedback when integrated into electronic prescribing systems. Box 2 shows the types of indicators used to assess prescribing quality.

What improvements can we expect in future?

Unified medical records, electronic prescribing with decision support, and instant feedback on prescribing have potential to reduce errors in prescribing and improve patients' care. Trials of new treatments, even if they include older people, currently tend to be highly selective, and the results do not easily generalise to a frail elderly population with multiple comorbidities. Ideally, such randomised controlled trials would include representative samples of frail older patients, but the practical problems with this are considerable.

Conclusions

Prescribing for elderly patients presents many challenges, most of which have not changed in the past 20 years.[38] Changes in pharmacodynamics and pharmacokinetics mean that these patients often need lower doses, and the presence of multiple medical problems and subsequent polypharmacy makes adverse drug reactions and interactions more common.

> **BOX 2 TYPES OF PRESCRIBING QUALITY INDICATORS[35]**
>
> **Quantitative indicators**
> Such as the mean number of drugs prescribed or the number classified in the *British National Formulary* as "black triangle" or "less suitable for prescribing."[11] These indicators are best used in conjunction with others
>
> **Qualitative indicators**
> These are drug specific indicators of unnecessary or ineffective prescribing (such as prescribing both an H2 receptor blocker and a proton pump inhibitor) or potentially harmful drugs (such as long acting hypoglycaemic agents)
>
> **Evidence based indicators**
> These measure the extent to which research evidence is put into practice, such as the use of antithrombotic therapy in atrial fibrillation, while allowing the prescriber to identify reasons why the evidence base should not be followed—for example, because a palliative care pathway is being followed or the patient has a history of an adverse reaction

---

> **ADDITIONAL EDUCATIONAL RESOURCES**
>
> *Information for patients*
> - Patient UK (www.patient.co.uk/dils.asp)—Free drug information site for patients
> - CKS (www.cks.library.nhs.uk/patient_information)—NHS sponsored patient information site
>
> *Information for health professionals*
> - National Service Framework: Medicine and Older People (www.hcsu.org.uk/index.php?option=com_docman&task=doc_download&gid=322%20)—Provides a format for detailed medication review

---

The evidence base for specific treatments in older people is increasing but, even when the evidence base does not extend to a particular age group, effective treatments should not be withheld purely on the basis of age, just as treatments would not be denied to specific ethnic groups who are under-represented in clinical studies.

Contributors: JM and IH-S searched the literature and wrote the article. SJ reviewed and revised the article. JM is guarantor.

Competing interests: None declared.

Provenance and peer review: Commissioned; externally peer reviewed.

1 Office for National Statistics. *Key population and vital statistics* . 2005. www.statistics.gov.uk/downloads/theme_population/KPVS32_2005/KPVS2005.pdf.

2 Department of Health. *Prescriptions dispensed in the community for 1993 to 2003*. England: DH, 2004.

3 Mallet L, Spinewine A, Huang A. Prescribing in elderly people 2: the challenge of managing drug interactions in elderly people. *Lancet* 2007;370:185-91.

4 Mangoni AA, Jackson SHD. Age-related changes in pharmacokinetics and pharmacodynamics: basic principles and practical applications. *Br J Clin Pharmacol* 2003;57:6-14.

5 Rollason V, Vogt N. Reduction of polypharmacy in the elderly: a systemic review of the role of the pharmacist. *Drugs Aging* 2003;20:817-32.

6 Information Centre (Health Care). *Prescriptions dispensed in the community. Statistics for 1996 to 2006: England*. 2007. www.ic.nhs.uk/webfiles/publications/PrescDispensed%2096to06/Bulletin%20220807%20version%20for%202006.pdf.

7 Campbell SE, Seymour DG, Primrose WR. A systematic literature review of factors affecting outcome in older medical patients admitted to hospital. *Age Ageing* 2004;33:110-5.

8 Frazier SC. Health outcomes and polypharmacy in elderly individuals. *J Gerontol Nursing* 2005;31:4-11.

9 Edwards RF, Harrison TM, Davis SM. Potentially inappropriate prescribing for geriatric inpatients: an acute care of the elderly unit compared to a general medicine service. *Consult Pharmacist* 2003;18:37-49.

10 Fick DM, Cooper JW, Wade WE, Waller JL, Maclean JR, Beers MH. Updating the Beers criteria for potentially inappropriate medication use in older adults. *Arch Intern Med* 2003;163:2716-24.

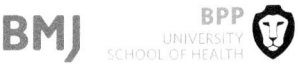

11 Mant J, Hobbs R, Fletcher K, Mant J, Hobbs FD, Fletcher K, et al; BAFTA investigators; Midland Research Practices Network (MidReC). Warfarin versus aspirin for stroke prevention in an elderly community population with atrial fibrillation (the Birmingham atrial fibrillation treatment of the aged study, BAFTA): a randomised controlled trial. *Lancet* 2007;370:493-503.

12 The National Collaborating Centre for Chronic Conditions. *Atrial fibrillation. National clinical guideline for management in primary and secondary care.* London: Royal College of Physicians, 2006.

13 Mangoni AA, Jackson SHD. The implications of a growing evidence base for drug use in elderly patients. Part 2. ACE inhibitors and angiotensin receptor blockers in heart failure and high cardiovascular risk patients. *Br J Clin Pharmacol* 2006;61:502-12.

14 Mangoni AA, Jackson SHD. The implications of a growing evidence base for drug use in elderly patients. Part 3. β-adrenoceptor blockers in heart failure and thrombolytics in acute myocardial infarction. *Br J Clin Pharmacol* 2006;61:513-20.

15 Mangoni AA, Jackson SHD. The implications of a growing evidence base for drug use in elderly patients. Part 1. Statins for primary and secondary cardiovascular prevention. *Br J Clin Pharmaol* 2006;61:494-501.

16 Dhesi JK, Allain TJ, Mangoni AA, Jackson SHD. The implications of a growing evidence base for drug use in elderly patients. Part 4. Vitamin D and bisphosphonates for fractures and osteoporosis. *Br J Clin Pharmacol* 2006;61:521-8.

17 Green JL, Hawley JN, Rask KJ. Is the number of prescribing physicians an independent risk factor for adverse drug events in an elderly outpatient population? *Am J Geriatr Pharmacother* 2007;5:31-9.

18 Department of Health. *Medicines and older people: implementing medicines-related aspects of the NSF for older people 2001.* 2001 www.hcsu.org.uk/index.php?option=com_docman&task=doc_download&gid=322%20.

19 Middlesborough Primary Care Trust. *Guidance to support the production of a repeat prescribing protocol.* www.npc.co.uk/repeat_prescribing/Policy%203%20-%20Sue%20Prout.pdf.

20 Rollason V, Vogt N. Reduction of polypharmacy in the elderly: a systemic review of the role of the pharmacist. *Drugs Aging* 2003;20:817-32.

21 Wu JYF, Leung WYS, Chang S, Lee B, Zee B, Tong PC, et al. Effectiveness of telephone counselling by a pharmacist in reducing mortality in patients receiving polypharmacy: randomised controlled trial. *BMJ* 2006;333:522-7.

22 Noyce PR. Providing patient care through community pharmacies in the UK: policy, practice, and research. *Ann Pharmacother* 2007;41:861-8.

23 Blenkinsopp A, Celino G, Bond C, Inch J. Medicines use reviews: the first year of a new community pharmacy service. *Pharm J* 2007;278:218-23.

24 Bond C, Matheson C, Williams S, Williams P, Donnan P. Repeat prescribing: a role for community pharmacists in controlling and monitoring repeat prescriptions. *Br J Gen Pract* 2000;50:271-5.

25 Duggan C, Feldman R, Hough J, Bates I. Reducing adverse prescribing discrepancies following hospital discharge. *Int J Pharm Pract* 1998;6:77-82.

26 Horrocks S, Anderson E, Salisbury C. Systematic review of whether nurse practitioners working in primary care can provide equivalent care to doctors. *BMJ* 2002;324:819-23.

27 O'Brien T, Oxman AD, Davis DA, Haynes RB, Freemantle N, Harvey EL. Educational outreach visits: effects on professional practice and health care outcomes. *Cochrane Database Syst Rev* 2000;(2):CD000409.

28 Freemantle N, Nazareth I, Eccles M, Wood J, Haines A; Evidence-based OutReach Trialists. A randomised controlled trial of the effect of educational outreach by community pharmacists on prescribing in UK general practice. *Br J Gen Pract* 2002;52:290-5.

29 Batty GM, Oborne CA, Hooper R, Jackson SHD. Investigating intervention strategies to increase the appropriate use of benzodiazepines in elderly medical inpatients. *Br J Clin Gov* 2001;6:252-8.

30 National Health Service. *ePrescribing.* 2008. www.connectingforhealth.nhs.uk/systemsandservices/eprescribing.

31 Lapane KL, Dubé C, Schneider KL, Quilliam BJ. Patient perceptions regarding electronic prescriptions: is the geriatric patient ready? *J Am Geriatr Soc* 2007;55:1254-9.

32 Franklin BD, O'Grady K, Donyai P, Jacklin A, Barber N. The impact of a closed-loop electronic prescribing and administration system on prescribing errors, administration errors and staff time: a before-and-after study. *Qual Safety Health Care* 2007;16:279-84.

33 Franklin BD, O'Grady K, Donyai P, Jacklin A, Barber N. The impact of a closed-loop electronic prescribing and automated dispensing system on the ward pharmacist's time and activities. *Int J Pharmacy Pract* 2007;15:133-9.

34 Batty GM, Grant RL, Aggarwal R, Lowe D, Potter JM, Pearson MG, et al. National clinical sentinel audit of evidence-based prescribing for older people. *J Eval Clin Pract* 2004;10:273-9.

35 Oborne CA, Batty GM, Maskrey V, Swift CG, Jackson SHD. Development of prescribing indicators for elderly medical patients. *Br J Clin Pharmacol* 1997;43:91-7.

36 Oborne CA, Hooper R, Swift CG, Jackson SHD. Explicit, evidence-based criteria to assess the quality of prescribing to elderly nursing home residents. *Age Ageing* 2003;32:102-8.

37 Batty GM, Grant RL, Aggarwal R, Lowe D, Potter JM, Pearson MG, et al. Using prescribing indicators to measure the quality of prescribing to elderly medical in-patients. *Age Ageing* 2003;32:292-8.

38 Swift CG. Prescribing in old age. *BMJ* 1988;296:913-5.

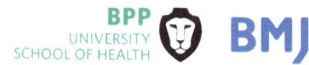

Assessing and helping carers of older people

I D Cameron, head[1], C Aggar, PhD student[2], A L Robinson, professor of primary care and ageing[3], S E Kurrle, head[4]

[1]Rehabilitation Studies Unit, Faculty of Medicine, University of Sydney, Ryde, NSW 1680, Australia

[2]Sydney Nursing School, University of Sydney

[3]Institute of Health and Society, Newcastle University, Newcastle, UK

[4]Curran Ageing Research Unit, Hornsby Ku-ring-gai Health Service, Hornsby, NSW, Australia

Correspondence to: I D Cameron ian.cameron@sydney.edu.au

Cite this as: BMJ 2011;343:d5202

DOI: 10.1136/bmj.d5202

http://www.bmj.com/content/343/bmj.d5202

This is the last in a series of four articles about assessing older people

Carers are an essential source of support to older people and take responsibility for most of their care needs. Although many carers find aspects of the caring role satisfying,[1] caring responsibilities can lead to a decline in their own physical and mental health[1 2 3]—especially when caring for those with dementia[4]—and adversely affect their employment and education prospects, financial position, and ability to participate in social and community life.[2] It is therefore important to identify people who have an important informal caring role. An assessment of the carer and his or her individual needs, and of the caregiving situation, can improve the health and wellbeing of the carer and ensure the provision of timely and appropriate support services.[1]

How do we identify carers?

Many carers do not formally recognise themselves as carers because they consider their input to be integral to their family duties. Therefore, whenever doctors have patients with serious long term illnesses or disabilities, they should identify the caring input of key family members. The rights of carers are widely recognised in policy and legislation, with carer policies focusing on benefits, services, employment, and the provision of carers with the right to request an assessment of their support needs.[5] In some countries, social (support) workers have a responsibility for providing support to carers. However, medical practitioners, especially general practitioners (family physicians), are the first point of access for patients in many countries and are well placed to identify and screen for people in an important caring role, detect those at risk of physical and mental health problems, and provide follow-up or referral as appropriate.[6] Carers may also present directly to their family doctor with physical or mental health problems as a result of their caring responsibilities, or to seek information, advice, and support.

How should a carer assessment be undertaken?

Although several high quality studies have recommended the need for carer assessments, less evidence is available on how the assessment should be structured and what domains it should cover. In addition, we do not believe that most medical practitioners have the time or expertise to complete a comprehensive carer assessment. We suggest that recognition of carers, a brief assessment of their needs, and, where indicated, referral should be the primary medical role. The referral could be to a staff member in the general practice with interest and training in carer issues.[7]

However, large observational studies of carers in Europe[8] and Australia show that key areas for assessment are:
- Any positive or satisfying components of providing care
- The suitability of the home environment
- The physical and psychological health of the carer and the care recipient
- The functional needs of the care recipient
- The levels of carer burden and carer stress
- The carer's cultural background, employment, and financial status
- The carer's information needs
- The presence of carer abuse.

Factors that have been shown to correlate with low wellbeing in carers include:
- Disturbed behaviour in the care recipient
- Being a female carer
- Rating the current relationship as poor
- Having no social support
- Having a narrow range of coping strategies.[9]

During an assessment, provide an opportunity for the carer to express his or her needs and allow collaborative decision making. We recommend using an assessment tool to guide the conversation and obtain vital information.[10 11] Many multidimensional and self reported carer assessment tools are available,[12] but there is little evidence to recommend one above the other, and few are designed to use within the time constraints of primary care. The figure provides a structured and detailed screening, assessment, and intervention template for use in practice, adapted from resources available to help medical practitioners identify and support carers.[10 11 12 13 14 15 16] Many assessment tools are available to measure aspects of the carer experience, particularly distress. The best known is the Zarit burden interview (ZBI) a 22 item questionnaire.[17] These tools are not in common use in primary medical practice but are regularly used in research settings. However, a recent review of six short form versions of the ZBI suggests that although the ZBI-12 is suitable for all caregiving populations,[18] asking the single question (item 22 on the ZBI)—"Overall how burdened do you feel?"—is useful for quick assessment.[19]

What are useful carer interventions?

Because caregiving situations, carer characteristics, and coping strategies are diverse and complex, interventions must have multiple components and be individually tailored, flexible, of sufficient frequency and duration (or ongoing), and developed in consultation with the carer.[20 21 22 23] The

SUMMARY POINTS

- Identifying carers is important because many do not recognise themselves as such, and care responsibilities can affect their health and financial and social aspects of their lives
- Comprehensive carer assessment may not be feasible but doctors can identify carers, briefly assess their needs, develop a care plan in collaboration with the carer, and refer where needed
- Key areas to ask about include physical and mental health needs of the carer and care recipient, information needs, financial status, levels of carer burden and stress, and the positive aspects of caring
- Asking the question "Overall how burdened do you feel?" is a useful, quick way to assess carer distress
- Provide specific interventions to carers where indicated, including education, information, counselling, and support
- To help the carer, provide the care recipient with specific interventions, including regular service provision, aids and equipment, and respite care
- Monitor carer on an ongoing basis and provide support after residential placement or bereavement

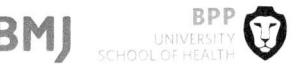

CASE SCENARIO I

Mr Brown is an 82 year old man with moderate dementia; he also has hypertension and lower limb osteoarthritis and has had a recent mild stroke, which caused a right hemiparesis and has slowed his walking. He lives at home with his 78 year old wife who is his carer. They have no children. Mrs Brown is a cognitively intact but increasingly frail woman with ischaemic heart disease and worsening cardiac failure. She now does the driving because her husband lost his driver's licence, and she has recently taken over management of the couple's financial affairs.

CASE SCENARIO II

Mrs Brown comes in one day for her usual prescriptions. You note her cardiac failure is not optimally controlled and she seems rather subdued. You advise changes to her drugs and ask how things are at home. She says her husband needs lots of attention and things can be difficult. You say you wonder if this is affecting her health and ask if she can come back later that week to check how the drugs are working and discuss the situation at home. She agrees but quickly adds "I do want to keep looking after him at home." You reassure her that you just want to help her stay well and support her care of her husband.

She is happy with this and returns a few days later, when you ascertain that her cardiac failure is better controlled, you ask who else helps her at home (see figure). It turns out that they have no immediate family or paid carers. When asked about her biggest difficulty in caring for him, she mentions that he sometimes gets angry and hits out at her, especially in the car as a passenger or when she has to shower him. When asked how else she helps him, Mrs Brown says he gets up several times to go to the toilet at night and needs help in getting back into bed. This interrupts her sleep. Informal discussion about managing household tasks revealed that she had difficulty keeping up with shopping and paying bills, and she said that she felt overwhelmed by her husband's care needs. She was unaware of the services that were available to her and had limited understanding of the progressive nature of her husband's dementia or how to manage his challenging behaviours.

figure shows interventions linked to assessment items. Referral pathways vary with health and social care systems. Many studies have looked at interventions specifically designed to help carers of patients with dementia and stroke.[23]Eagar and colleagues suggest that the support needs of carers looking after patients with various illnesses do not differ, other than the extra support needed to cope with the emotional pressures on carers dealing with the behavioural changes associated with dementia.[24]

Small but consistent benefits have been shown for multicomponent educational programmes and multicomponent psychological interventions for carers, and programmes with greater intensity are associated with a larger effect size.[10] [25] [26] In particular, cognitive behavioural therapy interventions have shown moderate effects on carer burden, anxiety, and depressive symptoms.[27] Although the benefits have been shown mainly for carers, there are also benefits for the care recipient in mood and behaviour, and the involvement of both care recipient and carer improves the effectiveness of these programmes.[25] Family support interventions and support groups have been shown to be effective mainly in the context of mental illness and dementia.[24]

Respite care can be provided regularly or sporadically and may occur in the home, in centre based care, or in institutional care.[24] A Cochrane review found no evidence of effectiveness for provision of respite care but cautioned that this might be because of a lack of high quality research.[28] A systematic review concluded that respite care had small effects, was beneficial only in subgroups in better controlled studies, did not delay entry to residential care, and did not negatively affect frail older people.[29] Despite the limited evidence of effectiveness, respite care should be considered if provided flexibly in response to the specific needs of carers.[30]

A recent systematic review of randomised controlled trials of case management for community living patients with dementia and their carers found weak evidence that it delayed admission to an institution, and inconclusive evidence of its effectiveness in organising formal care and services and reducing informal caring hours.[31] The effect of case management on carer burden and depression is mixed.[32] [33]

Evidence based clinical practice guidelines suggest an approach based on early and ongoing carer assessment

Carer Details

Name: .... Age: .... Sex: M/F Relationship.......................................

Carer Assessment

Intervention

Practicalities

Co-residence? Yes ☐ No ☐
Do you drive? Yes ☐ No ☐ Mode of transport........................

Transport assistance
Home visits

Carer health and wellbeing

How would you rate your health?
Excellent ☐ Good ☐ Fair ☐ Poor ☐
Do you have any health concerns?
Do you have regular health checks?
How stressed do you feel in caring for the care recipient?
Not stressed ☐ Somewhat stressed ☐ Very stressed
Do you feel angry or depressed with your caregiving situation?
Rarely ☐ Occasionally ☐ Most of the time

General health check

Mental Health Assessment
Referral for
Psycho-educational or
Cognitive behavioural therapy

Caregiving Details

How long have you been providing care?
What assistance do you provide?
How many hours a week/per day do you provide care?
Do you have support from family members or friends?
What caregiving activities cause you most concern?

Support Services

What support services are being utilised?
What support services do you feel you need to manage?

Care Recipient Details

What aspects of the care recipient's health are of concern?
Functional ☐ Memory ☐ Behavioural

Caregiving Concerns

Social isolation ☐ Financial strain ☐
Stress on relationships ☐ Time for self ☐

Support services
Transport/Home help/
Meals/Aged care service/
Community nursing service
Home modifications
Equipment/Aids
Practical Advice/Problem Solving
Nutrition supplements/
Sleep Disturbance/
Behavioural Problems
Respite
Short/long term
Residential/in home
Referral for Counselling
Individual, family or group
Information/Education
Care recipient illness/prognosis
Carer associations/
support centres/networks
Planning for emergencies
Emergency response
Systems/
Personal ID equipment

Financial barriers and concerns

Employment Status

Financial and Legal Issues

Financial assistance/advice
Government benefits,
charitable organisations
Legal support
Health care directives,
guardianship, power of
attorney

Carer assessment and recommended interventions template; adapted from various sources[10] [11] [12] [13] [14] [15] [16]

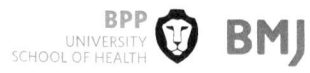

SOURCES AND SELECTION CRITERIA

As well as using our personal reference collections, we searched the Cochrane database and reviewed guidelines from the National Institute for Health and Clinical Excellence. Where appropriate we selected systematic reviews and meta-analyses. Observational studies and consensus guidelines were used to define elements of carer assessment.

CASE SCENARIO III

Mrs Brown was given help with bathing and personal care for her husband three days a week, and this reduced his aggressive behaviour towards her. Mr Brown refused to attend a day respite centre, but Mrs Brown did receive in-home respite for several hours twice each week, which allowed her to get to her medical appointments, do her shopping, and pay her bills. She was also able to attend a regular carer support group, which provided education about caring and dementia, and she found this helpful because of the information provided and the support available from staff and other carers. At review three months later Mrs Brown is still stressed but says she is coping with her husband much better. Her cardiac failure is well controlled and she sees you regularly for follow-up.

IMPROVING PRACTICE

Educational resources for carers

- CarersUK (www.carersuk.org/)—Carer organisation website that provides information and practical advice for carers; UK focus

- Family Caregiver Alliance (www.caregiver.org/caregiver/jsp/home.jsp)—Carer organisation website that provides information and advice for carers; USA focus

Educational resources for healthcare professional

- Royal Princess Trust for Carers (http://professionals.carers.org/)—Resource for professionals working with carers; UK focus

- Supporting Carers in General Practice e-learning programme (www.e-lfh.org.uk/projects/supportingcarersingeneralpractice)—Well designed continuing educational programme; requires registration and is available readily only to UK based health professionals

- Family Caregiver Alliance (www.caregiver.org/caregiver/jsp/content_node.jsp?nodeid=1695)—Carer organisation website for professionals working with carers; USA focus

- BMA. Working with carers: guidelines for good practice, 2009. www.bma.org.uk/healthcare_policy/community_care/Workingwithcarers.jsp. Excellent summary of issues for medical practitioners working with carers; UK focus

and flexible provision of interventions according to carer preference and assessed need.[10][27] Increased needs should be anticipated if there are major changes in health status of the care recipient or carer, or environmental changes for the carer. Support may still be needed for the carer after the care recipient moves to a residential care setting or after his or her death.

What are the challenges for carer assessment and intervention?

A major challenge facing clinicians is the limited time available for assessment. However, the broader benefits flowing from effective support of carers need to be recognised. Clinicians may find that family members do not identify with the term "carer" and are therefore less likely to seek assessment. Carers, spouses in particular, may decline to use support services or accept interventions for themselves because of a perceived lack of need or loss of control,[34] or the reluctance

of the care recipient to accept services.[35] Other barriers to service use include the inflexibility of service providers in what they will provide and the amount of time available, the complex application procedures needed to enable access, a limited understanding or knowledge of what is available, and the financial cost of the services.[36]

From the family doctor perspective, ongoing contact and support, the development of a therapeutic relationship with the carer, and a flexible approach are likely to be needed to encourage carers to accept help. One practical approach is to suggest a trial of a service for a limited period, with the option to stop after that time. Another approach is to involve other family members in discussing what services might be helpful. It is useful to emphasise to carers that they are the most important people providing care, so that their health and wellbeing must be maintained to allow them to continue in that role. Monitor carer on an ongoing basis and provide support after residential placement or bereavement.

Conclusion

Carer assessment and the provision of individually tailored interventions are essential elements in the healthcare of older people. The figure suggests ways to achieve this. Steven Zarit, one of the originators of carer research, has stated "the implications of research as well as principles of good practice unequivocally support the premise that assessing caregivers is a necessary and essential part of working with older clients in virtually every setting."[37]

IDC, SEK, CA, and ALR jointly wrote the paper. IDC is guarantor.

Funding: Preparation of the paper was supported by an Australian National Health and Medical Research Council Health Services Research Grant ID 402791. CA's salary is funded by a scholarship from the above grant, and IDC's salary is supported by an Australian National Health and Medical Research Council Practitioner Fellowship (ID 1002488).

Competing interests: All authors have completed the ICMJE uniform disclosure form at (available on request from the corresponding author) and declare: no support from any organisation for the submitted work, except from the Australian National Health and Medical Research Council Health Services Research Grant 402791; no financial relationships with any organisations that might have an interest in the submitted work in the previous three years, no other relationships or activities that could appear to have influenced the submitted work, except CA is a board member of Carers NSW (an organisation supporting carers) and SEK is a board member of Hammond Care (an organisation providing community and residential care services for older people and their carers).

Patient consent not required (patient anonymised, dead, or hypothetical).

1   Chappell NL, Dujela C. Caregiving: predicting at-risk status. *Can J Aging* 2008;27:169-79.
2   Horner B, Boldy DP. The benefit and burden of "ageing-in-place" in an aged care community. *Aust Health Rev* 2008;32:356-65.
3   Schulz R, Beach S. Caregiving as a risk factor for mortality: the Caregiver Health Effects Study. *JAMA* 1999;282:2215-9.
4   Bertrand RM, Fredman L, Saczynski J. Are all caregivers created equal? Stress in caregivers to adults with and without dementia. *J Aging Health* 2006;18:534-51.
5   Department of Health. Carers. 2011. www.dh.gov.uk/en/SocialCare/Carers/index.htm.
6   Guberman N, Nicholas E, Nolan M, Rembicki D, Lundh U, Keefe J. Impacts on practitioners of using research-based carer assessment tools: experiences from the UK, Canada and Sweden, with insights from Australia. *Health Social Care Commun* 2003;11:345-55.
7   Greenwood N, Mackenzie A, Habibi R, Atkins C, Jones R. General practitioners and carers: a questionnaire survey of attitudes, awareness of issues, barriers and enablers to provision of services. *BMC Fam Pract* 2010;11:100.
8   Eurofamcare. Services for supporting family carers of older dependent people in Europe: characteristics, coverage, and usage—The Trans-European survey report. In: Eurofamcare, ed. Institute for Medical Sociology, 2006. www.uke.de/extern/eurofamcare/documents/deliverables/teusure_web_080215.pdf.
9   Oyebode J. Assessment of carers' psychological needs. *Adv Psychiatr Treat* 2003;9:45-53.
10 Family Caregiver Alliance. Selected caregiver assessment measures: a resource inventory for practitioners. FCA, 2002.

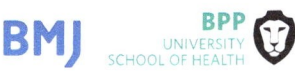

11 Family Caregiver Alliance. Caregivers count too! A tool kit to help practitioners assess the needs of family caregivers. FCA, 2006.

12 Deekin J, Taylor K, Mangan P, Yabroff K, Ingham J. Care for the caregivers: a review of self-reported instruments developed to measure the burden, needs and quality of life of informal caregivers. *J Pain Sympt Manage* 2003;26:922-53.

13 National Collaborating Centre for Mental Health. A NICE-SCIE guideline on supporting people with dementia and their carers in health and social care. National clinical practice guideline 42 (updated version). 2011. www.nice.org.uk/nicemedia/live/10998/30320/30320.pdf.

14 American Medical Association. Caregiver self-assessment questionnaire. How are you? www.snocare.org/kit/04CaregiverSelfAssessmentQuestionaire.pdf.

15 Princess Royal Trust for Carers. Supporting carers: an action guide for general practitioners and their teams. Sheffield University. http://static.carers.org/files/prtc-introductory-section-3660.pdf.

16 BMA. Working with carers: guidelines for good practice, 2009. www.bma.org.uk/healthcare_policy/community_care/Workingwithcarers.jsp.

17 Zarit burden interview (ZBI). www.rgpc.ca/best/GiiC%20Resources/GiiC/pdfs/3%20Caregiver%20Support%20-%20The%20Zarit%20Burden%20Interview.pdf.

18 Bédard M, Molloy DW, Squire L, Dubois S, Lever JA, O'Donnell M. The Zarit burden interview. *Gerontologist* 2001;41:652-57.

19 Higginson IJ, Gao W, Jackson D, Murray J, Harding R. Short-form Zarit caregiver burden interviews were valid in advanced conditions. *J Clin Epidemiol* 2010;63:535-42.

20 Schulz R, Martire L, Klinger J. Evidence-based caregiver interventions in geriatric psychiatry. *Psychiatr Clin North Am* 2005;28:1007-38.

21 Zarit S, Femia E, Kim K, Whitlatch C. The structure of risk factors and outcomes for family caregivers: implications for assessment and treatment. *Aging Ment Health* 2010;14:220-31.

22 Cameron M, Massuch L, Wishart D. Research-based recommendations for effective caregiver interventions: University of Michigan, 2008. www.dementiacoalition.org/pdfs/Recomm_Eff_CG_Interventions_3_6_08.pdf.

23 Lee J, Soeken K, Picot S. A meta-analysis of interventions for informal stroke caregivers. *West J Nurs Res* 2007;29:344-56.

24 Eagar K, Owen A, Wiliams K, Westera A, Marosszeky N, England R, et al. Effective caring: a synthesis of the international evidence on carer needs and interventions. Centre for Health Service Development-CHSD. Paper 27, 2007. www.health.gov.au/internet/main/publishing.nsf/Content/035CFE9F19D3745CCA25746400216027/$File/CHSDEffecCaringV2Final.pdf.

25 Brodaty H, Green A, Koschera A. Meta-analysis of psychosocial interventions for caregivers of people with dementia. *J Am Geriatr Soc* 2003;51:657-64.

26 Pinquart M, Sörensen S. Helping caregivers of persons with dementia: which interventions work and how large are their effects? *Int Psychogeriatr* 2006;18:577-95.

27 Parker D, Mills S, Abbey J. Effectiveness of interventions that assist caregivers to support people with dementia living in the community: a systematic review. *Int J Evidence Based Health* 2008;6:137-72.

28 Lee H, Cameron M. Respite care for people with dementia and their carers. *Cochrane Database Syst Rev* 2004;2:CD004396.

29 Mason A, Weatherly H, Spilsbury K, Golder S, Arksey H, Adamson J, et al. The effectiveness and cost-effectiveness of respite for caregivers of frail older people. *J Am Geriatr Soc* 2007;55:290-9.

30 Shaw C, McNamara R, Abrams K, Cannings-John R, Hood R, Longo M, et al. Systematic review of respite care in the frail elderly. *Health Technol Assess* 2009;13:1-246.

31 Pimouguet C, Lavaud T, Dartigues J, Helmer C. Dementia case management effectiveness on health care costs and resource utilization: a systematic review of randomized controlled trials. *J Nutr Health Aging* 2010;14:669-76.

32 Lam L, Lee J, Chung J, Lau A, Woo J, Kwok T. A randomised controlled control to examine the effectiveness of case management model for community dwelling older persons with mild dementia in Hong Kong. *Int J Geriatr Psychiatry* 2009;25:395-402.

33 Specht J, Bossen A, Hall GR, Zimmerman B, Russell J. The effects of a dementia nurse care manager on improving caregiver outcomes *Am J Alzheimers Dis Other Demen* 2009;24:193-207.

34 Sussman T. The influence of service factors on spousal caregivers' perceptions of community services. *J Gerontol Social Work* 2009;52:406-22.

35 Long SK, Liu K, Black K, O'Keeffe J, Molony S. Getting by in the community. Lessons from frail elders. *J Aging Social Policy* 2005;17:19-44.

36 Liu K, Manton KG, Aragon C. Changes in home care use by disabled elderly persons: 1982-1994. *J Gerontol Ser B Psychol Sci Social Sci* 2000;55B:S245-53.

37 Family Caregiver Alliance. Caregiver assessment: voices and views from the field. Report from a National Consensus Development Conference (Vol I). San Francisco, 2006. www.caregiver.org/caregiver/jsp/content_node.jsp?nodeid=1630.

Related links

bmj.com/archive
- Fall assessment in older people (2011;343:d5153)
- Cognitive assessment of older people (2011;343:d5042)
- Functional assessment in older people (2011;343:d4681)

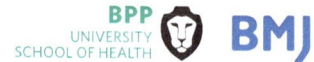

Post-acute care and secondary prevention after ischaemic stroke

K S McArthur, clinical research fellow, T J Quinn, lecturer in geriatric medicine,
P Higgins, clinical research fellow, P Langhorne, professor of stroke care

Institute of Cardiovascular and
Medical Sciences, University
of Glasgow, Western Infirmary,
Glasgow G11 6NT, UK

Correspondence to: K S McArthur
kate.mcarthur@glasgow.ac.uk

Cite this as: BMJ 2011;342:d2083

DOI: 10.1136/bmj.d2083

http://www.bmj.com/content/342/
bmj.d2083/rapid-responses

In the first part of this two part review (BMJ 2011;342:d1938) we discussed acute diagnosis and management of cerebrovascular events. Much of the focus of recent research, public health initiatives, a nd health policy has been around acute and hyperacute management of stroke. However, important goals of stroke care are to maximise functional recovery and prevent recurrent events. Here we draw on evidence from randomised trials and meta-analyses to discuss models of care, rehabilitation, and secondary prevention in stroke.

An important aspect of post-acute stroke care is rehabilitation. Rehabilitation research remains a "young" science, although an evidence base is emerging. As we make progress in this field, we need a common language to describe this important intervention. In the box we offer our own definition of stroke rehabilitation, although others may offer differing suggestions. Many questions remain unanswered regarding timing, optimal components, and frequency and intensity of rehabilitation. Further discussion of rehabilitation as a concept or rehabilitation theory specific to stroke is beyond the scope of this article, but recent high quality publications on the subject are available.[w1 w2]

This review will focus on the early period after stroke. Effective early intervention may affect longer term outcomes,[w3] with combined analysis of three UK stroke cohorts (n=7710 patients) showing that long term survival is predicted by functional outcome at six months.[w4] Most interventional research in stroke has focused on these first days to months after a stroke event, whereas health needs and management of stroke survivors outside of this period has received little attention. This is unfortunate in a cohort with high incidence of residual disability and often complex comorbidity, and more work is needed to inform practice and policy.

How should I assess a patient who has survived a stroke?

Assessment in the first days after stroke will guide subsequent management. The aims are to ascertain the pathology and mechanism of the stroke, identify post-stroke complications, and describe initial impairments.

"Acute" brain imaging was discussed in the first part of this review and will not be covered here. Further investigation to identify a possible origin and guide treatment may include assessment of extracranial carotid arteries, heart structure, or arrhythmia. The potential deleterious effects of deranged "physiology" (temperature, blood pressure, glycaemic control) were also discussed in the previous review. Evidence for intervention remains inconclusive, although routine frequent monitoring of these parameters in the first 72 hours remains usual practice.

Regular (at least daily) assessments of neurological function are important in planning effective ongoing medical care and early rehabilitation. Longitudinal cohort studies suggest that early measures of disability predict longer term outcomes.[w5] In the first days after stroke, neurological findings are dynamic. The National Institutes of Health Stroke Scale[w6] and Glasgow Coma Scale[w7] are often used initially as global measures. Deterioration suggests that further investigation is needed to exclude hemispheric oedema or haemorrhage. Therapists will plan intervention on the basis of early functional assessments of visuospatial awareness, sitting balance, and mobility. Later the focus of assessment will move to activity measures, using validated tools such as the Barthel index[w8] or modified Rankin scale.[w9]

Post-stroke dysphagia is common—occurring in up to half of patients—and is associated with an increased risk of aspiration pneumonia and poor outcomes related to disability, increased length of stay, and death.[w10] Meanwhile, withholding oral intake presents a risk of dehydration and malnutrition. Routine early assessment of swallow is recommended by national guidelines.[1 2] Assessment should be frequent; most patients with early dysphagia will regain swallow by the second week.[w11] A bedside water swallow test (where a patient is asked to swallow a small volume of water) is a reasonable screening test[w12] and will determine the need for formal assessment of swallowing. Such assessment is performed by speech and language therapists and is often complemented by functional imaging, such as video fluoroscopy.

What kind of care should be delivered in hospital?

Evidence of benefit of stroke units
In the past two decades many single centre trials highlighted poor outcomes associated with generic care compared with care undertaken in dedicated stroke units. A Cochrane review from 2007 of 31 trials (n=6936 participants) confirmed the benefits of organised specialist care for patients with stroke.[3] Compared with general wards, the number needed to treat in a specialist unit was 22 to prevent one death and 16 to prevent one patient losing their independence, which compares favourably with other interventions for stroke (tables 1 and 2). The benefits of being cared for in a stroke unit extend to all ages, subtypes, and severities of stroke, and studies with longer follow-up suggest that benefits endure.[w3, w13] An economic analysis alongside a

SUMMARY POINTS

- The management of stroke patients within dedicated stroke units prevents disability and saves lives for patients of all ages, with all types and severities of stroke
- Venous thromboembolism prophylaxis with compression stockings is not routinely recommended and may cause harm.
- Early mobilisation and physiotherapy are recommended by guidelines and appear to be safe, although definitive data on efficacy are awaited
- Medical complications after stroke are common and affect functional outcomes as well as mortality; infection, delirium, and dysphagia are potentially treatable
- Early artificial feeding with percutaneous gastrostomy tube has not shown longer term benefit for stroke survivors with impaired swallow and nasogastric feeding is recommended for initial management
- Secondary prevention with anti-hypertensive, anti-thrombotic, and lipid lowering drugs reduces likelihood of recurrent stroke

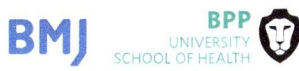

STROKE REHABILITATION—A WORKING DEFINITION

Stroke rehabilitation is not (usually) a single intervention; rather, it is an active process with a holistic, individualised focus. It usually involves teams made up of various professionals, the patient, and other relevant parties (such as carers), all with a final common goal of enhancing functioning to enable patients and carers to live their lives to the fullest potential.

Based on Quinn and Langhorne, Oxford Desk Reference Geriatric Medicine, 2011.

---

randomised trial found that care in a dedicated stroke unit was cost effective.[w14] The evidence clearly suggests that such a service should be available for all patients who experience a stroke.

What makes a stroke unit?

To tease out the components of an effective complex intervention can be a challenge.[4] Although a systematic review has highlighted the importance of monitoring and treating complications,[5] traditional medical input is unlikely to be the sole factor contributing to the success of a stroke unit. A survey of recent trials suggests that an essential component is the multidisciplinary team with a specialist interest in stroke, who provide an organised package of care coordinated through regular team meetings. The setting and achievement of goals requires collaboration of medical, nursing, and therapy staff in hospital and in the community and should be guided by the patient and carers.

Within this generic description, care in the stroke unit varies, and the definition of the "ideal" stroke unit is flexible. Many countries are pushing towards direct admission to stroke units, although other models of care were included in the Cochrane review[3] Although the benefits of immediate admission to stroke care seem intuitive (early specialist input, prompt intervention), robust supporting evidence is not available.

Recent research has focused on opening the "black box" of stroke unit care. The individual components that have been investigated and shown to be beneficial, potentially beneficial, or of uncertain benefit are summarised in the figure. Robust evidence is emerging for specific areas of stroke care and those with recent data have been selected for further discussion here.

Prevention of venous thrombosis

Stroke survivors are at substantially increased risk of developing deep vein thrombosis because they are immobile and often dehydrated.[w15 w16] An open label randomised trial compared prophylactic low molecular weight heparin and unfractionated heparin for the prevention of venous thromboembolism after acute ischaemic stroke, and showed that enoxaparin was effective and relatively safe in reducing ultrasound detected deep vein thrombosis, although whether a clinical benefit exists is uncertain.[6] The trial did not compare heparin with placebo. The available data do not allow definitive advice on use of heparin, and further research about targeting this treatment to those at greatest risk is needed.[w17]

The recently published Clots in Legs Or sTockings after Stroke (CLOTS) trials provided pragmatic data about use of thromboembolic prevention stockings. Compared with no stockings, thigh or knee length stockings did not significantly reduce the risk of deep vein thrombosis.[7] There was a trend towards increased deep vein thrombosis in the group that used knee length stockings, and substantial rates of skin complications were reported with both types of stocking.[8] Although the clinical implications of the CLOTS

Opening the 'black box' of stroke unit care

Important components of stroke unit care

Staff with specialist interest	Early discharge planning
Early mobilisation	Multidisciplinary team
Prompt investigation	Goal setting approach
Prompt pharmacotherapy	Positioning and handling
Physiological monitoring	

Potentially important components

Management of:	Oral care
Pyrexia	Assessment of dysphagia
Hyperglycaemia	Bladder and bowel care
Hypoxia	Information provision
Hypertension	Involvement of carers
Hydration/nutrition	

Components with no evidence of efficacy

Routine use of compression stockings
Early percutaneous gastronomy feeding
Routine use of nutritional supplements

Components of effective stroke unit care subject to randomised trials (based on Langhorne et al[5])

---

trials continue to be debated, routine use of stockings cannot be recommended on the basis of current evidence.

Feeding patients

The Feed Or Ordinary Diet (FOOD) family of large randomised trials assessed different aspects of nutrition after stroke. The first assessed routine oral supplementation in stroke survivors with intact swallow (n=4023)[9] compared with normal diet, and found that routine supplementation did not improve outcomes or reduce complications (absolute risk reduction in mortality 0.7%, 95% confidence interval -1.4 to 2.7; overall mortality rates were 12% in groups receiving supplements and 13% in those with no supplements). However, these findings do not preclude the targeted use of supplements where there is evidence or risk of malnutrition. The second and third studies examined the relative merits of early feeding by nasogastric tube (n=859) or percutaneous gastrostomy tube (n=321) after stroke.[10] Early tube feeding was associated with a trend towards reduction in risk of death (absolute risk reduction 5.8%, 95% confidence interval -0.8 to 12.5). By contrast, early feeding by percutaneous gastrostomy tube was associated with a trend towards increased risk of death or poor outcome (7.8%, 0 to 15.5). This finding is partly explained by the severity of stroke that requires artificial feeding; however, use of percutaneous gastrostomy tube is not a benign intervention and has associated short and longer term morbidity.[w18 w19] Patients' preferences and quality of life after percutaneous gastrostomy tube feeding are poorly researched, but available data suggest no improvement in quality of life.[w20] Based on these findings, early placement of percutaneous gastrostomy tubes is not advisable. Options for long term feeding are limited and percutaneous gastrostomy tube feeding may have a role in selected individuals, after discussion with the patient, relatives, and multidisciplinary team.

Mobilisation: how soon?

UK guidelines recommend by consensus that patients should sit out of their bed and become mobile as soon as their clinical condition permits. It seems intuitive that early mobilisation should reduce the sedentary complications of stroke (muscle wasting, thrombosis, pressure sores, hypostatic pneumonia) but there is limited evidence to support the practice. A Very Early Rehabilitation Trial (AVERT)

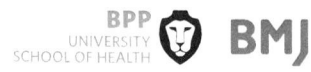

Table 1 Potential population impact of acute stroke interventions for a hypothetical population of one million with 2500 strokes per year[34]

Treatment	Efficacy (extra independent survivors (n))*	Eligibility (proportion stroke population)	Effectiveness (number of extra independent survivorst)
Aspirin in acute ischaemic stroke	25	80%	20
Thrombolysis in ischaemic stroke			
rt-PA within 3 hours	280	10%	28
rt-PA within 3-4.5 hours	125	10%	12
Basic stroke unit care	125	80%	100
Early supported discharge teams and home rehabilitation	120	35%	42

rt-PA=tissue plasminogen activator. Calculations indicate number of extra independent survivors (modified Rankin score 0-2) resulting from an intervention during a one year period. *Assuming all stroke patients are eligible for treatment. †Taking into account population eligible for treatment.

Table 2 Summary of patient outcomes in the stroke unit trials[3]

Outcome	Stroke unit	Conventional care	Extra events per 100 patients (95% CI)
Home (independent)	44 %	38%	5 (1 to 8)*
Home (dependent)	16%	16%	0 (−2 to 3)
Institutional care	18%	20%	−2 (−5 to 0)*
Dead	22%	26%	−3 (−6 to −1)*

Proportion (%) of patients with various outcomes at the end of scheduled follow-up (median one year), based on data from Stroke Unit Review (n=6900).
* P<0.05 for difference between groups.

is currently assessing the value of early mobilisation in a multicentre randomised controlled trial. Fears that early mobilisation may be harmful seem to be unfounded; initial results suggest that mobilisation within the first day is well tolerated and may prevent complications.[w21]

Facilitating discharge

Patients and their carers have reported feeling afraid and unsupported at the time of discharge, and an interview questionnaire study has shown that inadequate provision of information is associated with poor satisfaction for stroke survivors and carers.[w22] However, a recent systematic review and meta-analysis of randomised controlled trials that evaluated dedicated stroke liaison services found no evidence of efficacy compared with standard care in improving measures of extended activities of daily living and patient/carer subjective health status.[11]

A prolonged inpatient stay is costly, and services are increasingly encouraged to facilitate an early return to the community. A 2005 meta-analysis of data from studies of early supported discharge concluded that a multidisciplinary, appropriately trained early supported discharge service can significantly reduce days in bed for stroke survivors with mild to moderate impairments, with no corresponding increase in readmission or morbidity[12] and with overall cost benefit.[w23]

In view of the sound evidence base for stroke unit admission and early supported discharge for selected patients, it is unfortunate that recent UK audit data suggest continuing inequity of access to these services. It seems reasonable to speculate that universal delivery of evidence based post-acute stroke care would, through its impact on disability, result in lower incidence of stroke survivors needing institutional or additional domiciliary care, and ultimately would offer cost savings.

Antithrombotic following ischaemic stroke

The preventive efficacy of aspirin, clopidogrel, dipyridamole, and the coumarin anticoagulant warfarin have been evaluated, as monotherapy and (because of their differing mechanisms of action) in combination. (table 3)

For monotherapy, a large meta-analysis showed a 15% reduction in risk of vascular events with aspirin compared with placebo over two years.[w41] A randomised trial showed a modest benefit of clopidogrel over aspirin in reducing

vascular events, in a population that included patients with stroke related disease.[w42] Dipyridamole has similar efficacy to aspirin but is associated with frequent adverse effects, mainly headache and gastrointestinal disturbance.[w43]

A meta-analysis of trials showed that the combination of aspirin and modified release dipyridamole is better than aspirin monotherapy[15] and equivalent to clopidogrel monotherapy for stroke prevention.[16] Dipyridamole has little effect on non-stroke vascular events, suggesting that it has specific cerebrovascular efficacy. Combinations of aspirin and clopidogrel have been studied in two large trials, both of which found that any reduction in vascular events was outweighed by increased haemorrhagic adverse events.[17 18] Bleeding rates with aspirin and clopidogrel in combination are similar to those with warfarin and the risks should not be underestimated.[w44] Some patients at high risk may benefit from short term combination antiplatelet therapy; in a trial of 107 patients with carotid stenosis and active embolisation, dual antiplatelet therapy was associated with reduced embolic burden and a trend towards reduced events.[19]

Interpretation of antiplatelet trial data to guide clinical practice is complex. While current Scottish guidance suggests aspirin and modified release dipyridamole as routine therapy, the most recent National Institute for Health and Clinical Excellence assessment recommends clopidogrel because of its better tolerability. For example, in one large study, premature discontinuation of aspirin plus extended release dipyridamole was substantially higher than with clopidogrel (1650 patients [16.4%] versus 1069 [10.6%], P<0.001).[w45]

Warfarin has been studied in patients with sinus rhythm and with atrial fibrillation. For those with sinus rhythm a series of trials has shown that any benefit of anticoagulation is outweighed by an increased risk of bleeding for all levels of stroke risk.[20] Patients with cardioembolic stroke face a particularly high risk of recurrence. Stroke risk in patients with atrial fibrillation can be stratified and scoring systems have been developed (webfigure) to guide choice of therapy. Regardless of the scoring system used, where a patient has sustained a cerebrovascular event, the risk of subsequent stroke is sufficiently high to warrant the use of warfarin where possible. In patients with atrial fibrillation treated with aspirin, the risk of first stroke is 2.7% per annum and risk of recurrent stroke 10%. Treatment with warfarin has been shown to reduce these risks to 1.5% and

Table 3 Evidence for antiplatelets in stroke prevention[w57-w59]

Antiplatelet and comparison		Comparator	Result for stroke	Comments
Aspirin	›	Placebo	RR 0.78 95% CI 0.61 to 0.99	AT secondary prevention analysis
Dipyridamole	›	Placebo	RR 0.88(95% CI 0.81 to 0.95)	SR (n=23.19 with ischaemic stroke)
Aspirin + dipyridamole MR	›	Thienopyridines (clopidogrel)	RR 0.76 95% CI 0.65 to 0.89	SR 4 RCT (n=1611)
Aspirin	‹	Clopidogrel	OR 0.91, 95% CI 0.84 to 0.98	SR 4 RCT (n=86 865)
Aspirin + dipyridamole MR	●	Aspirin	HR 1.01 (95% CI 0.92 to 1.11)	RCT (n=20 332)
Aspirin + clopidogrel	●		RR 0.93 (95%CI 0.83 to 1.05)	SR (n=15 603 with risk factors)
Aspirin + clopidogrel	● *	Clopidogrel	RRR 6.4% 95% CI −4.6 to 16.3)	RCT (n=7599 with risk factors)
(Aspirin +) dipyridamole + clopidogrel		–	–	On-going multicentre trials

Data are for ischaemic stroke secondary prevention unless otherwise stated; references for individual trials and analysis within main body of text.

› indicates greater efficacy than; ‹ indicates lesser efficacy than; ● indicates equivalent efficacy; RR=relative risk; OR=odds ratio; HR=hazard ratio; RRR=relative risk reduction; AT=antiplatelet trialists; SR=systematic review; RCT=randomised controlled trial.

*Increased risk of life threatening or major bleeding seen with addition of aspirin.

4% respectively in a meta-analysis.[21] A Cochrane review confirmed the benefit of warfarin compared with aspirin (odds ratio 0.49, 95% confidence interval 0.33 to 0.72), calculating 60 fewer annual recurrent strokes per 1000 patients treated with warfarin.[22]

The timing of anticoagulant initiation after stroke is unclear. Large infarcts or major clinical deficits raise concerns about haemorrhage and decisions should be based on individual patients' characteristics. Some guidelines suggest starting therapy within 14 days. Although this is a reasonable general approach, patients must be considered individually—these data are from a single study (n=225) where less than half of the participants started warfarin within the first two weeks.[w46]

Despite its clear efficacy, clinicians may avoid warfarin, perhaps fearing risk of haemorrhage and problems with monitoring and adherence. Risk of warfarin related bleeding complications can also be stratified (webfigure). Oral anticoagulation shows the classic "inverse care law", with those at greatest risk of stroke least likely to receive therapy. For example, older cohorts have a raised prevalence of atrial fibrillation and greater risk of stroke, yet underuse of anticoagulation remains prevalent,[w47] despite compelling evidence from a UK general practice based study that showed the efficacy and relative safety of warfarin in selected older patients.[23] A new generation of oral anticoagulants are showing promise in clinical trials and may widen delivery of anticoagulation.[24]

How are common complications treated after stroke?

Common complications in the longer term after stroke include delirium, infection, depression, post-stroke pain, falls, and incontinence. All these complications may be underdiagnosed and have little evidence available to guide treatment, although they affect rehabilitation negatively and are strong predictors of poor functional outcome and mortality.[13] [w24]

Delirium is a common complication after stroke; observational studies suggest an incidence of around 13-48% of patients[w25] but assessment is complicated by the prevalence of concomitant communication deficits and dementia. The stroke insult itself may cause delirium, but infection is often a precipitant. The rate of nosocomial infection after stroke can be as high as 30%.[w26] Pneumonia and urinary tract infections remain the most common infections, although they may be prevented by regular assessment of swallow and avoidance of urinary catheters.[w27]

Post-stroke depression has been reported in a third of patients[w28] but the validity of estimates is questionable because the best method for screening or diagnosis is uncertain. A systematic review found that drug treatment can improve mood and reduce excessive emotions but had frequent side effects, and there was no robust evidence of benefit for non-drug treatments.[w29]

Post-stroke pain is multifactorial in origin, with important components including neuropathic pain and spasticity. Treatments that have been assessed for specific causes of pain include tricyclics, anticonvulsants, and botulinum toxin; evidence of their benefit is emerging but high costs and side effects may limit their widespread use. Shoulder pain in a paretic limb is increasingly recognised.[w30] Robust evidence to guide management of such pain is lacking,[w31] although suggestions are available for best practice in assessment and intervention.[w32]

Falls are common both in the acute setting and in the longer term after stroke.[w33] Putative risk factors include dementia, depression, polypharmacy, and sensory impairment.[w34] The incidence of fracture is substantial (twofold increase in risk of hip/femur fracture[w35]) in the post-stroke population.[w36] Interventions to reduce risk of fracture are extrapolated from studies in older people that were not limited to those who had had a stroke; no stroke specific data are available. Preventive treatments may include bisphosphonates and preparations of calcium vitamin D, and multidisciplinary prevention packages that focus on personal and environmental factors. A recent systematic review and meta-analysis has highlighted the need for future randomised controlled trials in this area; it found evidence only to support vitamin D supplementation in a female population in hospital.[w37]

Prevalence of urinary incontinence is estimated at 40-60% in an acute stroke population, with 15% remaining incontinent at one year.[w38] Causes may include abnormalities of normal central control of voiding, lower urinary tract infection, and functional incontinence. A Cochrane review evaluated the limited evidence on physical interventions such as bladder retraining and pelvic floor exercises, and drug treatment, which may have a role in selected patients.[w39]

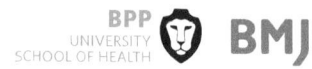

SOURCES AND SELECTION CRITERIA

This review is based on the authors' clinical and research experience and informed by a search of published literature. Electronic databases (Medline and Embase) were searched from inception to December 2010 inclusive, using truncated keywords: "stroke or cerebrovascular"; "rehabilitation"; "prevention". In addition key reference works, national and international guidelines, and journals were searched for relevant papers. Particular attention was given to large randomised controlled trials, systematic reviews, and meta-analyses. The intention was not to offer comprehensive systematic review but to give a narrative overview and critique of published work.

ADDITIONAL EDUCATIONAL RESOURCES

Resources for healthcare professionals

- Stroke Association Professional Training (www.stroke. org.uk/professionals/training_and_development/index. html)— A selection of training and education programmes offered by the stroke association, suitable for all healthcare professionals
- European Stroke Organisation (www.eso-stroke.org)— Comprehensive access to European stroke guidelines and educational resources for health professionals and lay people
- UK Stroke Research Network (www.uksrn.ac.uk)—Provides an infrastructure to facilitate stroke research and improve communication between academics, stroke clinicians, stroke service users, and research funders
- Stroke Training and Awareness Resources (STARS) project (www.stroketraining.org)—Commissioned by the Scottish Government to provide an e-learning resource for all healthcare professionals and social care staff working with patients affected by stroke

Resources for patients

- The Stroke Association (www.stroke.org.uk)—Produces a number of publications to help educate and inform and increase awareness of stroke, including patient leaflets, and *Stroke News* (a quarterly magazine)
- Act FAST campaign (www.nhs.uk/actfast/Pages/stroke. aspx)—Public awareness campaign to improve community recognition of stroke symptoms and encourage those affected to seek urgent medical help
- Connect (www.ukconnect.org/index.aspx)—communication disability charity for patients and carers affected by aphasia
- Carers UK (www.carersuk.org)—charity providing support for home carers

What measures help to prevent another stroke?

The risk of recurrent vascular events after a stroke or TIA is substantial. Recurrent stroke has been reported in 17.3% of patients after TIA and 18.5% after minor stroke at three months.[w40] National guidelines suggest that secondary preventive strategies be commenced early and continue indefinitely.[1] [14]

Management of carotid disease

International guidelines recommend that survivors of stroke are investigated for large artery atherosclerosis, particularly ipsilateral extracranial carotid artery disease.[25] Where imaging confirms stenotic carotid disease, patients with non-disabling events may benefit from surgical carotid endarterectomy. As a general rule, all patients with greater than 50% symptomatic internal carotid stenosis should be considered for intervention in the setting of a neurovascular multidisciplinary team. The benefits of intervention vary with degree of stenosis and time since event. A pooled analysis of data from randomised controlled trials of endarterectomy for symptomatic carotid stenosis (6092 patients) showed that for severe symptomatic stenosis (>70%), surgery afforded a 15.6% absolute risk reduction in ipsilateral ischaemic stroke over five years versus medical treatment alone, with a smaller 4.5% absolute risk reduction for moderate (50-69%) stenosis.[26] Surgery carried no benefit in less severe disease or in cases of complete occlusion. Greater benefit is seen with early surgery. Treatment within two weeks of symptoms afforded an absolute risk reduction of 23%, by comparison with absolute risk reduction of 7.4% for those treated after 12 weeks. In order to prevent one ipsilateral stroke at five years, the number needed to treat is five within two weeks and 125 if surgery is delayed beyond 12 weeks.[27] The benefits of early treatment are particularly pronounced in women, where significant efficacy of revascularisation is seen only in the first two weeks.[w48]

Percutaneous stenting of carotid vessels has been proposed as a less invasive method of revascularisation, but studies have failed to show that stenting has the long term benefits of traditional endarterectomy. Risk and benefit may change as technical expertise develops but present guidelines do not recommend stenting outside clinical trials.[28]

How to manage hypertension

Management of hypertension in the acute phase was discussed in the first part of this review. Long term management of hypertension significantly reduces the risk of recurrent events. Meta-analysis of secondary prevention trials showed a 24% reduced odds of recurrent stroke with antihypertensive treatment (odds ratio 0.76, 95% confidence interval 0.63-0.92; absolute rate of recurrent stroke 10%).[w49] Risk reduction is related to change in blood pressure and substantial benefit is seen even with a modest change in pressure. An overview of published reviews including more than 188 000 participants, showed that for each 10 mm Hg reduction in systolic pressure, risk was reduced by one third. This finding was consistent across sex, region, and stroke subtypes.[29]

Evidence clearly indicates that all patients should be considered for antihypertensive therapy to prevent recurrent stroke. UK guidelines suggest a target blood pressure of 130/80 mm Hg; for most patients this will require at least two agents, one of which should be a diuretic.[28]

The large PROGRESS trial has been pivotal in guiding post-stroke blood pressure management.[30] Treatment with the ACE inhibitor perindopril, in combination with the thiazide indapamide, showed a 26% reduced risk of stroke (95% confidence interval 16% to 34%) compared with placebo. Patients were considered for inclusion regardless of baseline blood pressure and benefits were seen even in those traditionally defined as normotensive.

Choice of antihypertensive agent may be important. In one pooled analysis the strongest evidence was for diuretic based therapy (odds ratio 0.63, 95% confidence interval 0.55 to 0.73).[w50] Theoretical benefits of angiotensin receptor antagonists in stroke prevention have not been supported by large scale trials.[w51] [w52]

Treating high cholesterol, diabetes and lifestyle risks

The stroke related benefits of statin treatment were originally described through sub-analyses data relating to ischaemic heart disease. In a large pooled analysis

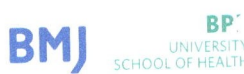
TIPS FOR NON SPECIALISTS

- Refer all patients with suspected stroke to the local dedicated stroke unit
- Stroke survivors with ipsilateral carotid disease may benefit from revascularisation. Outcomes are best when intervention is performed early; liaise with a vascular multidisciplinary team
- Look out for common post-stroke complications such as infection, delirium, depression, pain, incontinence, and falls
- Treat hypertension aggressively and ensure that patients receive long term thromboprophylaxis
- Consider anticoagulation for all stroke survivors with atrial fibrillation, remembering that age alone is not a contraindication to anticoagulation

QUESTIONS FOR FUTURE RESEARCH

- What is the optimal model for deep vein thrombosis prophylaxis for patients with ischaemic stroke?
- What is the optimal timing and intensity of multidisciplinary intervention? Can this be targeted?
- Is there a role for screening stroke survivors for common complications; do we have adequate tools to inform a screening approach?
- Can we develop novel drugs to minimise recurrent disease and provide alternative strategies for intolerant patients; are novel anticoagulation treatments cost effective?
- What is the role of short duration, high potency antithrombotic therapy following ischaemic stroke?
- What happens to stroke survivors' functional status in the longer term (years) post-event; is there a role for ongoing or opportunistic intervention and rehabilitation?

of data from coronary disease trials, statin treatment significantly reduced the risk of incident stroke (odds ratio 0.79, 95% confidence interval 0.73 to 0.85).[31] The SPARCL trial (n=4731), a stroke specific placebo controlled study of statins (atorvastatin 80 mg), showed a reduction in incident ischaemic stroke (number needed to treat 45 over five years) and other vascular events, but a rise in incident haemorrhagic stroke (number needed to harm 107 over five years).[w53] UK guidelines recommend treating to a total cholesterol of less than 4.0 mmol/L and LDL less than 2.0 mmol/L.[28] Statins are not recommended after intracerebral haemorrhage unless indicated for other vascular disease.

Observational studies have suggested a high prevalence of occult diabetes in stroke cohorts, which suggests that screening for diabetes may be useful after stroke. Although diabetes is an important risk factor for vascular events, no specific guidelines are available for optimal therapy in patients with stroke. A subgroup analysis of the PROactive trial described a reduced incidence of stroke with pioglitazone in selected patients[32] but the findings must be interpreted in the light of other risks associated with thiazolidinediones. Several large randomised controlled trials have compared aggresive glycaemic control with standard therapy. Although these studies were not designed to measure stroke outcomes, they did not show reduced incidence of stroke with tight glycaemic control.[w54]

No data from randomised controlled trials are available to guide lifestyle modification in patients with stroke. Compelling observational data support cessation of smoking.[w55] The relation between alcohol and cerebrovascular risk is controversial. Meta-analysis of 84 observational studies described a "J-shaped curve" where lowest vascular risk was associated with modest intake, but

one unit daily.[w56] Controlled weight reduction in overweight patients and physical activity have been associated with improvements in blood pressure, cholesterol, and diabetes. There are no stroke specific data on dietary modification, although routine vitamin supplementation probably has no benefit.[33]

Contributors: All authors contributed to writing the manuscript and have approved the final version. KSMcA is guarantor.

Competing interests: All authors have completed the Unified Competing Interest form at www.icmje.org/coi_disclosure.pdf (available on request from the corresponding author) and declare: no external support for the submitted work; KSMcA, PH, PL have no relationships with companies that might have an interest in the submitted work in the previous three years. TJQ has received modest speakers' fees and travel assistance from Bristol Myers Squibb, Sanofi, and Pfizer; no non-financial interests that may be relevant to the submitted work.

Provenance and peer review: Commissioned, externally peer reviewed.

1   National Collaborating Centre for Chronic Conditions. Stroke: national clinical guideline for diagnosis and initial management of acute stroke and transient ischaemic attack (TIA). Royal College of Physicians, 2008.
2   Scottish Intercollegiate Guideline Network. Management of patients with stroke: identification and management of dysphagia. A national clinical guideline. 2010.
3   Stroke Unit Trialists' Collaboration. Organised inpatient (stroke unit) care for stroke. Cochrane Database Syst Rev 2007;4:CD000197.
4   Govan L, Langhorne P, Weir CJ, Stroke Unit Trialists' Collaboration. Does the prevention of complications explain the survival benefit of organized inpatient (stroke unit) care? Further analysis of a systematic review. Stroke 2007;38:2536-40.
5   Langhorne P, Pollock A, Stroke Unit Trialists' Collaboration. What are the components of effective stroke unit care? Age Ageing 2002;31:365-71.
6   Sherman DG, Albers GW, Bladin C, Fieschi C, Gabbai AA, Kase CS, et al. The efficacy and safety of enoxaparin versus unfractionated heparin for the prevention of venous thromboembolism after acute ischaemic stroke (PREVAIL Study): an open-label randomised comparison. Lancet 2007;369:1347-55.
7   CLOTS Trials Collaboration, Dennis M, Sandercock PA, Reid J, Graham C, Murray G, et al. Effectiveness of thigh-length graduated compression stockings to reduce the risk of deep vein thrombosis after stroke (CLOTS trial 1): a multicentre, randomised controlled trial. Lancet 2009;373:1958-65.
8   CLOTS Trial Collaboration. Thigh-length versus below-knee stockings for deep venous thrombosis prophylaxis after stroke. Ann Intern Med 2010;153:553-62.
9   Routine oral nutritional supplementation for stroke patients in hospital (FOOD): a multicentre randomised controlled trial. Lancet 2005;365:755-63.
10 Effect of timing and method of enteral tube feeding for dysphagic stroke patients (FOOD): a multicentre randomised controlled trial. Lancet 2005;365:764-72.
11 Ellis G, Mant J, Langhorne P, Dennis M, Winner S. Stroke liaison workers for stroke patients and carers: an individual patient data meta-analysis. Cochrane Database Syst Rev 2010;5:CD005066.
12 Langhorne P, Taylor G, Murray G, Dennis M, Anderson C, Bautz-Holter E, et al. Early supported discharge services for stroke patients: a meta-analysis of individual patients' data. Lancet 2005;365:501-6.
13 Quinn TJ, Paolucci S, Sunnerhagen KS, Sivenius J, Walker MF, Toni D, et al. Evidence-based stroke rehabilitation: an expanded guidance document from the European Stroke Organisation (ESO) guidelines for management of ischaemic stroke and transient ischaemic attack 2008. J Rehab Med 2009;41:99-111.
14 Scottish Intercollegiate Guidelines Network. Management of patients with stroke or TIA: assessment, investigation, immediate management and secondary prevention. A national clinical guideline. 2008.
15 Verro P, Gorelick PB, Nguyen D. Aspirin plus dipyridamole versus aspirin for prevention of vascular events after stroke or tia: a meta-analysis. Stroke 2008;39:1358-63.
16 Sacco RL, Diener HC, Yusuf S, Cotton D, Ounpuu S, Lawton WA, et al. Aspirin and extended-release dipyridamole versus clopidogrel for recurrent stroke. N Engl J Med 2008;359:1238-51.
17 Bhatt DL, Fox KA, Hacke W, Berger PB, Black HR, Boden WE, et al. Clopidogrel and aspirin versus aspirin alone for the prevention of atherothrombotic events. N Engl J Med 2006;354:1706-17.
18 Diener HC, Bogousslavsky J, Brass LM, Cimminiello C, Csiba L, Kaste M, et al. Aspirin and clopidogrel compared with clopidogrel alone after recent ischaemic stroke or transient ischaemic attack in high-risk patients (MATCH): randomised, double-blind, placebo-controlled trial. Lancet 2004;364:331-7.
19 Markus HS, Droste DW, Kaps M, Larrue V, Lees KR, Siebler M, et al. Dual antiplatelet therapy with clopidogrel and aspirin in symptomatic carotid stenosis evaluated using doppler embolic signal detection: the clopidogrel and aspirin for reduction of emboli in symptomatic carotid stenosis (CARESS) trial. Circulation 2005;111:2233-40.

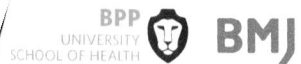

20 Algra A, De Schryver EL, van GJ, Kappelle LJ, Koudstaal PJ. Oral anticoagulants versus antiplatelet therapy for preventing further vascular events after transient ischaemic attack or minor stroke of presumed arterial origin. *Cochrane Database Syst Rev* 2006;3:CD001342.

21 van WC, Hart RG, Singer DE, Laupacis A, Connolly S, Petersen P, et al. Oral anticoagulants vs aspirin in nonvalvular atrial fibrillation: an individual patient meta-analysis. *JAMA* 2002;288:2441-8.

22 Saxena R, Koudstaal P. Anticoagulants versus antiplatelet therapy for preventing stroke in patients with nonrheumatic atrial fibrillation and a history of stroke or transient ischemic attack. *Cochrane Database Syst Rev* 2004;4:CD000187.

23 Mant J, Hobbs FD, Fletcher K, Roalfe A, Fitzmaurice D, Lip GY, et al. Warfarin versus aspirin for stroke prevention in an elderly community population with atrial fibrillation (the Birmingham Atrial Fibrillation Treatment of the Aged Study, BAFTA): a randomised controlled trial. *Lancet* 2007;370:493-503.

24 Connolly SJ, Ezekowitz MD, Yusuf S, Eikelboom J, Oldgren J, Parekh A, et al. Dabigatran versus warfarin in patients with atrial fibrillation. *N Eng J Med* 2009;361:1139-51.

25 European Stroke Organisation (ESO) Executive Committee, ESO Writing Committee. Guidelines for management of ischaemic stroke and transient ischaemic attack 2008. *Cerebrovasc Dis* 2008;25:457-507.

26 Rothwell PM, Eliasziw M, Gutnikov SA, Fox AJ, Taylor DW, Mayberg MR, et al. Analysis of pooled data from the randomised controlled trials of endarterectomy for symptomatic carotid stenosis. *Lancet* 2003;361:107-16.

27 Rothwell PM, Gutnikov SA, Warlow CP. Reanalysis of the final results of the European Carotid Surgery Trial. *Stroke* 2003;34:514-23.

28 Intercollegiate Stroke Working Party. National clinical guideline for stroke. Third ed. Royal College of Physicians, 2008.

29 Lawes CM, Bennett DA, Feigin VL, Rodgers A. Blood pressure and stroke: an overview of published reviews. *Stroke* 2004;35:776-85.

30 PROGRESS Collaborative Group. Randomised trial of a perindopril-based blood-pressure-lowering regimen among 6105 individuals with previous stroke or transient ischaemic attack. *Lancet* 2001;358:1033-41.

31 Amarenco P, Labreuche J, Lavalle P, Touboul PJ. Statins in stroke prevention and carotid atherosclerosis: systematic review and up-to-date meta-analysis. *Stroke* 2004;35:2902-9.

32 Dormandy JA, Charbonnel B, Eckland DJ, Erdmann E, Massi-Benedetti M, Moules IK, et al. Secondary prevention of macrovascular events in patients with type 2 diabetes in the PROactive Study (PROspective pioglitAzone Clinical Trial In macroVascular Events): a randomised controlled trial. *Lancet* 2005;366:1279-89.

33 VITATOPS Trial Study Group. B vitamins in patients with recent transient ischaemic attack or stroke in the VITAmins TO Prevent Stroke (VITATOPS) trial: a randomised, double-blind, parallel, placebo-controlled trial. *Lancet Neurology* 2010;9:855-65.

34 Langhorne P, Sandercock P, Prasad K. Evidence-based practice for stroke. *Lancet Neurology* 2009;8:308-9.

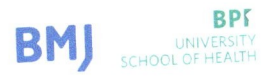

Investigation and management of unintentional weight loss in older adults

Jenna McMinn, foundation year 2, medicine[1], Claire Steel, specialist trainee year 6 in medicine for the elderly[2], Adam Bowman, consultant physician[3]

[1]Queen Elizabeth National Spinal Injuries Unit, Southern General Hospital, Glasgow G51 4TF, UK

[2]Department of Medicine for the Elderly, Monklands Hospital, Airdrie, UK

[3]Department of Medicine for the Elderly, Glasgow Royal Infirmary, Glasgow, UK

Correspondence to: J McMinn, Department of Medicine, Southern General Hospital jennamcminn@gmail.com

Cite this as: BMJ 2011;342: d1732

DOI: 10.1136/bmj.d1732

http://www.bmj.com/content/342/bmj.d1732

Unintentional weight loss occurs in 15-20% of older adults (those over 65) and is associated with increased morbidity and mortality.[1] Clinical and epidemiological studies have reported even higher prevalence in certain populations, with as many as 27% of community dwelling elderly people and 50-60% of nursing home residents being affected.[1 2 w1]

Weight loss may be the presenting problem or an incidental finding during a consultation for other reasons. There are no published guidelines on how to investigate and manage patients with unintentional weight loss, and responses range from doing nothing (if it is viewed as a normal part of the ageing process) to extensive blind investigation because of the fear that it represents underlying cancer. Observational studies have shown that in as many as 25% of cases no identifiable cause is found, despite extensive investigation.[3 4] It is not clear how far clinicians should go to investigate older patients with unintentional weight loss in the absence of an obvious medical cause.

We review the available evidence (mainly epidemiological and observational studies) and outline a structured approach to investigation and management of the older patient with unintentional weight loss.

When is unintentional weight loss clinically important?

Age related physiological changes occur in elderly people and contribute to the so called "anorexia of ageing." These include a reduction in lean body mass, bone mass, and basal metabolic rate; reduced sense of taste and smell; and altered gastric signals leading to early satiation.[5] However, observational studies of healthy older adults report this normal age related weight loss to be only 0.1-0.2 kg a year,[6] and most elderly patients maintain weight over a reasonably long period of 5-10 years.[7] Substantial weight loss should not be dismissed as natural age related change and should be investigated.

Although no universally accepted definition of clinically important weight loss exists, most observational studies define it as a 5% or more reduction in body weight over 6-12 months.[3 4 8] To take into account the variability of baseline weight, weight loss is best expressed as a percentage rather than an absolute value; a loss of 2-3 kg is less important in a 90 kg patient than in a frail elderly patient who is underweight already.

Reported mortality within 1-2.5 years of clinically important weight loss ranges from 9% to 38%,[1 w2] and those particularly at risk include frail elderly people,[w1] those with low baseline body weight,[w3] and elderly patients recently admitted to hospital.[1 7]

Substantial weight loss has been shown to be associated with an increased risk of in-hospital and disease related complications,[9] increased disability and dependency,[7] higher rates of admission to residential home or nursing home,[w1] and poorer quality of life.[w4] At the extreme, cachexia (the disproportional loss of skeletal muscle rather than body fat, which leads to skeletal and cardiac muscle wasting, loss of visceral protein, and alterations in physiological functions including impaired immunity and a systemic inflammatory response) contributes to adverse outcomes through increased rates of infection, poor wound healing, pressure sores, reduced response to medical treatment, and increased risk of mortality.[10 w5]

Weight loss in elderly people significantly increases the rate of hip bone loss and the risk of hip fracture. In a prospective cohort study of 6785 elderly women, weight loss—both intentional and unintentional—of 5% or more from baseline weight (regardless of whether baseline weight was low or normal) almost doubled the risk of subsequent hip fracture (odds ratio 1.8, 95% confidence interval 1.43 to 2.24) compared with those with stable or increasing weight.[11]

What can cause unintentional weight loss in older adults?

Although involuntary weight loss in younger adults often has a medical cause, in older patients causes are more diverse, with psychiatric and socioeconomic factors playing an important part.

Prospective and retrospective studies from Germany, Belgium, Israel, the United States, and Spain have looked at patients who were investigated for involuntary weight loss to determine the common causes and their relative frequency (table 1).[3 4 8 12 13 w6] The studies varied considerably in terms of country, age of patients (most were not confined to the elderly), length of follow-up, and the type of patients recruited. However, cancer, non-malignant gastrointestinal disease, and psychiatric problems (particularly dementia and depression) were consistently among the most common causes of unintentional weight loss).

Several aids have been devised to enable doctors to consider the many possible causes of unintentional weight loss in older patients. These include the "9 Ds of weight loss in the elderly"[14] and "meals on wheels"[15] mnemonics (box 1). Our approach is to group the possible causes of weight loss into organic (malignant and non-malignant), psychosocial, and unknown causes.

Organic causes
Organic causes of weight loss include cancer, non-malignant medical disorders, and side effects of drugs (table 2).

SUMMARY POINTS

- Unintentional weight loss is common in elderly people and is associated with considerable morbidity and mortality
- Weight loss is clinically relevant if more than 5% of body weight is lost over 6-12 months, although smaller losses may be important in frail elderly people
- Causes can be classified as organic (malignant and non-malignant), psychological, social, or unknown
- Drugs should be reviewed because side effects often contribute to weight loss
- All patients should be assessed by a dietitian and screened for depression and cognitive impairment
- If initial history, examination, and investigations are normal, three months of "watchful

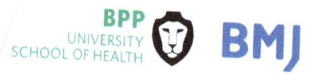

Table 1 Observational studies of causes of unintentional weight loss

Study	Follow-up (months)	Mean age of patients (years)	Most common cause of weight loss	Unknown cause of weight loss
Prospective German study of 158 men and women in secondary care[3]	25-36	68 (SD 14)	Cancer (24%) especially gastrointestinal (53% of cancers)	16%
			Non-malignant gastrointestinal disorders (19%)	
			Endocrine disease (11.4%)	
			Psychological (10.8%)	
			Cardiopulmonary disease (10.1%)	
Prospective Belgian study of 101 men and women in secondary care[4]	≥6	64 (SD 13)	Malignancy (22%) especially gastrointestinal (45% of cancers)	28%
			Psychological (16%)	
			Non-malignant GI disorders (15%)	
			Infectious diseases (8%)	
			Systemic inflammatory disorders (4%)	
Prospective study from the US of 91 men, mostly inpatients[8]	12	58 (SD 18)	Malignancy (19%)	26%
			Non-malignant gastrointestinal disorders (14%)	
			Psychiatric disorders (9%)	
			Cardiovascular disease (9%)	
			Alcohol related disease (8%)	
Retrospective Israeli study of 154 male and female inpatients[12]	30	64 (range 27-88)	Malignancy (36%)	23%
			Non-malignant gastrointestinal disorders (17%)	
			Psychiatric disorders (10%)	
			Endocrine disease, infectious disease, renal disease (4% each)	
Retrospective study of 50 male and female outpatients in the US[w6]	24	>63	Psychiatric (20%)	24%
			Malignancy (16%)	
			Non-malignant gastrointestinal disorders (11%)	
			Endocrine disease (9%)	
			Neurological disease (7%)	
Retrospective study of 236 inpatients and 92 outpatients in the US[13]	>12	65 (SD 17)	Malignancy (35%)	6% (although 30 patients were lost to follow-up)
			Psychiatric (24%)	
			Non-malignant gastrointestinal disorders (8.8%)	
			Endocrine disease (7%)	
			Rheumatic disease (7%)	

SD=standard deviation.

Psychosocial

Published observational studies (summarised in table 1) report that psychiatric problems, particularly dementia and depression, are the main cause of unexplained weight loss in 10-20% of elderly patients. This figure rises to 58% in nursing home residents.[17]

Cognitive impairment

Patients with cognitive impairment who are agitated or have a tendency to "wander" can expend substantial energy. Others may forget that they have to eat or become suspicious and paranoid about food.[1] Self feeding skills are lost with the progression of Alzheimer's disease and dysphagia may develop.[w9]

Depression

Depression can lead to weight loss because of loss of appetite or reduced motivation to...

in elderly people than in younger adults,[w10] and it was associated with increased mortality in a systematic review of elderly patients (>65 years) living in the community (estimated odds ratio for mortality with depression of 1.73, 1.53 to 1.95).[18]

Reported rates of depression in the community vary dramatically according to a systematic review of 34 community based studies of the prevalence of depression in later life (>55 years), but they can be as high as 35%, depending on the criteria used to define depression.[19] Even higher prevalences have been reported in institutionalised elderly patients[w7 w10]

Socioeconomic factors

Poverty or social isolation may contribute to weight loss in elderly people through inadequate food intake and malnutrition.[20] Physical...

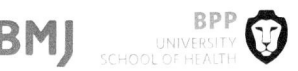

BOX 1 MNEMONICS FOR CAUSES OF UNINTENTIONAL WEIGHT LOSS IN ELDERLY PEOPLE

9 Ds of weight loss in elderly[14]

- Dementia
- Depression
- Disease (acute and chronic)
- Dysphagia
- Dysgeusia
- Diarrhoea
- Drugs
- Dentition
- Dysfunction (functional disability)
- (Don't know was later added as a 10th "D")[w7]

Meals on wheels[15]

- M: Medication effects
- E: Emotional problems (especially depression)
- A: Anorexia nervosa, alcoholism
- L: Late life paranoia
- S: Swallowing disorders
- O: Oral factors (such as poorly fitting dentures, caries)
- N: No money
- W: Wandering and other dementia related behaviours
- H: Hyperthyroidism, hypothyroidism, hyperparathyroidism, hypoadrenalism
- E: Enteric problems
- E: Eating problems (such as inability to feed self)
- L: Low salt, low cholesterol diet
- S: Stones, social problems (such as isolation, inability to obtain preferred foods)

or feed themselves may further contribute to insufficient food intake because they may rely on family members or carers, who may visit at erratic times.

Unknown

The cause of weight loss remained unknown in 16-28% of patients in published prospective and retrospective observational studies, despite extensive investigation over periods ranging from six months to three years.[3] [4] [8] [12] [13] This may be because elderly patients often have multiple comorbidities rather than one serious illness, are on multiple drugs, and may have psychological or social problems. Each individual factor might not be sufficient to cause substantial weight loss, but the cumulative effect of all the factors might result in clinically important weight loss.

All studies that have assessed prognosis in elderly patients with unintentional weight loss have found that patients who fall into this category of "unknown cause" have a much better prognosis than those diagnosed with cancer,[3] [12] and no worse than that of patients diagnosed with non-malignant causes.[3] Cancers diagnosed in the setting of involuntary weight loss usually have a poor prognosis because they are often advanced by the time weight loss becomes apparent.[4]

How is unintentional weight loss in older adults investigated?

We present our approach to investigation, which is based on an extensive literature review (fig 1. We know of no clinical guidelines or standardised system for investigating this common and complex problem.

Table 2 Organic causes of unintentional weight loss in elderly people[1] [3] [4] [8] [12] [13] [w6]*

Causes	Comments
Cancer (16-36%)*	
Gastrointestinal malignancy	About 50% of cancers that present with weight loss are gastrointestinal in origin[3] [4]
Other cancers (most often lung, lymphoma, prostate, ovarian, or bladder)	Non-gastrointestinal cancers present less commonly with involuntary weight loss, which tends to be a later feature
Non-malignant organic disorders	
Gastrointestinal disorders (11-19%):	
These include motility or swallowing disorders, peptic ulcers, gallstones, mesenteric ischaemia, and malabsorption disorders such as coeliac disease	Mechanisms contributing to weight loss include dysphagia, chronic nausea, pain related to eating (leading to food avoidance), and malabsorption
Other chronic diseases:	
These include congestive cardiac failure and other cardiac diseases (2-9%), chronic obstructive pulmonary disease and other respiratory diseases (6%), endocrine disease (4-11%), neurological disorders (2-7%), end stage renal failure (4%), connective tissue diseases (2-4%), and chronic or /recurrent infection (2-5%)	Any disease that increases metabolic demand or leads to a catabolic state can lead to weight loss despite a normal food intake; weight loss is often an indicator of disease severity in chronic disease[1]; elderly patients often do not fully regain weight lost because of acute stressful events, so a history of recurrent infections may lead to serious weight loss
Oral and dental problems:	
Poor dentition, ill fitting dentures, xerostomia (dry mouth)—often as a result of drugs	Often overlooked by the medical profession, but can lead to serious weight loss as a result of inadequate energy intake; the number of oral and dental problems has been shown to be an important predictor of weight loss at one year[w8]
Side effects of drugs†	
Anorexia (antibiotics, digoxin, opiates, selective serotonin reuptake inhibitors, anticonvulsants, antipsychotics, amantadine, metformin, benzodiazepines), nausea and vomiting (antibiotics, bisphosphonates, digoxin, dopamine agonists, levodopa, opiates, selective serotonin reuptake inhibitors, tricyclics), dry mouth (anticholinergics, loop diuretics, antihistamines), altered taste or smell (angiotensin converting enzyme inhibitors, calcium channel blockers, propranol, spironolactone, iron, anti-parkinsonian drugs (levodopa, pergolide, selegiline), opiates, gold, allopurinol), dysphagia (bisphosphonates, antibiotics, levodopa, gold, iron, non-steroidal anti-inflammatory drugs, potassium)	This is a particular problem in elderly patients because of the prevalence of polypharmacy, which in itself is known to interfere with taste and cause anorexia[16]; drugs such as sedatives and opiate analgesics may interfere with cognition and affect the patient's ability to eat

*Percentages are based on the published studies referenced above.

†Drugs listed are only a few examples of commonly used drugs that cause these side effects and this is not intended to be a comprehensive list.

Initial evaluation of the patient involves a detailed history, clinical examination, and baseline investigations. The findings should be used to guide further investigation.

History

Try to establish the exact amount of weight loss over a specified time. Questions about appetite may help elucidate whether the weight loss is caused by inadequate energy intake or has occurred despite an adequate intake. A corroborative history from relatives or carers may help in patients with cognitive impairment.

Previous and current medical history may identify conditions that could have led to weight loss (see table 2) and drugs that may contribute via their side effects.

Social history may elicit information on alcohol intake (which might contribute to malnutrition or vitamin deficiency) and smoking (a risk factor for cancer and other organic diseases). It is important to elucidate the patient's social circumstances. Who does he or she live with? Who buys and prepares the food? Is there any home help or help from family members?

A history that includes a review of systems may elicit additional symptoms that might direct further investigation.

In addition, screen all patients for cognitive impairment and depression using standardised assessment tools.[21] [22] [W11]

Some authors recommend a nutritional assessment only when no evidence of organic disease is found.[1] [8] We believe, however, that all elderly patients presenting with unintentional weight loss should undergo nutritional assessment by a dietitian. This is because malnutrition has a high prevalence in elderly people and might still be present even when an organic cause of the weight loss is found.

We suggest that patients seen in primary care (by general practitioners)—where facilities (and time) for assessing cognitive function, mood, and nutritional status are not always readily available—should be referred to specialists in the care of older people.

Physical examination

In patients with unintentional weight loss a full physical examination should aim to exclude major cardiovascular and respiratory illnesses, as well as abdominal masses, organomegaly, prostate enlargement, and breast masses that may indicate cancer. Palpable lymphadenopathy could indicate infection, cancer, or haematological disease. Examine the mouth to exclude any obvious dental problems, poor oral hygiene, dry mouth, or lesions that may make chewing and swallowing difficult or painful.

Baseline investigations

Baseline investigations for all patients should include bloods tests (full blood count, urea and electrolytes, liver function tests, thyroid function tests, C reactive protein, glucose, and lactate dehydrogenase), chest radiography, urinalysis, and faecal occult blood testing.[1] [4] [12] [13] [23] The rationale behind these baseline tests is explained in box 2.

Tumour markers are not useful diagnostic tests; they should not be used as part of the initial evaluation and may be misleading.[1] [24] Their role is in monitoring response to treatment in patients with cancer or detecting tumour recurrence early after treatment. Abnormal findings on initial evaluation should be used to guide further investigations into the cause of the weight loss.

If the history, examination, and baseline investigations are all normal, published evidence suggests that further investigation is not warranted immediately and that three months' "watchful waiting" is advisable, rather than a blind pursuit of additional, more invasive or expensive investigations. Because organic disease is found only rarely in patients with normal results from physical examination and laboratory tests, this waiting period is unlikely to have an adverse outcome.[3] [4]

Although three scoring systems have been developed to help clinicians identify which patients with weight loss are likely to have a physical or malignant cause rather than a psychological or social cause,[8] [13] [23] none of these has been validated in independent populations presenting with weight loss.

Should a negative baseline reassure?

The claim that a negative baseline evaluation should reassure the clinician of the lack of serious underlying disease is based on only small non-randomised studies. Most of these are also not limited to elderly patients (in the UK defined as >70 years of age). However, most authors agree that in elderly patients with clinically relevant unintentional weight loss, major organic (and especially malignant) diseases are highly unlikely when a thorough baseline evaluation is normal, and that in this setting a watchful waiting approach may be preferable to undirected and invasive testing.[1] [3] [4] [13] [23]

There is currently no evidence that blind computed tomography scanning is helpful in investigating such patients. Disadvantages of blind computed tomography scanning include high costs (with low yield) and the likelihood of finding "incidental-omas."

Several studies have used abdominal ultrasound as part of their initial evaluation, although they did not comment on its usefulness in this role, noting only that 27% of patients with underlying cancer had hepatomegaly on examination

History
History of weight loss
Previous medical history
Current drugs
Social history (alcohol, smoking, social circumstances)
Review of systems (symptoms that may help direct further investigation)

↓

Examination
Cardiovascular
Respiratory
Gastrointestinal (including mouth and per rectal examination)
Breast
Examine for lymphadenopathy

↓

Baseline Investigations
Blood tests (full blood count, urea and electrolytes, liver function tests, thyroid function tests, C reactive protein and erythrocyte sedimentation rate, glucose, lactate dehydrogenase)
Chest radiography
Urinalysis
Faecal occult blood testing

↓

Abnormal findings → Further appropriate investigations → Treat any cause found

No abnormal findings → 3 month period of "watchful waiting"

In addition, for all patients:

Nutritional assessment | Appropriate dietary/ social interventions

Evaluation of unintentional weight loss in elderly people

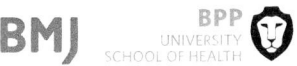
BOX 2 BASELINE TESTS FOR INVESTIGATING UNEXPLAINED WEIGHT LOSS IN OLDER PEOPLE

Blood tests

Full blood count

- Anaemia is suggestive of an organic cause of weight loss,[13] and it should prompt further investigations, which will depend on the type of anaemia (microcytic, macrocytic, etc). A raised white cell count may also suggest organic disease (malignant, infectious, or inflammatory processes) and was felt to be an important variable in several observational studies that assessed likelihood of a malignant or other organic cause of unintentional weight loss[4][13]

Urea and electrolytes

- Although the published studies do not seem to find this a particularly helpful test in predicting an organic versus non-organic cause for weight loss,[4][13] it is a reasonable investigation to perform at this stage and abnormal results may point towards an organic cause

Liver function tests, including γ-glutamyl transpeptidase and albumin

- Normal liver function tests make serious organic causes for weight loss less likely, particularly cancer, which is usually advanced by the time weight loss occurs.[4] Alkaline phosphatase is particularly useful because it can be raised when liver or bone disease is present. One observational study found that alkaline phosphatase >300 IU/L increased the likelihood of a malignant cause of weight loss (odds ratio 14.7) and serum albumin >35 g/L reduced the likelihood (0.11)[13]

Thyroid function tests

- Hyperthyroidism is a common endocrinal cause of weight loss

C reactive protein and erythrocyte sedimentation rate

- Normal test results make a serious organic cause for the weight loss less likely. In one observational study, C reactive protein was raised in 91% of patients subsequently diagnosed with malignancy, and in 69% of patients with non-malignant organic disease.[4] In another study,[13] a raised erythrocyte sedimentation rate was associated with an increased likelihood of malignancy (2.9, 1.7 to 5.1). Erythrocyte sedimentation rate can also be raised in other organic disorders including systemic inflammatory disorders. A raised erythrocyte sedimentation rate or C reactive protein would therefore point towards a possible organic cause for the weight loss

Serum glucose

- Uncontrolled diabetes is a common endocrinal cause of weight loss

Lactate dehydrogenase

- Lactate dehydrogenase >500 IU/L is associated with an increased likelihood of a malignant cause of involuntary weight loss (26.9)[13]

Chest radiography

- Chest radiography should be performed in all patients to identify respiratory disease, including malignant and non-malignant causes[1][4]

Urinalysis

- Urinalysis is included in almost all studies as part of the initial evaluation and is non-invasive and inexpensive; however, the published studies do not specify its diagnostic benefit as part of the initial evaluation of elderly patients with unintentional weight loss, only that it is of less value than other investigations[4]

Faecal occult blood analysis

- Because of the high proportion (about a third) of patients with an underlying gastrointestinal disorder,[3] whether malignant or non-malignant, such analysis is a reasonable first line investigation. It is non-invasive (compared with endoscopy), and although it is not particularly sensitive or specific, a positive result would prompt further investigation of the gastrointestinal tract (such as endoscopy or colonoscopy)

---

and a similar percentage had palpable masses.[4] Abnormal findings on examination (or abnormal liver function tests) would have prompted further investigation anyway.

Gastrointestinal disorders (malignant and non-malignant) account for about a third of all causes of unexplained weight loss in studies of adults of all ages, so some authors advocate upper gastrointestinal endoscopy in patients as a first line investigation.[3] However, because endoscopy is invasive and not without risk (particularly for elderly patients), we think that it should be reserved for patients in whom it is indicated on the basis of history, examination, or baseline investigations (such as a history of gastrointestinal bleeding or evidence of iron deficiency anaemia).

In one study where patients with a normal baseline evaluation underwent further investigation s including computed tomography and endoscopy, only one additional diagnosis was made (a patient diagnosed with lactose intolerance).[4]

Managing unexplained weight loss in elderly people

The primary principle of management is to identify and treat any underlying causes. Optimal management often requires multidisciplinary assessment (doctors, dentists, dietitians, speech therapists, physiotherapists, occupational therapists, social services).[20][w12] We strongly suggest reviewing drugs in an attempt to eliminate those whose side effects may contribute to weight loss.

If a psychiatric cause of weight loss, such as depression, is suspected we recommend assessment by a psychogeriatrician or psychologist. In such cases, consider treatment with an antidepressant because depression is a potentially reversible cause of weight loss.[w12]

If the initial baseline evaluation is negative, we suggest that patients are reassessed after three months to establish if any further symptoms or signs have developed and to check their weight. In the interim, because evidence to support any drug treatment is lacking,[1][20] a variety of non-drug based interventions can be used (outlined in box 3).

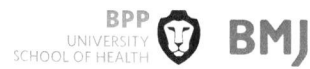

BOX 3 NON-DRUG BASED INTERVENTIONS FOR UNEXPLAINED WEIGHT LOSS IN ELDERLY PATIENTS

Optimise food intake

- Encourage the patient to eat smaller meals more often
- Encourage the patient to eating favourite foods and snacks, and minimise dietary restrictions (which are often energy poor and less palatable, therefore cause increased risk of weight loss in elderly patients)[2] [w13] [w14]
- High energy foods should be eaten at the main meal of the day (elderly people, particularly those with dementia, tend to consume most of their daily energy at breakfast)[25]
- Optimise and vary dietary texture—this is of particular benefit in patients with dementia[26]
- Eating in company or with assistance is useful. Eating in company has been suggested to improve enjoyment of meals and therefore increase intake.[2] Many elderly people have physical or cognitive disabilities that impair their ability to feed themselves without assistance or prompting
- Community nutritional support services (such as "meals on wheels" programmes) are recommended for elderly patients in the community to improve dietary intake

Oral nutritional supplements if recommended by the dietitian

- Oral nutritional supplements (such as high energy drinks) have been shown to increase daily energy intake and weight gain, although evidence that they result in long term benefit in terms of health, functional ability, and survival in undernourished elderly patients is limited
- Supplements should be taken between meals to avoid appetite suppression and decreased intake of food at meal times[20]

Daily multivitamin tablet

- There is little evidence that this leads to a reduction in weight loss. However, it is recommended by some authors because of the high prevalence of nutritional deficiencies in elderly people

Ensure adequate oral health

- Problems with dentition and oral health are commonly overlooked causes of weight loss[w15]

Regular exercise or physiotherapy

- Regular exercise (particularly resistance training) is also recommended for frail elderly patients because it stimulates appetite and prevents sarcopenia. Physiotherapy may help achieve this in some patients

---

SOURCES AND SELECTION CRITERIA

We searched the literature for current clinical or best practice guidelines, trials, reviews, and relevant publications. We used online resources including the Cochrane and TRIP databases, Medline, and Google in addition to specific sites such as the Scottish Intercollegiate Guidelines Network (SIGN),[1] the National Institute for Health and Clinical Excellence (NICE), and the British Geriatrics Society.

We then performed Medline and Google searches, using keywords "unintentional", "weight loss", and "elderly". The term "unintentional" was also substituted with "involuntary" and "unexplained" to expand our search. We later performed further specific searches to explore particular aspects of this article.

Contributors: AB had the idea for the article and is guarantor; JM and CS searched the literature; JM wrote the article, and AB and CS helped with editing.

Competing interests: All authors have completed the Unified Competing Interest form at www.icmje.org/coi_disclosure.pdf (available on request from the corresponding author) and declare: no support from any organisation for the submitted work; no financial relationships with any organisations that might have an interest in the submitted work in the previous three years; no other relationships or activities that could appear to have influenced the submitted work.

Provenance and peer review: Not commissioned; externally peer reviewed.

TIPS FOR NON-SPECIALISTS

- General practitioners and non-specialist hospital doctors should perform the initial history, examination, and baseline investigations
- Refer any abnormality suggesting a possible organic cause for the weight loss to the appropriate specialty
- If no obvious cause is found, the referrer can undertake the three months of watchful waiting or refer to secondary care (medicine for the elderly), where facilities for multidisciplinary assessment are often better
- If the initial evaluation and watchful waiting are undertaken by primary care, repeat the history, examination, and investigations at the end of this period. If no cause is identified and the patient is still losing weight, refer to secondary care

FURTHER RESEARCH AND UNANSWERED QUESTIONS

- Most published studies are based on small numbers of patients, focus on unintentional weight loss in adults of all ages, and many are more than 10 years old
- Studies focusing on elderly people are needed—ideally multicentre studies with large numbers of patients and with longer follow-up periods to see whether additional diagnoses are made and whether these patients continue to lose weight
- If the patient is referred to secondary care, weight loss persists or progresses but no cause has been identified after three months of watchful waiting, what then?
- Should we continue to assess at regular three monthly intervals? Should we consider blind investigations?

1   Alibhai S.M.H, Greenwood C, Payette H. An approach to the management of unintentional weight loss in the elderly. *CMAJ* 2005;172:773-80.
2   Bouras EP, Lange SM, Scolapio JS. Rational approach to patients with unintentional weight loss, *Mayo Clin Proc* 2001;76:923-9.
3   Lankish PG, Gerzmann M, Gerzmann JF, Lehnick D. Unintentional weight loss: diagnosis and prognosis. The first prospective follow-up study from a secondary referral centre. *J Intern Med* 2001;249:41-6.
4   Metalidis C, Knockaert DC, Bobbaers H, Vanderschueren S. Involuntary weight loss. Does a negative baseline evaluation provide adequate reassurance? *Eur J Intern Med* 2008;19:345-9.
5   Clarkston WK, Pantano MM, Morley JE, Horowitz M, Littlefield JM, Burton FR. Evidence for the anorexia of aging—gastrointestinal transit and hunger in healthy elderly vs young adults. *Am J Physiol* 1997;41:R243-8.
6   Wallace JI, Schwartz RS. Epidemiology of weight loss in humans with special reference to wasting in the elderly. *Int J Cardiol* 2002;85:15-21.
7   Newman A, Yanez D, Harris T, Duxbury A, Enright PL, Fried LP. Weight change in old age and its association with mortality. *J Am Geriatr Soc* 2001;49:1309-18.
8   Marton KI, Sox HC Jr, Krupp JR. Involuntary weight loss: diagnostic and prognostic significance. *Ann Intern Med* 1981;95:568.

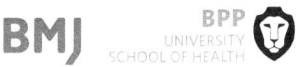

9   Chapman KM, Nelson RA. Loss of appetite: managing unwanted weight loss in the older patient. *Geriatrics* 1994;49:54-9.

10 Ryan C, Bryant E, Eleazer P, Rhodes A, Guest K. Unintentional weight loss in long-term care: predictor of mortality in the elderly. *South Med J* 1995;88:721-4.

11 Ensrud KE, Ewing SK, Stone KL, Cauley JA, Bowman PJ, Cummings SR. Intentional and unintentional weight loss increase bone loss and hip fracture risk in older women. *J Am Geriatr Soc* 2003;51:1740-7.

12 Rabinovitz M, Pitlik SD, Leifer M, Garty M, Rosenfeld JB. Unintentional weight loss: a retrospective analysis of 154 cases. *Arch Intern Med* 1986;146:186.

13 Hernandez JL, Riancho JA, Matorras P, Gonzalez-Macias J. Clinical evaluation for cancer in patients with involuntary weight loss without specific symptoms. *Am J Med* 2003;114:631-7.

14 Robbins LJ. Evaluation of weight loss in the elderly. *Geriatrics* 1989;44:31-4.

15 Morley JE, Silver AJ. Nutritional issues in nursing home care. *Ann Intern Med* 1995;123:850-9.

16 Carr-Lopez SM, Phillips SK. The role of medications in geriatric failure to thrive. *Drugs Aging* 1996;8:221-5.

17 Morley J.E, Kraenzie D. Causes of weight loss in a community nursing home. *J Am Geriatr Soc* 1994;42:583-5.

18 Saz P, Dewey ME. Depression, depressive symptoms and mortality in persons aged 65 and over living in the community: a systematic review of the literature. *Int J Geriatr Psychiatry* 2001;16:622-30.

19 Beekman AT, Copeland JR, Prince MJ. Review of community prevalence of depression in later life. *Br J Psychiatry* 1999;174:307-11.

20 Smith KL, Greenwood C, Payette H, Alibhai SMH. An approach to the nonpharmacologic and pharmacologic management of unintentional weight loss among older adults. *Geriatr Aging* 2007;10:91-8.

21 Folstein MF, Folstein SE, McHugh PR. "Mini-mental state". A practical method for grading the cognitive state of patients for the clinician. *J Psychiatr Res* 1975;12:189-98.

22 Yesavage JA, Brink TL, Rose TL, Lum O, Huang V, Adey M, et al. Development and validation of a geriatric depression screening scale: a preliminary report. *J Psychiatr Res* 1983;17:37-49.

23 Bilbao-Gara J, Barba R, Losa-Garcia JE, Martin H, Garcia de Casasola G, Castilla V. Assessing clinical probability of organic disease in patients with involuntary weight loss: a simple score. *Eur J Intern Med* 2002;13:240-5.

24 Sturgeon CM, Lai LC, Duffy MJ. Serum tumour markers; how to order and interpret them. *BMJ* 2009;339:b3527.

25 Young KW, Greenwood CE. Shift in diurnal feeding patterns in nursing home residents with Alzheimer's disease. *J Gerontol A Biol Sci Med Sci* 2001;56:M656-61.

26 Boylston E, Ryan C, Brown C, Westfall B. Increasing oral intake in dementia patients by altering food texture. *Am J Alzheimer's Dis* 1995;10:37-9.

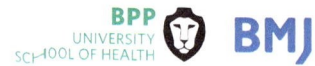

Management of chronic pain in older adults

M Carrington Reid, associate professor of medicine[1], Christopher Eccleston, director[2], Karl Pillemer, professor of human development and of gerontology in medicine[3]

[1]Division of Geriatrics and Palliative Medicine, Weill Cornell Medical College, New York, NY 10065, USA

[2]Centre for Pain Research, University of Bath, Bath, UK

[3]Department of Human Development, Cornell University, Ithaca, NY, USA

Correspondence to: M C Reid mcr2004@med.cornell.edu

Cite this as: BMJ 2015;350:h532

DOI: 10.1136/bmj.h532

Chronic pain is one of the most common conditions encountered by healthcare professionals, particularly among older (.65 years) patients.[1] Pain is associated with substantial disability from reduced mobility, avoidance of activity, falls, depression and anxiety, sleep impairment, and isolation.[1][2][3] Its negative effects extend beyond the patient, to disrupt both family and social relationships. Chronic pain poses a significant economic burden on society.[1] Prevalence rates for pain are expected to increase as populations continue to age—by 2035 an estimated one quarter of the population in the European Union will be 65 or older—thereby increasing the public health impact of pain. Healthcare providers, irrespective of specialty, should develop competencies to assess and manage chronic pain in their older patients. In this review we summarize recent evidence on the assessment and management of pain in older patients. Evidence is taken from systematic reviews, meta-analyses, individual trials, and clinical guidelines.

What is chronic pain and how is it caused?

Although no universally accepted definition exists for chronic pain, it is often defined as pain that persists beyond the expected time of healing (typically 12 weeks) and may or may not be associated with an identifiable cause or actual tissue damage.[3][4] Musculoskeletal disorders are common in later life, and increasingly common are painful neuropathies from diabetes, herpes zoster, chemotherapy, and surgery. Other types of pain are also prevalent among older adults, including pain due to cancer as well as cancer treatments.[5][6] Pain is also common in the advanced stages of many chronic diseases, including congestive heart failure, end stage renal disease, and chronic obstructive pulmonary disease.[7] Furthermore, millions of joint repair and replacement surgeries are performed annually, and an important minority of patients undergoing these procedures report chronic pain despite surgery.[8] Finally, vertebral compression fractures are highly prevalent and cause substantial pain and discomfort, particularly among older women.[9] Box 1 lists other common diseases where pain is a major symptom.

Who gets it?

Chronic pain in later life is a worldwide problem. In one nationwide survey of older adults (n=7601) in the United States, 52.8% reported experiencing bothersome pain in the preceding month.[10] Similar findings have been reported in studies conducted in Europe, Asia, and Australia[11][12][13] and in both developed and less developed countries.[14] Risk factors include advancing age, female sex, lower socioeconomic status, lower educational level, obesity, tobacco use, history of injury, history of a physically strenuous job, childhood trauma, and depression or anxiety.

Factors predicting poor outcomes (that is, higher pain scores, disability, depression) among people with chronic pain include higher levels of pain severity and disability, longer duration of pain, multiple pain sites, history of anxiety or depression, maladaptive coping strategies (for example, worry, avoidance), and low social support at the time of diagnosis. In one study of older adults (n=403) with musculoskeletal pain, three brief items assessed at the initial clinical encounter—degree of interference from pain, pain in multiple body sites, and duration of pain—predicted lack of patient improvement at six months and helped general practitioners predict this outcome above clinical judgment alone.[15] Simple risk stratification approaches like this could help to tailor care.

How are older patients with chronic pain assessed?

A comprehensive pain assessment can increase the likelihood of identifying a specific diagnosis for the pain, guide selection of treatments most likely to benefit the patient, and identify targets for intervention (for example, unrealistic treatment goals) besides pain relief. Office based assessment can be challenging, however, because of constraints on time. Having patients complete parts of the assessment before the visit (or in the office over multiple visits) can be helpful.

Clinicians often struggle with the question of how comprehensive the assessment needs to be to establish a specific cause of pain. Unfortunately the literature provides little guidance on this but does indicate that a specific cause is not found in a large number of patients, despite comprehensive evaluation. Potential benefits to identifying a cause of pain include earlier initiation of an appropriate treatment and providing reassurance as patients often worry about the cause of their pain. These putative benefits must be weighed against the risks of extensive investigations, which often uncover incidental findings, are expensive, and can increase patient worry.

History

Chronic pain is more than just a sensory event; it has affective (emotional responses to pain), cognitive (attitudes and beliefs about pain), behavioral (for example, behaviors manifested in response to pain by patients and their family members or caregivers), as well as sensory components (for example, quality, location, temporal pattern). Assessing for the presence and severity of pain captures only a small part of the pain experience. All older patients with chronic pain should undergo a comprehensive pain assessment (box 2 outlines the key elements).

Box 3 lists these and other core elements of the assessment along with sample questions that can be

---

THE BOTTOM LINE

- Chronic pain in later life is a worldwide problem
- All older adults with chronic pain should undergo a comprehensive geriatric pain assessment
- A comprehensive assessment can guide selection of treatments most likely to benefit the patient and identify targets for intervention besides pain relief
- A multimodal approach that includes both drug and non-drug modalities for pain is recommended
- Given the limited reach of cognitive behavioral and exercise approaches to manage pain in later life, patients should be encouraged to engage in and adopt these techniques
- Involve and engage family members and paid caregivers and seek out other resources that can help to reinforce adherence to treatment and maintain gains from treatment

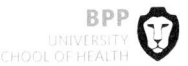

employed during the interview. Additional guidance about assessment approaches can be found in UK and US guidelines[17] [18] and in an international consensus report on this topic.[19]

Examination

A physical examination should be conducted, focusing on the musculoskeletal (is there evidence of inflammation?) and neurologic (is there evidence of weakness or neuropathy?) systems. Because many older adults with chronic pain report the presence of weakness, it is important to distinguish pain induced weakness from true motor weakness. This can be done by documenting abnormal results from nerve conduction studies or by treating pain successfully and seeing if the muscle weakness improves. Tackling physical functioning and risk of falls is critically important, given that pain is associated with these outcomes. This part of the assessment should include self report and performance based measures such as gait speed, timed up and go test, balance. The results provide a baseline against which the functional impact of treatment can be evaluated.

Imaging

Diagnostic imaging is often overused and does not indicate better care.[20] In one study of Portuguese adults (n=5094) more than half of all respondents with chronic pain reported undergoing a diagnostic imaging procedure in the previous six months.[21] Such imaging often uncovers incidental findings, leading to more testing, costs, and worry for patients. An additional concern is the low correlation between pathologic findings identified by imaging and the extent to which patients report experiencing pain.[22] Many patients with major disease identified by imaging report no pain, whereas others without major disease often report severe pain.[22] Diagnostic imaging is appropriate when the history or physical examination identifies abnormalities that suggest a specific diagnosis for the pain. Imaging procedures should also be strongly considered in the presence of "red flags," to include worsening pain in patients with a history of cancer, risk factors for infection (injecting drug use, immunosuppressive therapy), and worrisome constitutional

signs or symptoms such as unexplained weight loss, fever, or loss of appetite.

Assessing pain in older patients with major cognitive impairment

Patients with limited verbal or cognitive abilities require modified approaches to assessment. A hierarchy of techniques is recommended, the first including an attempt to obtain self report data followed by a search for potential causes of the pain, observing patient behavior (for example, facial expressions, vocalizations, guarding), obtaining proxy data from family members or caregivers who know the patient well and can report on whether changes in behavior or activity are very different from baseline, and conducting an analgesic trial to see whether the behavior resolves with treatment.[23] Several tools for behavioral pain assessment have been developed to assess for pain in non-verbal patients and are reviewed elsewhere.[19] [23]

What is the approach to management?

Management of pain in later life can be complex; problems with both nociceptive and neuropathic pain are common and often coexist. Nociceptive pain arises from actual or threatened damage to non-neural tissue through activation of nociceptors, whereas neuropathic pain occurs as a consequence of abnormalities in the central or peripheral somatosensory nervous system.[4] Management is further

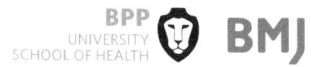

Table 1 Standardized tools for pain assessment

Measure (No of items)	Domains assessed
Multidimensional measures:	
Brief pain inventory-short form (n=9)[w1]	Sensory (intensity, location); pain related interference or disability; treatments, degree of relief provided by treatments; affect
Geriatric pain measure (n=24)[w2]	Sensory (intensity, temporal pattern); pain related interference or disability; affect
Pain disability index (n=7)[w3]	Pain related interference or disability
Short-form McGill pain questionnaire (n=15)[w4]	Sensory; exacerbating or ameliorating factors; affect
PROMIS* pain interference, behavior, intensity items[w5]	Pain related interference or disability; pain behaviors; pain intensity
WOMAC (n=24)[w6]	Sensory (intensity); pain related interference or disability; joint stiffness
Roland Morris disability questionnaire† (n=24)[w7]	Pain related interference or disability; affect
Unidimensional measures:	
Numeric rating scale (n=1)[w8]	Sensory (intensity)
Verbal rating scale (n=1)[w9]	Sensory (severity)
Visual analog scale (n=1)[w9]	Sensory (intensity)
Faces pain scale (n=1)[w10]	Sensory (intensity)
LANSS pain scale (n=7)[w11]	Sensory (assessment of possible neuropathic pain)
DN4 (n=4)[w12]	Sensory (assessment of possible neuropathic pain)

WOMAC=Western Ontario and McMaster Universities osteoarthritis index; LANSS=Leeds assessment of neuropathic symptoms and signs; DN4=Douleur Neuropathique 4 questions.

*Available in long and short form versions: long version for pain interference has 40 items; there are five short form versions for pain interference where the number of questions varies from 4 to 8; long form version for pain behavior has 39 items, short form version has 7. PROMIS pain intensity measure has three items.

†Originally developed as tool to measure perceived disability in patients with back pain. Increasingly used to measure perceived disability due to pain from any cause.

complicated by age related physiologic changes, which lead to altered drug absorption and decreased renal excretion, sensory and cognitive impairments, polypharmacy, and multimorbidity, particularly chronic conditions such as disorders of gait and balance, and kidney, lung, and cardiovascular disease.[16] Other barriers to management include a limited evidence base to guide decisions, physician concerns about the potential for treatment related harm, as well as older adults' beliefs about pain and treatments for the pain. However, it is important to note that these barriers are not universally present in older adults; an important tenet of geriatric medicine is that chronologic age does not equal biologic age.

Chronic pain in older patients most often occurs in the setting of multiple comorbidities, limiting treatment options. A comprehensive management approach should deal with common sequelae such as depression, isolation, and physical disability, and include both drug and non-drug treatments. UK and US guidelines on the management of pain in later life strongly endorse this approach.[2][3] Recent data provide support for multimodal treatment approaches. In one randomized clinical trial (n=454) of overweight or obese older adults with osteoarthritis of the knee, intensive weight reduction combined with exercise training produced significant improvements in pain, functional status, and physical performance over an 18 month period when compared with exercise only (and diet only) control groups.[24]

In terms of care delivery, collaborative approaches have proved efficacy in the primary care setting.[25][26][27] One recent randomized clinical trial involving older primary care patients (n=250) with chronic musculoskeletal pain found that a telephone based collaborative care management intervention delivered by a nurse care manager, physician pain specialist, and the patient's primary care provider led to improved patient outcomes at 12 months, largely through optimizing non-opioid analgesics by using a stepped care approach.[25] Given the complexities of managing most older patients with chronic pain, a multidisciplinary approach that includes physician, nursing, and social work perspectives is strongly recommended.

Social aspects of management

Clinicians are advised to take family responses and dynamics into account when formulating treatment plans. Older patients' chronic pain often affects their close relatives and caregivers.

Spouses typically play an important role in caring for older patients, often times delivering emotional and instrumental support. However, when an older spouse experiences chronic pain, problems of communication and commitment to the marriage can occur.

Therapeutic interventions directed at patients with chronic pain increasingly involve the family, most often by including relatives in cognitive behavior therapy (CBT) or self management training. Although evidence is mixed, several well conducted, randomized trials suggest that spousal participation in the treatment process can yield measurable benefits for patients, including enhanced emotional wellbeing and reduced pain levels.[28][29]

Home visits

We are not aware of any literature that has examined the value of home visits for older adults with chronic pain. Despite a lack of evidence supporting the use of home visits, clinicians should consider them on a case by case basis because of several potential benefits, which include clarifying reasons for non-adherence to drug and behavioral interventions, gathering proxy data that may not be available during an office visit, and preventing the use of old prescription drugs often stored by patients. Perhaps the most important benefit is a strengthening of the doctor-patient relationship. From the physician's perspective, observing the patient's environment often offers intangible but valuable insights into the patient's condition. From the patient's perspective, most feel enormously supported by a physician who cares enough to make a home visit.

What drug interventions are available?

Table 2 summarizes current UK and US guideline recommendations,[2][3] highlights key safety concerns about analgesics, and provides guidance on specific drug treatments for both nociceptive and neuropathic pain

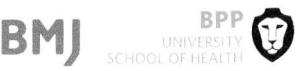

BOX 3 ELEMENTS OF A COMPREHENSIVE GERIATRIC PAIN ASSESSMENT

Sensory

- Please tell me all of the places you experience pain or discomfort. What does it feel like? What words come to mind?
- Is your pain or discomfort with you all of the time or does it come and go? How long has it been present? What makes it better, what makes it worse?

Emotional impact

- Has pain affected your mood, sense of wellbeing, energy level?
- Are you worried about your pain or what may be causing it?

Functional impact

- Has pain affected your ability to do every day activities? To do things you enjoy?
- How about relating with others? If so, how?

Sleep

- Has pain affected your sleep?
- Do you have trouble falling asleep or need to take drugs to help you sleep on account of your pain?

Attitudes and beliefs

- Do you have any thoughts or opinions about experiencing pain at this point in your life that you believe would be important for me to know?
- Do you have any thoughts or opinions about specific pain treatments that you believe would be important for me to know?

Coping styles

- What things do you do to help you cope with your pain? This could be listening to your favorite music, praying, sitting still, or isolating yourself from others

Treatment expectations and goals

- What do you think is likely to happen with the treatment I have recommended?
- What are the most important things you hope will happen as a result of the treatment?

Resources

- Is there anyone at home or in the community that you can turn to for help and support when your pain is really bad?

disorders. The use of drug combinations often results in enhanced analgesic effectiveness, with lower toxicity than is seen with the use of a single agent at higher doses, and is encouraged.[30]

Paracetamol

Because of its favourable safety profile, paracetamol (acetaminophen) is the preferred treatment for older patients with mild or moderate pain. In one meta-analysis of seven randomized controlled trials comparing paracetamol with placebo, paracetamol (up to 4 g daily) was found to be modestly effective in reducing pain, which decreased on average by 4 points on a scale of 0-100. The number needed to treat ranged from 4 to 16. Paracetamol did not improve physical function or stiffness when compared with placebo..[31] While it is not associated with significant cardiovascular, renal, or gastrointestinal effects,[3] unintentional overdose of paracetamol is an important cause of hepatotoxicity. Patients should be counseled to not exceed the maximum recommended daily dose.

Non-steroidal anti-inflammatory drugs

Oral non-steroidal anti-inflammatory drugs (NSAIDs) have established gastrointestinal, cardiovascular, and renal risks, which increase with age. Oral NSAIDs can be effective in some patients but are safest when used for pain flares (transient increases in pain that typically persist for hours to days). The current evidence base provides little guidance about the NSAID for safest use in this patient population. A network meta-analysis examined the cardiovascular safety of various NSAIDs and found that naproxen was the least harmful compared with other non-selective (for example, ibuprofen) and selective (for example, celecoxib) NSAIDs.[32] These data indicate that naproxen is most appropriate (compared with other NSAIDs) for patients with cardiovascular risk factors. Risk of renal and gastrointestinal injury must also be weighed, however, before initiating any trial involving NSAIDs. If a trial of an NSAID is undertaken, have the patient return to the office within two weeks to ask about treatment benefit and gastrointestintal side effects, check blood pressure, and carry out renal function tests.

Topical NSAIDs represent an alternative to oral NSAIDs, are generally well tolerated, and should be considered, especially for patients with localized pain.

Opioids

Opioids may be considered when an older patient's pain has not responded to other treatments or when major functional impairment persists despite treatment. The short term efficacy of opioid use (≤12 weeks) among older adults has been established.[33] In a retrospective cohort study of (n=133) older patients (mean age 82) newly started on an opioid because of pain due to chronic musculoskeletal conditions, reductions in pain were recorded in 66% of participants.[34] However, opioids were discontinued in 48% of the participants, mostly as a result of poorly tolerated side effects, including constipation, changes to mental status, and nausea. Given the established risks associated with opioid use,[35] the potential negative effects must be weighed against the consequences of untreated or partially treated pain. A recent systematic review found limited evidence in support of long term opioid treatment, and the risk for serious harm increased in line with opioid dose.[35] If an opioid trial is undertaken, it is important to closely monitor (that is, biweekly during the initiation and dose titration phase of treatment) whether treatment goals are being met. If not, the drug should be tapered and discontinued.

There is no evidence to support the use of one weak opioid (for example, hydrocodone, codeine) over another when the response to paracetamol or a NSAID is lacking. Selection of a specific opioid depends on the clinician's clinical experience and knowledge, the patient's previous experiences, and availability of the drug in local pharmacies. Strong opioids (for example, morphine, hydrocodone) should not be given to patients who have never used opioids. Efforts to reduce opioid related risks are particularly appropriate given dramatic increases in and complications associated with opioid use. These include the use of screening tools (for example, the screener and opioid assessment for people with pain, opioid risk tool) that can be used to assess risk for the likelihood of opioid misuse, as well as guide decisions about the extent of monitoring neede d if an opioid trial is undertaken. Such monitoring might extend to the use of urine toxicology screens on a periodic basis. Before older patients are prescribed opioid analgesics, physicians should be satisfied with arrangements for safe storage of the drug,

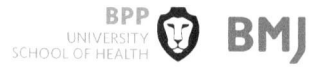

Table 2 Guideline recommendations for drug management of chronic pain

Analgesic class	Recommendation*	Safety concerns	Quality of evidence†
Paracetamol (acetaminophen)	Use for mild to moderate pain	Liver toxicity a concern at higher doses, particularly from unintentional overdose	High
Oral NSAIDs	Use for shortest time possible; may be appropriate when other treatments have failed	Selective and non-selective NSAIDs associated with adverse gastrointestinal, renal, and cardiovascular side effects	High
Topical NSAIDs	Use as alternative to oral NSAIDs, particularly when pain is localized	Safety of topical NSAIDs in patients receiving anticoagulation or with renal impairment remains unknown	Moderate
Tramadol	Consider for use in patients who do not respond to paracetamol/NSAIDs	Increased risk of seizures or serotonin syndrome when used with antidepressants; side effect profile similar to that of opioids	Not reported
Opioids	Use for moderate to severe pain or with substantial impairments in functioning or quality of life and when other treatments have been unsuccessful	Side effects limit use (constipation, sedation, nausea)	Low
Tricyclic antidepressants	Avoid tertiary tricyclics (for example, amitriptyline) because of concerns over adverse side effects; consider trial of secondary amine (nortriptyline) for neuropathic pain	Side effects limit use, electrocardiographic monitoring required owing to risk of QTc prolongation; serum level monitoring also recommended	Moderate
Anticonvulsants (for example, pregabalin, gabapentin)	Use for neuropathic pain	Side effects limit use (for example, sedation, peripheral edema); dose adjustment necessary in those with renal impairment	Moderate

NSAIDs=non-steroidal anti-inflammatory drugs.
*Recommendations present in both UK and US guidelines.[2][3]
†Quality of evidence ratings are from the 2009 American Geriatrics Society guideline.

given the risk for drug diversion (that is, use of the drug for a purpose other than pain reduction). In terms of initiating a given opioid trial, no special dosing guidelines exist for older patients. Beginning at the lowest possible dose and titrating upwards based on tolerability and efficacy is recommended, given that age is associated with a greater incidence of treatment related adverse effects. This risk is increased by the presence of multiple comorbidities, polypharmacy, and physiologic vulnerability. Careful surveillance is necessary after beginning an analgesic trial. Frequent telephone or email contact is recommended to assess for and deal with any adverse effects.

What psychological interventions are available?
There is optimism about the role of psychological interventions as treatment for older patients with chronic pain.[36]

Cognitive behavioral therapy
The use of CBT is promising.[37] CBT is used to enhance patients' control over pain, based on the premise that an individual's beliefs, attitudes, and behaviors play a central role in the experience of pain. Standard CBT protocols instruct patients in the use of specific cognitive and behavioral techniques, teach them how certain thoughts, beliefs, attitudes, and emotions influence pain, and highlight the patient's own role in controlling and adapting to chronic pain. CBT techniques are underutilized, particularly among older adults with chronic pain. Few providers have been trained to deliver the protocols for pain, particularly in less developed countries.[38] Early innovation in remote therapy that makes use of communication technology may help to overcome this barrier. Although the quality of the early trials in this area is poor, the use of ehealth and mhealth technologies can improve access to treatments and could improve the treatments.[39] Particularly promising

are efforts to train non-psychologists in CBT delivery and related therapies, which could increase the reach of these treatments.[40] In addition, two recent high quality trials broaden the scope of treatment to include sustainable self management practices in primary care.[41][42] In one trial, investigators evaluated a CBT based self management program for use by older patients with chronic pain in primary care.[41] Significant improvements in distress from the pain, disability, and self efficacy were found in patients who received CBT training compared with an exercise only and wait list control group. Communicating with older patients—particularly those who are reluctant to try behavioral treatments—that using non-drug as well as drug treatments is the standard of care can be helpful. Routinely inquiring about and dealing with patient barriers to engagement with treatment (for example, belief that non-drug treatments are ineffective) is also recommended.

Self management programs
Self management programs merge physical, psychological, and social dimensions and adopt a largely educational approach, teaching patients specific strategies to reduce pain by changing their behavioral, cognitive, and emotional responses to pain and building self efficacy for managing pain and its sequelae. These programs combine education about pain and its consequences and training in relaxation and communication skills. Among the best known of these programs is the Arthritis Foundation self help program (http://patienteducation.stanford.edu/programs/asmp.html). Evidence about the value of self management programs for pain is mixed. Several reviews have reported positive treatment outcomes,[43][44] whereas others have not.[45][46] Despite the conflicting data, we believe it is reasonable to encourage patient participation in self management, and a clearer matching of tailored treatment content to specific outcomes.[47]

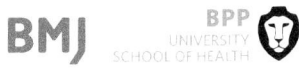

What rehabilitative and exercise approaches are available?

Exercise interventions for older adults with chronic pain are evidenced based, underutilized, and should be a core component of any long term treatment plan. Primary components include training in balance, flexibility, endurance, and strengthening, the mix of which should be tailored to best meet the needs of each patient. Clinicians can refer patients to physiotherapists to develop an exercise program. Physiotherapists can also reinforce related concepts to include coaching on risk of falls, balance training, body mechanics, and pacing. Simple physician advice to remain physically active despite pain, in the absence of a specific exercise routine, is ineffective.

Community based programs include the evidence based Arthritis Foundation exercise program (www.cdc.gov/arthritis/interventions/physical_activity.htm), which is delivered in a group format. Classes are held 1-3 times a week for eight weeks. Health or fitness trainers (such as exercise therapists) lead the groups, which focus on specific exercises appropriate for patients with arthritis or arthritis related diseases. In a recent uncontrolled study (n=110) of a group based exercise training program for older adults with arthritis, participation led to significant improvements in physical functioning.[48] Tai Chi and yoga programs should also be considered, with the caveat that the instructor should be properly qualified.[18] Exercise based programs are low cost and accessible in many communities.[49] Healthcare providers should familiarize themselves with these resources.

Practitioners should consider the preferences of individual patients when prescribing exercise, including the preferred location (for example, gym, home) as well as type of exercise. Older patients with chronic pain may not have access to facilities for exercise or may lack the motivation to engage. It is important to address these barriers or adherence will be low. In support of this approach is a randomized controlled trial of community dwelling older adults (n=56) with chronic pain.[50] In this study, participants randomized to an eight week group based exercise program that included motivational interviewing techniques delivered by a physiotherapist showed significant improvements in pain intensity, self efficacy, anxiety level, and mobility compared with a group based activity control group.[50]

When should patients be referred to a pain specialist?

Practitioners should refer patients when pain is unresponsive (or poorly responsive) to standard treatments, a psychiatric condition (for example, active substance use disorder, excluding nicotine) or medical condition (for example, hepatic or renal dysfunction) would complicate management, there are concerns about misuse of opioids, and procedures (for example, nerve block) may help to clarify a diagnosis or are indicated for the treatment of a given pain disorder.

What is the role of mobile health technology?

Recent advances in mobile health technologies suggest these devices may play a role in the near future by facilitating the collection and transmission of information for the assessment of pain.[51] [52] These devices could potentially improve patient care through more effective monitoring of treatment outcomes, enhanced patient-provider communication, and by providing new ways to deliver treatment.[51] For example, a recent SMS text message based social support intervention delivered by mobile phone was found to reduce pain and pain interference levels among patients with chronic pain.[52]

QUESTIONS FOR FUTURE RESEARCH

- What are the implications of ethnic and cultural diversity on the experience of pain among older people, and the effectiveness of interventions?
- What are the best ways to measure outcomes in geriatric pain research, including both observable and subjective dimensions?
- Can access to psychological therapies be improved by training non-psychologists in delivering them and by using mhealth and ehealth solutions?
- What effect does pain have on cognitive ability and motivation in older people, and how can this be best managed with cognitive behavioral therapy?
- How can the evidence base in trials of pharmacologic, physical, and psychological treatments be improved for older people?
- Should the inclusion of older people in the design of novel interventions be mandatory?
- What evidence based approaches work best to maximize treatment adherence?

TIPS FOR NON-SPECIALISTS

- Pain is more than just a sensory event; assessing for the presence and severity of pain captures only a small part of the pain experience
- Diagnostic imaging is often overused and does not equal better care
- Consider specialist referral for older patients who have complicated psychiatric histories, debilitating pain, or pain that does not respond to customary treatments
- Use combinations of analgesic drugs to enhance analgesic effectiveness
- Non-drug approaches to include exercise and cognitive behavioral approaches are underutilized. Educate older patients about these approaches and identify local practitioners or agencies that provide them
- Implement surveillance plan to assess treatment efficacy, tolerability, and adherence with each new treatment

What limitations exist in the evidence base about treatment?

Although the number of well designed studies evaluating drug or non-drug treatments for older adults with chronic pain is growing, there are important limitations in the existing evidence base. Factors limiting the generalizability of findings include the use of various outcome measures, which make it difficult to compare across studies, short duration of most trials (≤12 weeks), lack of diversity in study populations (inclusion of mostly white, non-Hispanic patients), and greater enrolment of young-old participants (with few participants aged .80) without major comorbidity. Questions about treatment adherence, as well as the long term safety and efficacy of these modalities in older populations remain inadequately defined. In terms of behavioral treatments, patient factors that positively (or negatively) impact treatment outcomes remain inadequately

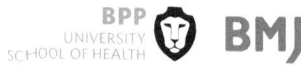

ADDITIONAL EDUCATIONAL RESOURCES

Resources for healthcare professionals

- International Association for the Study of Pain (www. iasp-pain.org/)—Offers extensive resources for healthcare professionals, including listings of educational opportunities, resources on management and treatment, and clinical updates (many countries have affiliates of IASP)
- American Geriatrics Society (www.americangeriatrics. org/health_care_professionals/clinical_practice/clinical_ guidelines_recommendations/2009/)—Provides resources and guidelines for clinicians in providing care to older adults with pain
- European Pain Federation (www.efic.org)—Promotes research, education, clinical management, and professional practice on pain, with training and educational opportunities

Resources for patients

- British Pain Society (www.britishpainsociety.org/)—Provides extensive information for people with pain, including suggested readings, frequently asked questions, and free downloadable publications on various aspects of pain management
- American Chronic Pain Association (www.theacpa.org/)—Offers education and support for people in pain, including educational online resources and a network of support groups in the United States, United Kingdom, and other countries
- Arthritis Foundation (www.arthritis.org/)—Offers programs, practical tips, and education to help people to better manage arthritis related pain

A PATIENT'S PERSPECTIVE

I have lived with chronic back pain for over 30 years. Early on I had surgery on my back that helped for maybe six months, but then the pain returned and has been with me ever since. It has affected my life in many ways: I don't have as much energy as I would like, I can only do housework for short periods before my back starts to hurt, and my kids only know me as a person with chronic back pain. I use different techniques to help me manage it. First off, having a supportive spouse and family is very important. I also find massage, which I get several times a week, to be incredibly helpful. I also go to the gym where I do stretches, walk on the treadmill, and do the exercise bike and elliptical for short periods (five minutes each) before my back starts to bother me. I do take pain medications; I will take ibuprofen for short periods. I also take hydrocodone when the pain is really bad but don't like taking it regularly because my mother had an addiction problem, which is a concern. I would say I have learned to live with the pain and won't let it defeat me.   Sally Smith, New York City

defined. Identifying optimal strategies for the delivery of behavioral treatment (for example, individual versus group based and online versus mobile health approaches) warrant further attention.[36]

Despite these knowledge gaps, we recommend that healthcare providers educate older patients about diverse treatment approaches and encourage their use, to include both drug and non-drug modalities, as a way of broadening their "pain management portfolio." Lack of evidence does not mean evidence of no effect; clinicians must make treatment decisions based on the interaction of individual needs and existing evidence. Given low rates of use of many non-drug management approaches in older patients, encouraging engagement in and adoption of these modalities, to include cognitive behavioral therapy and exercise is particularly recommended.

Contributors: All authors conceived and designed the article, participated in its drafting and revision, and approved the final version. MCR is guarantor.

Competing interests: We have read and understood the BMJ policy on declaration of interests and declare that: MCR has received funding from the National Institute on Ageing (P30AG022845), the Agency for Healthcare Quality and Research (R01HS020648), Howard and Phyllis Schwartz Philanthropic Fund, and Endo Pharmaceuticals. KP has received research funding from the National Institute on Ageing (P30AG022845). CE has received a grant from the UK National Institute for Health Research Cochrane Program.

Patient consent obtained.

Provenance and peer review: Commissioned; externally peer reviewed.

1   Institute of Medicine (US) Committee on Advancing Pain Research, Care, and Education. Relieving pain in America: a blueprint for transforming prevention, care, education, and research. National Academies Press (US), 2011.
2   Abdulla A, Adams N, Bone M, Elliott AM, Gaffin J, Jones D, et al. Guidance on the management of pain in older people. Age Ageing 2013;42 (Suppl 1):1-57.
3   American Geriatrics Society Panel on Persistent Pain in Older Persons. Pharmacological management of persistent pain in older persons. J Am Geriatr Soc 2009;57:1331-46.
4   International Association for the Study of Pain. IASP taxonomy. 2012. www.iasp-pain.org/Taxonomy?navItemNumber=576.
5   Solano JP, Gomes B, Higginson IJ. A comparison of symptom prevalence in far advanced cancer, AIDS, heart disease, chronic obstructive pulmonary disease, and renal disease. J Pain Symptom Manage 2006;31:58-69.
6   Enck RE. Postsurgical chronic pain. Am J Hosp Palliat Care 2010;27:301-2.
7   Smith AK, Cenzer IS, Knight SJ, Puntillo KA, Widera E, Williams BA, et al. The epidemiology of pain in the last 2 years of life. Ann Intern Med 2010;153:563-9.
8   Wyldea V, Hewlett S, Learmonth ID. Persistent pain after joint replacement: prevalence, sensory qualities, and postoperative determinants. Pain 2011;152:457-76.
9   Cooper G, Lane JM, Lin J. Medscape: overview of osteoporotic compression fractures. 2013. www.emedicine.com/pmr/byname/ nonoperative-treatment-of-osteoporotic-compression-fractures.htm.
10 Patel KV, Guralnik JM, Dansie EJ, Turk DC. Prevalence and impact of pain among older adults in the United States: findings from the 2011 National Health and Aging Trends Study. Pain 2013;154:2649-57.
11 Leadley RM, Armstrong N, Lee YC, Allen A, Kleijnen J. Chronic diseases in the European Union: the prevalence and health cost implications of chronic pain. J Pain Palliat Care Pharmacother 2012;26:310-25.
12 Henderson JV, Harrison CM, Britt HC, Bayram CF, Miller GC. Prevalence, causes, severity, impact, and management of chronic pain in Australian general practice patients. Pain Med 2013;14:1346-61.
13 Jackson T, Chen H, Iezzi T, Yee M, Chen F. Prevalence and correlates of chronic pain in a random population study of adults in Chongqing, China. Clin J Pain 2014;3:346-52.
14 Tsang A, Von Korff M, Lee S, Alonso J, Karam E, Angermeyer MC, et al. Common chronic pain conditions in developed and developing countries: gender and age differences and comorbidity with depression-anxiety disorders. J Pain 2008;9:883-91.
15 Mallen CD, Thomas E, Belcher J, Rathod T, Croft P, Peat G. Point-of-care prognosis for common musculoskeletal pain in older adults. JAMA Intern Med 2013;173:1119-25.
16 Makris UE, Abrams RC, Gurland B, Reid MC. Management of persistent pain in the older patient: a clinical review. JAMA 2014;312:825-36.
17 Royal College of Physicians, British Geriatrics Society, and British Pain Society. The assessment of pain in older people: national guidelines. Concise guidance to good practice series, No 8. Royal College of Physicians, Oct 2007.
18 American Geriatrics Society Panel on Persistent Pain in Older Persons. The management of persistent pain in older persons. J Am Geriatr Soc 2002;50(Suppl 6):205-24.
19 Hadjistavropoulos T, Herr K, Turk DC, Fine PG, Dworkin RH, Helme R, et al. An interdisciplinary expert consensus statement on assessment of pain in older persons. Clin J Pain 2007;23(Suppl 1):1-43.
20 Chou R, Qaseem A, Owens DK, Shekelle P. Clinical Guidelines Committee of the American College of Physicians. Diagnostic imaging for low back pain: advice for high-value health care from the American College of Physicians. Ann Intern Med 2011;154:181-9.
21 Azevedo LF, Costa-Pereira A, Mendonça L, Dias CC, Castro-Lopes JM. Chronic pain and health services utilization: is there overuse of diagnostic tests and inequalities in nonpharmacologic treatment methods utilization? Med Care 2013;51:859-69.
22 Dansie EJ, Turk DC. Assessment of patients with chronic pain. Br J Anaesth 2013;111:19-25.
23 Herr K, Coyne PJ, McCaffery M, Manworren R, Merkel S. Pain assessment in the patient unable to self-report: position statement with clinical practice recommendations. Pain Manag Nurs 2011;12:230-50.
24 Messier SP, Mihalko SL, Legault C, Miller GD, Nicklas BJ, DeVita P, et al. Effects of intensive diet and exercise on knee joint loads, inflammation, and clinical outcomes among overweight and obese

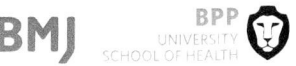

adults with knee osteoarthritis: the IDEA randomized clinical trial. *JAMA* 2013;310:1263-73.

25 Kroenke K, Krebs EE, Wu J, Yu Z, Chumbler NR, Bair MJ. Telecare collaborative management of chronic pain in primary care: a randomized clinical trial. *JAMA* 2014;312:240-8.

26 Dobscha SK, Corson K, Perrin NA, Hanson GC, Leibowitz RQ, Doak MN, et al. Collaborative care for chronic pain in primary care: a cluster randomized trial. *JAMA* 2009;301:1242-52.

27 Lin EHB, Katon W, Von Korff M, Tang L, Williams JW Jr, Kroenke K, et al. Effect of improving depression care on pain and functional outcomes among older adults with arthritis: a randomized controlled trial. *JAMA* 2003;290:2428-9.

28 Keefe FJ, Blumenthal J, Baucom D, Affleck G, Waugh R, Caldwell DS, et al. Effects of spouse-assisted coping skills training and exercise training in patients with osteoarthritic knee pain: a randomized controlled study. *Pain* 2004;110:539-49.

29 Martire LM, Schulz R, Keefe FJ, Rudy TE, Starz TW. Couple-oriented education and support intervention for osteoarthritis: effects on spouses' support and responses to patient pain. *Fam Syst Health* 2008;26:185-95.

30 Gilron I, Bailey JM, Tu D, Holden RR, Weaver DF, Houlden RL. Morphine, gabapentin, or their combination for neuropathic pain. *N Engl J Med* 2005;352:1324-34.

31 Towheed TE, Maxwell L, Judd MG, Catton M, Hochberg MC, Wells G. Acetaminophen for osteoarthritis. *Cochrane Database Syst Rev* 2006;1:CD004257.

32 Trelle S, Reichenbach S, Wandel S, Hildebrand P, Tschannen B, Villiger PM, et al. Cardiovascular safety of non-steroidal anti-inflammatory drugs: network meta-analysis. *BMJ* 2011;342:c7086.

33 Papaleontiou M, Henderson CR Jr, Turner BJ, Moore AA, Olkhovskaya Y, Amanfo L, et al. Outcomes associated with opioid use in the treatment of chronic noncancer pain in older adults: a systematic review and meta-analysis. *J Am Geriatr Soc* 2010;58:1353-69.

34 Reid MC, Henderson CR Jr, Papaleontiou M, Amanfo L, Olkhovskaya Y, Moore AA, et al. Characteristics of older adults receiving opioids in primary care: treatment duration and outcomes. *Pain Med* 2010;11:1063-71.

35 Chou R, Turner JA, Devine EB, Hansen RN, Sullivan SD, Blazina I, et al. The effectiveness and risks of long-term opioid therapy for chronic pain: a systematic review for a National Institutes of Health pathways to prevention workshop. *Ann Intern Med* 2015; published online 13 Jan.

36 McGuire BE, Nicholas MK, Asghari A, Wood BM, Main CJ. The effectiveness of psychological treatments for chronic pain in older adults: cautious optimism and an agenda for research. *Curr Opin Psychiatry* 2014;27:380-4.

37 Lunde LH, Nordhus I, Pallesen S. The effectiveness of cognitive and behavioural treatment of chronic pain in the elderly: a quantitative review. *J Clin Psychol Med Settings* 2009;16:254-62.

38 Draguns JG. Cross-cultural and international extensions of evidence-based psychotherapy: toward more effective and sensitive psychological services everywhere. *Psychologia* 2013;56:74-88.

39 Eccleston C, Fisher E, Craig L, Duggan GB, Rosser BA, Keogh E. Psychological therapies (Internet-delivered) for the management of chronic pain in adults. *Cochrane Database Syst Rev* 2014;2:CD010152.

40 Riddle DL, Keefe FJ, Ang D, Khaled J, Dumenci L, Jensen MP, et al. A phase III randomized three-arm trial of physical therapist delivered pain coping skills training for patients with total knee arthroplasty: the KASTPain protocol. *BMC Musculoskelet Disord* 2012;13:149.

41 Nicholas MK, Asghari A, Blyth FM, Wood BM, Murray R, McCabe R, et al. Self-management intervention for chronic pain in older adults: a randomized controlled trial. *Pain* 2013;154:824-35.

42 Broderick JE, Keefe FJ, Bruckenthal P, Junghaenel DU, Schneider S, Schwartz JE, et al. Nurse practitioners can effectively deliver pain coping skills training to osteoarthritis patients with chronic pain: a randomized, controlled trial. *Pain* 2014;155:1743-54.

43 Reid MC, Papaleontiou M, Ong A, Breckman R, Wethington E, Pillemer K. Self-management strategies to reduce pain and improve function among older adults in community settings: a review of the evidence. *Pain Med* 2008;9:409-24.

44 Du S, Yuan C, Xiao X, Chu J, Qiu Y, Qian H. Self-management programs for chronic musculoskeletal pain conditions: a systematic review and meta-analysis. *Patient Educ Couns* 2011;85:e299-310.

45 Chodosh J, Morton SC, Mojica W, Maglione M, Suttorp MJ, Hilton L, et al. Meta-analysis: chronic disease self-management programs for older adults. *Ann Intern Med* 2005;143:427-38.

46 Warsi A, Wang PS, LaValley MP, Avorn J, Solomon DH. Self-management education programs in chronic disease. A systematic review and methodological critique of the literature. *Arch Intern Med* 2004;164:1641-9.

47 Morley S, Williams A, Eccleston C. Examining the evidence of psychological treatments for chronic pain: time for a paradigm shift? *Pain* 2012;154:1929-31.

48 Levy SS, Macera CA, Hootman JM, Coleman KJ, Lopez R, Nichols JF, et al. Evaluation of a multi-component group exercise program for adults with arthritis: Fitness and Exercise for People with Arthritis (FEPA). *Disabil Health J* 2012;5:305-11.

49 Tobias KR, Lama SD, Parker SJ, Henderson CR Jr, Nickerson AJ, Reid MC. Meeting the public health challenge of pain in later life: what role can senior centers play? *Pain Manag Nurs* 2014;15:760-7.

50 Tse MM, Vong SK, Tang SK. Motivational interviewing and exercise programme for community-dwelling older persons with chronic pain: a randomized controlled study. *J Clin Nurs* 2013;22:1843-56.

51 Richardson JE, Reid MC. The promises and pitfalls of leveraging mobile health technology for pain care. *Pain Med* 2013;14:1621-6.

52 Guillory J, Chang P, Henderson CR Jr, Shengelia R, Lama S, Warmington M, et al. Piloting a text message-based social support intervention for patients with chronic pain: establishing feasibility and preliminary efficacy. *Clin J Pain* 2015; published online 6 Jan.

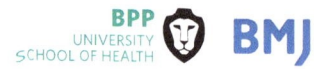

The management of chronic breathlessness in patients with advanced and terminal illness

Magnus P Ekström, postdoctoral research fellow[1] [2], Amy P Abernethy, professor[3], David C Currow, professor[2]

[1]Department of Clinical Sciences, Division of Respiratory Medicine & Allergology, Lund University, Lund, Sweden

[2]Discipline of Palliative and Supportive Services, Flinders University, Adelaide, Australia

[3]Division of Medical Oncology, Department of Medicine, Duke University Medical Center, Durham, NC, USA

Correspondence to: M P Ekström, The Respiratory Unit, Department of Medicine, Blekinge Hospital, Karlskrona, Sweden pmekstrom@gmail.com

Cite this as: *BMJ* 2015;350:g7617

DOI: 10.1136/bmj.g7617

http://www.bmj.com/content/349/bmj.g7617/related

Breathlessness—the sensation of discomfort with breathing—is a major cause of impaired activity and suffering worldwide and is common among elderly people in the community and in people with advanced disease.[1] [w1] Proper evaluation and treatment of breathlessness is vital to improve patients' quality of life.

Importantly, the sensation of breathlessness that persists despite disease specific treatment can be relieved for many people. This review focuses on the management of refractory breathlessness, defined as breathlessness at rest or on limited exertion that persists despite optimal treatment of the underlying conditions, in advanced chronic disease, or towards the end of life.[2] [w4]

What is breathlessness?

Breathlessness is defined by the American Thoracic Society as the "subjective experience of breathing discomfort that consists of qualitatively distinct sensations that vary in intensity."[w1] According to the present neurophysiological model, breathlessness is the awareness of a mismatch between the ventilator drive (the need to breathe) and the achieved ventilation (the ability to breathe).[w1]

Importantly, breathlessness is a sensation and not a physiological variable. The presence and severity of breathlessness cannot be predicted sufficiently for an individual from variables such as oxygen saturation, respiratory rate, and forced expiratory volume in one second.[w2] [w3] Distressing breathlessness may be present despite a normal breathing rate and can be absent in patients with severe respiratory compromise. Patients should be asked about their symptoms.

How common is it in advanced and terminal illness?

Chronic breathlessness, often defined as breathlessness for more than 4-8 weeks, is highly prevalent in the community and especially in people with advanced disease, and it often intensifies near death. In a study from South Australia, 9% of the population and 17% aged more than 65 years had chronic breathlessness.[1] In a similar Norwegian study, 13% of the general population were limited by breathlessness and 5% reported severe breathlessness.[w5] Among 1556 patients admitted to five tertiary hospitals in the United States, about 50% reported breathlessness.[w6]

In a review of advanced and terminal disease, the prevalence of breathlessness was high across all diagnoses: cancer (16-77%), chronic heart failure (18-88%), and renal disease (11-82%), and particularly high in chronic obstructive pulmonary disease (56-98%).[3]

In a prospective study, the prevalence of breathlessness among 5862 patients attending specialized palliative care increased from 50% to 65% during the last three months of life.[4] Patients with cancer had less breathlessness overall than patients with non-malignant disease but the breathlessness increased more before death, whereas patients with other diagnoses on average had more severe and constant breathlessness, often for many years. Despite receiving specialized palliative care, 26% of the patients reported severe breathlessness during the last three months of life.[4] Patients with advanced illnesses need to be monitored closely as the clinical trajectories are highly variable.[w7] An estimated 60% of all people dying in high income countries are in need of palliative care at some point.[w8]

What is the impact of breathlessness?

Both patients and carers report breathlessness as a distressing symptom.[w9] To reduce breathlessness, patients limit their physical activity.[w1] Several observational studies link breathlessness to a more sedentary lifestyle,[w10] deconditioning (decreased physical fitness),[w11] increased anxiety and depression,[w11] [w12] impaired quality of life,[w11] [w13] loss of the will to live near death,[w14] increased likelihood of admission to hospital,[w15] and earlier death.[5] [w13] Breathlessness can worsen in a spiral of interacting symptoms—it may, for example, both cause anxiety and worsen as a consequence of the anxiety.[w16]

How is it measured?

The ideal method for measuring breathlessness is by patients' self report.[w1] In a recent cross sectional study of patients with lung cancer, agreement between patients and doctors on ratings of breathlessness was only 45%.[w13]

Several instruments exist for measuring different aspects of breathlessness, such as intensity, unpleasantness, and functional impact.[w1] Patients should use a simple tool, such as a numerical rating scale, to rate the severity of their breathlessness. They could be asked to rate the severity of their breathlessness "right now" or as an average over the past 12 or 24 hours, depending on the clinical setting. A numerical rating scale—a categorical 11 point

---

THE BOTTOM LINE

- Breathlessness is the subjective sensation of discomfort with breathing
- It is a common cause of major suffering in people with advanced and terminal disease
- Breathlessness should be measured routinely in patients with advanced disease and can be reduced by appropriate treatment
- The preferred treatments for refractory breathlessness are pulmonary rehabilitation and oral low dose opioids
- Evidence for use of benzodiazepines and supplemental oxygen (in the absence of severe hypoxemia) is lacking or inconsistent and these interventions are not recommended for refractory breathlessness
- Consider early referral to specialist care (including palliative care) if the cause remains unclear or if the response to treatment is insufficient

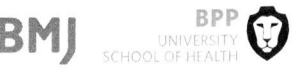

scale between 0 (no breathlessness) to 10 (worst possible breathlessness)—is reliable and valid for measuring changes in breathlessness in individual patients.[w1 w17] The same tool should be used to measure changes over time and response to treatment. According to a recent pooled analysis of trials on opioids for chronic breathlessness, a difference of 1 point on a numerical rating scale was identified as a clinically meaningful change in chronic breathlessness by patients.[6]

In people with critical illness who are unable to self report, the severity of breathlessness can be estimated using the validated respiratory distress observation scale based on eight observer rated clinical variables.[7]

How is it evaluated?

Breathlessness may be the first presentation of a disease or may represent worsening of a pre-existing condition. The evaluation of breathlessness should identify all contributing causes that are amenable to treatment,[w1] along with taking a medical history, carrying out a physical examination, and requesting basic tests.[2 8] The extent of the evaluation needs to be guided by the patient's wishes, expected benefits and harms from investigations and subsequent interventions, and the stage of disease.

In a study of 129 patients aged 60 years or older in primary care, chronic breathlessness was mainly associated with respiratory disease (53%), heart disease (21%), obesity (16%), and deconditioning (4%).[8] Differential diagnoses (table) include asthma, chronic obstructive pulmonary disease, interstitial lung disease, heart failure, ischemic heart disease, anemia, chronic pulmonary embolism, pleural effusion, obesity, and neuromuscular disease.[2 8 w1]

[w18] In any advanced disease, breathlessness will increase with worsening cachexia.[8]

In one study a thorough history and medical examination was shown to correctly identify 55% of definitive causes of unexplained breathlessness.[2] The table lists the clinical features suggestive of different underlying causes. A history of wheezing, productive cough (sputum), and palpitations suggests a cardiopulmonary disease.[w18] Breathlessness described as "chest tightness" is suggestive of bronchospasm due to asthma.[w1 w18] Breathlessness that is precipitated by lying down (orthopnea) is non-specific and seen in patients with heart failure, chronic obstructive pulmonary disease, obesity, and neuromuscular impairment.[w18]

A structured diagnostic algorithm including basic laboratory tests, electrocardiography, chest radiography, spirometry, and additional investigations as indicated, can establish a underlying cause of breathlessness in most patients.[2] At least 20% of patients have several contributing causes.[2 w1 w18] If the cause of chronic breathlessness remains unclear, or if patients have severe distress or complicating factors, early referral to a cardiologist, pulmonologist, or breathlessness clinic could be considered.[9]

What is the approach to management?

The treatment of breathlessness involves interventions such as psychosocial support and walking aids, optimized treatment of underlying diseases and complications, relief of coexisting symptoms such as pain contributing to breathlessness, and treatment directed against deconditioning and the sensation of breathlessness itself (figure). There is level I evidence for the use of pulmonary

Main conditions	Frequency (%)	Symptoms and signs[w1 w15]
All conditions		All diagnoses are associated with breathlessness initially on exertion; and on minimal exertion or at rest in severe disease
Respiratory		
Asthma	29 (20)	Intermittent (provoked) wheezing, chest tightness, cough (often worst at night/in the morning)
Chronic obstructive pulmonary disease	13 (9)	Productive cough (bronchitis), wheezing, prolonged expiration, decreased breath sounds/hyper-resonance (emphysema). Smoking, but about 20% of patients with chronic obstructive pulmonary disease are never smokers. Leg swelling can be seen in respiratory failure
Asthma/chronic obstructive pulmonary disease	13 (9)	Concomitant signs of the two conditions
Interstitial lung disease	12 (8)	Nonproductive cough, fine basal inspiratory crackles can be an early sign, extra-pulmonary signs in underlying systemic disease, progressive breathlessness and hypoxemia at exertion
Pulmonary artery hypertension	3 (2)	Insidious, unspecific, progressive breathlessness, lethargy, and hypoxemia at especially on exertion; right heart failure in severe disease
Other	8 (5)	
Heart and vascular disease		
Heart disease:		
Heart failure		Heart failure: lethargy, exercise intolerance, edema, abdominal symptoms (for example, loss of appetite); most have orthopnea and an abnormal electrocardiogram
Ischemic heart disease	9 (6)	Suggested by episodes of chest discomfort; may be provoked by for example exertion, eating, or stress; often unspecific symptoms in elderly patients and people with diabetes
Valvular heart disease	5 (3)	Heart murmur, signs of cardiac ischemia or heart failure.
Anemia	5 (3)	Pallor, lethargy, blood loss, symptoms of underlying insufficiency (iron, vitamin B12, folate) or disease; symptoms of precipitated cardiac disease
Other	4 (3)	
Non-cardiopulmonary		
Obesity/deconditioning	26 (18)	Signs of underlying conditions if secondary deconditioning
Hyperventilation/psychogenic	15 (10)	Fluctuating and unspecific symptoms, including tingling, anxiety, and loss of control; exclusion of underlying disease
Other	5 (3)	

Main underlying diagnoses from a study with detailed data of 123 patients referred for unexplained breathlessness of at least eight weeks' duration to a pulmonary outpatient clinic.[2] The main diagnosis groups were consistent with a study in primary care[8]

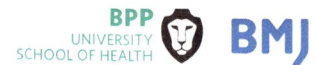

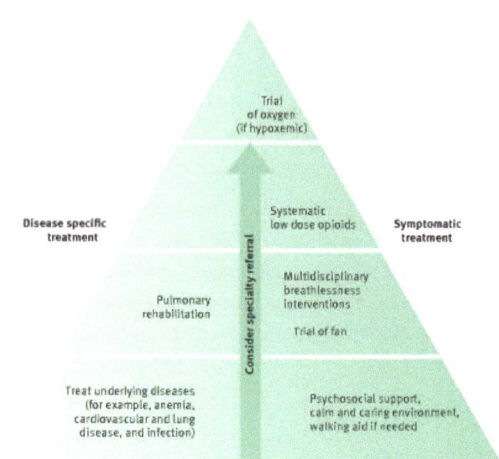

Principles of breathlessness management. Treatment is given for the underlying causes as well as the sensation of breathlessness itself, and is escalated depending on symptom severity, availability, and cost of treatments, as well as the beneficial and adverse effects for individual patients

rehabilitation, especially in people with chronic obstructive pulmonary disease, and for systemic, low dose, sustained release opioids in patients with advanced disease.[10] [11] [12] [w1] Supplemental oxygen, in the absence of severe hypoxemia, and benzodiazepines are not recommended for breathlessness owing to inconsistent or no evidence of a net clinical benefit.[13] [14] [15]

Symptomatic under-treatment remains an important problem.[16] In a population based study of patients with cancer, 9% had to visit the emergency department during the last six months of life and 5% during the last two weeks.[w19] The main reasons included pain, malaise, nausea, constipation, and breathlessness—causes that may be avoidable with appropriate symptomatic treatment and follow-up.[w19] The management should, importantly, address wishes, expectations, fears and concerns of the patient and family and carers. Patients may have concerns about the side effects of drugs, addiction, tolerance, and approaching the end of life.

One approach is to develop a treatment model that tackles underlying causes whenever possible and that simultaneously treats the symptom itself (see web extra figure). If the cause of the breathlessness is unclear, if the symptoms are causing considerable distress, or there is insufficient treatment response on breathlessness, consider referral to specialty care (including palliative care).

What non-drug interventions are available for refractory breathlessness?

Pulmonary rehabilitation
Strong evidence suggests that pulmonary rehabilitation decreases breathlessness, increases exercise capacity, and improves quality of life in patients with symptomatic cardiopulmonary limitation.[11] A Cochrane analysis of 12 studies (323 patients) showed a clinically meaningful improvement in breathlessness on the chronic respiratory questionnaire (mean 1.1 points, 95% confidence interval 0.9 to 1.3) compared with usual care.[17] Eligible patients include those who become breathless at least when hurrying on the level or walking up a slight hill.[11] Most evidence pertains to chronic obstructive pulmonary disease, but there is some evidence of benefit also in interstitial lung disease and cancer.[11] Multidisciplinary rehabilitation should be

offered for at least six weeks and includes endurance and strength training, improved breathing techniques, and an opportunity for smoking cessation, optimized treatment of underlying conditions, and nutritional and psychosocial support.[11] Pulmonary rehabilitation is beneficial and safe in patients with stable comorbidity, including cardiovascular disease and respiratory failure.[11] [18] Real world data are needed on the long term effects and how to improve uptake and feasibility of tailored rehabilitation programs in patients with advanced disease.

Multidisciplinary support services
In a recent single blinded randomized trial of 105 consecutive patients with advanced disease (54% with chronic obstructive pulmonary disease, 20% with cancer, and 18% with interstitial lung disease), the patients' "mastery" of breathlessness was improved by an multidisciplinary breathlessness support service, involving respiratory medicine, physiotherapy, occupational therapy, and palliative care management. On the mastery domain of the chronic respiratory questionnaire the mean difference was 0.58 (95% confidence interval 0.1 to 1.15) over six weeks compared with usual care, which could be clinically important for patients.[19] Interestingly, the multidisciplinary intervention was also associated with improved survival.[19]

Non-invasive ventilation
In a recent randomized trial of 200 patients with advanced solid cancers and acute respiratory failure, non-invasive ventilation was associated with a decrease in breathlessness compared with oxygen therapy and the need for morphine; a mean decrease of 0.58 points (95% confidence interval 0.23 to 0.92) on the Borg scale (12 point ordinal scale between 0 "nothing at all" and 10 "maximal" breathlessness).[20] Non-invasive ventilation improves breathlessness in acute hypercapnic respiratory failure due to chronic obstructive pulmonary disease.[w24] In the setting of palliative care, non-invasive ventilation should only be used if it is tolerated by the patient and provides symptomatic relief; further studies of efficacy and feasibility are needed.[21]

Other non-drug interventions
A Cochrane analysis of non-drug interventions for the relief of breathlessness reported moderate evidence for use of walking aids (for example, the rollator, a wheeled walking frame) as needed.[w21] Evidence supported the use of chest wall vibration and neuroelectrical muscle stimulation,[w21] although the utility of these two modalities may be limited in clinical practice. A handheld fan directed toward the mouth and nose may relieve breathlessness and might be tried especially in relatively immobilized patients.[w21] [w22] Although the efficacy of fan use is the subject of ongoing studies, it is inexpensive and has no reported side effects.[22]

What drug interventions are available for refractory breathlessness?

Opioids
The preferred treatment for the relief of chronic refractory breathlessness is a systemic (oral or parenteral) low dose opioid (level I evidence).[10] [12] The effect of opioids seems to be mediated mainly by a central reduction of the ventilator demand and altered perception of breathlessness.[23] [w1] In a meta-analysis of nine small, randomized studies (116 patients) and an adequately powered randomized crossover trial (48 outpatients), systemic opioids reduced

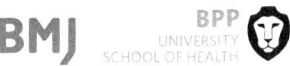

SOURCES AND SELECTION CRITERIA

We searched Medline, the Cochrane Database of Systematic Reviews, reference lists of major reviews, guidelines and consensus documents, and personal records using the terms "dyspnea" and "breathlessness". We focused on systematic reviews, meta-analyses, randomized controlled trials, and high quality observational studies in patients with advanced or terminal disease.

SUGGESTIONS FOR FURTHER RESEARCH

- Underlying mechanisms of breathlessness and treatment effects
- Burden and causes of breathlessness, including in low income and middle income countries
- Predictors of long term beneficial and adverse effects of opioids to individualize treatment, including pharmacogenetic studies
- Increasing the evidence base for effect of opioids during rehabilitation and for new treatments for breathlessness

TIPS FOR NON-SPECIALISTS

- Assess the severity of breathlessness routinely in patients with advanced disease
- Always consider the presence and optimal treatment of underlying conditions
- Consider pulmonary rehabilitation and low dose systemic opioids for refractory breathlessness in advanced disease
- Judicious use of low dose opioids is safe
- Give prophylaxis for constipation and follow up the patient's clinical condition and response to treatment
- Consider referral to specialty care (including palliative care) in the setting of unclear cause, considerable distress, or insufficient treatment response on breathlessness

ADDITIONAL EDUCATIONAL RESOURCES

Resources for healthcare professionals

- American Academy of Family Physicians. ACCP releases statement on dyspnea treatment in patients with advanced lung or heart disease (www.aafp.org/afp/2010/1015/p999.pdf)—American guideline informing breathlessness management in primary care
- Canadian Thoracic Society. Managing dyspnea in patients with advanced chronic obstructive pulmonary disease. (www.respiratoryguidelines.ca/sites/all/files/CTS%20COPD%20Dyspnea%20Slide-Kit%202011_Final.pdf)—Canadian guideline focusing on management of breathlessness in chronic obstructive pulmonary disease
- Registered Nurses of Ontario. Nursing care of dyspnea: the 6th vital sign in individuals with chronic obstructive pulmonary disease (http://rnao.ca/sites/rnao-ca/files/Nursing_Care_of_Dyspnea_-The_6th_Vital_Sign_in_Individuals_with_Chronic_Obstructive_Pulmonary_Disease.pdf)—resource for breathlessness management for nurses
- Kamal AH, Maguire JM, Wheeler JL, Currow DC, Abernethy AP. Dyspnea review for the palliative care professional: assessment, burdens, and etiologies. *J Palliat Med* 2011;14:1167-72
- Kamal AH, Maguire JM, Wheeler JL, Currow DC, Abernethy AP. Dyspnea review for the palliative care professional: treatment goals and therapeutic options. *J Palliat Med* 2012;15:106-14

Resources for patients

- American Academy of Physicians. Chronic obstructive pulmonary disease: a clinical practice guideline (http://annals.org/article.aspx?articleID=479663)
- UpToDate. Patient information: shortness of breath (dyspnea) (beyond the basics) (www.uptodate.com/contents/shortness-of-breath-dyspnea-beyond-the-basics)
- ATS. Patient information series: breathlessness (http://patients.thoracic.org/information-series/en/resources/ATS_Patient_Ed_Breathlessness.pdf)
- Patient.co.uk. Breathlessness (www.patient.co.uk/doctor/Breathlessness.htm)
- UK NHS. Patient information factsheet: controlling your breathing when feeling breathless (www.uhs.nhs.uk/Media/Controlleddocuments/Patientinformation/Medicinestherapiesandanaesthetics/Controllingyourbreathingpatientinformation.pdf)

the mean chronic breathlessness by approximately 20% over baseline.[10][12] Nebulized opioids are not recommended, given the current evidence.[12]

Which patients should be treated with opioids?

Trials included mainly patients with severe chronic obstructive pulmonary disease (and a few with restrictive pulmonary disease, cancer, or heart failure) and breathlessness at rest or minimal exertion limiting daily activities despite optimized treatments. In a pooled analysis, the benefit from opioids was stronger in younger patients and in those with severe breathlessness.[24] Data in severe chronic heart failure are limited,[25][26] but evidence that the benefit depends on the type of underlying disease is inconsistent.[6]

Which opioid dose is needed to relieve chronic breathlessness?

In an observational dose titration study of oral opioids 64% of the 83 patients reported a reduction in breathlessness.[27] Of these, 70% responded to 10 mg regular, sustained release morphine daily and more than 90% responded to 20 mg morphine or less daily.[27] The opioid effect seemed to increase during the week after each dose increment.[w20] After three months, 53% of responders had sustained benefit from opioids without the need for doses to be increased.[27]

Importantly, regular, low dose, sustained release opioids seem to be safe in patients with advanced and terminal disease. Side effects are mainly nausea in the first two days of starting opioids, and constipation.[10][12][27] No cases of respiratory depression or other serious adverse effects resulting in admission to hospital or death have been reported in studies of low dose sustained release opioids.[10][12][27] In a recent large observational study of patients with chronic respiratory failure associated with chronic obstructive pulmonary disease, low dose opioids were not associated with increased risk of admission to hospital or death.[28] Data are needed on long term effects and on the net clinical benefit of opioids for breathlessness in less severe disease.

How is opioid treatment initiated and managed in practice?

The approach for chronic breathlessness is similar to that for opioid treatment of pain. Available evidence suggests that regular sustained release opioid is initiated in a dose equivalent to 10 mg oral morphine daily, and titrated upward, preferably once weekly, balancing beneficial and adverse effects.[w20] All patients should receive prophylaxis and treatment against constipation.

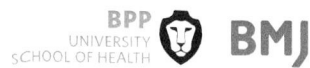

Oxygen

Oxygen is often given in the hope of relieving breathlessness, but the evidence for efficacy is inconsistent.[13] [14] [29] There are no studies of oxygen for breathlessness in severe resting hypoxemia (arterial oxygen pressure <7.4 kPa), and a large double blind randomized trial in 239 patients with milder or no hypoxemia reported no change in breathlessness from oxygen compared with air.[13] Oxygen therapy is costly and may impose an unnecessary burden on some patients. A recent crossover trial found that oxygen did not relieve breathlessness in patients in the last days or hours of life and concluded that for most patients near death oxygen seems not to be beneficial.[14] If tried, oxygen should be given only to patients with moderate to severe levels of breathlessness and hypoxemia, and it should be withdrawn if the patient does not report relief of breathlessness within a few days.[14]

Other drugs

Benzodiazepines—although benzodiazepines are often used and may relieve anxiety,[28] a recent Cochrane meta-analysis of seven studies (200 patients) found that benzodiazepines did not relieve breathlessness and increased the risk of drowsiness.[15] These studies were, however, heterogeneous and the sample sizes were small.

Antidepressants—current evidence for antidepressants decreasing breathlessness is inconsistent.[w1]

Saline—a randomized single blind trial of 40 people with an exacerbation of chronic obstructive pulmonary disease showed no consistent relief of breathlessness from nebulized isotonic saline compared with placebo.[30]

Furosemide (frusemide)—in exploratory studies, the results for efficacy of inhaled furosemide (frusemide) on breathlessness have been conflicting.[w23] Efficacy needs to be confirmed in large clinical trials.[w1]

We thank Duke University employees Donald T Kirkendall (medical editor) and Laura Roe (graphics designer) for their assistance in preparing this article.

Contributors: All authors conceived and designed the paper, revised it for important intellectual content, and approved the final version to be published. MPE drafted the first version of the paper. APA planned the content and participated in writing the paper and revisions, and accepts full responsibility for the work, had access to the included data, and controlled the decision to publish. She is the guarantor.

Competing interests: We have read and understood the BMJ policy on declaration of interests and declare the following interests: DCC is on the clinical trials advisory board for Helsinn Pharmaceuticals, is a clinical trials consultant for MaynePharma, and has received research funding from Mundipharma. APA is on the scientific advisory boards for Bristol-Myers Squibb, is a consultant for Bristol-Myers Squibb, Novartis, and Pfizer, has received research funding from National Institute of Nursing Research, National Cancer Institute, Agency for Healthcare Research and Quality, DARA, Glaxo Smith Kline, Celgene, Helsinn, Dendreon, and Pfizer and is due to receive research funding from Genentech, Bristol Myers Squibb, Insys, and Kanglaite. APA has a paid leadership role with American Academy of Hospice & Palliative Medicine (president) and corporate leadership responsibility in Athena Health (health IT company), Advoset (an education company that has a contract with Novartis), and Orange Leaf Associates LLC (an IT development company).

Provenance and peer review: Commissioned; externally peer reviewed.

1 Currow DC, Plummer JL, Crockett A, Abernethy AP. A community population survey of prevalence and severity of dyspnea in adults. *J Pain Symptom Manage* 2009;38:533-45.
2 Pratter MR, Abouzgheib W, Akers S, et al. An algorithmic approach to chronic dyspnea. *Respir Med* 2011;105:1014-21.
3 Moens K, Higginson IJ, Harding R. Are there differences in the prevalence of palliative care-related problems in people living with advanced cancer and eight non-cancer conditions? a systematic review. *J Pain Symptom Manage* 2014;48:660-77.
4 Currow DC, Smith J, Davidson PM, et al. Do the trajectories of dyspnea differ in prevalence and intensity by diagnosis at the end of life? A consecutive cohort study. *J Pain Sympt Manage* 2010;39:680-90.
5 Nishimura K, Izumi T, Tsukino M, et al. Dyspnea is a better predictor of 5-year survival than airway obstruction in patients with COPD. *Chest* 2002;121:1434-40.
6 Johnson MJ, Bland JM, Oxberry SG, et al. Clinically important differences in the intensity of chronic refractory Breathlessness. *J Pain Symptom Manage* 2013;46:957-63.
7 Campbell ML, Templin T, Walch J. A respiratory distress observation scale for patients unable to self-report dyspnea. *J Palliat Med* 2010;13:285-90.
8 Pedersen F, Mehlsen J, Raymond I, et al. Evaluation of dyspnoea in a sample of elderly subjects recruited from general practice. *Int J Clin Pract* 2007;61:1481-91.
9 Schwartzstein RM, Adams L. Dyspnea. In: Mason RJ, Broaddus VC, Martin TR, et al., eds. Murray and Nadel's textbook of respiratory medicine. 5th ed. Saunders-Elsevier, 2010.
10 Abernethy AP, Currow DC, Frith P, Fazekas BS, McHugh A, Bui C. Randomised, double blind, placebo controlled crossover trial of sustained release morphine for the management of refractory dyspnoea. *BMJ* 2003;327:523-8.
11 Bolton CE, Bevan-Smith EF, Blakey JD, Crowe P, Elkin SL, Garrod R, et al. British Thoracic Society guideline on pulmonary rehabilitation in adults. *Thorax* 2013;68:ii1-30.
12 Jennings AL, Davies AN, Higgins JP, Gibbs JS, Bradley KE. A systematic review of the use of opioids in the management of dyspnoea. *Thorax* 2002;57:939-44.
13 Abernethy AP, McDonald CF, Frith PA, et al. Effect of palliative oxygen versus room air in relief of breathlessness in patients with refractory dyspnoea: a double-blind, randomised controlled trial (NCT 00327873). *Lancet* 2010;376:784-93.
14 Campbell ML, Yarandi H, Dove-Medows E. Oxygen is nonbeneficial for most patients who are near death. *J Pain Symptom Manage* 2013;45:517-23.
15 Simon ST, Higginson IJ, Booth S, et al. Benzodiazepines for the relief of breathlessness in advanced malignant and non-malignant diseases in adults. *Cochrane Database Syst Rev* 2010;1:CD007354.
16 Pratter MR, Curley FJ, Dubois J, et al. Cause and evaluation of chronic dyspnea in a pulmonary disease clinic. *Arch Intern Med* 1989;149:2277-82.
17 Lecasse Y, Goldstein R, Lasserson TJ, Martin S. Pulmonary rehabilitation for chronic obstructive pulmonary disease. *Cochrane Database Syst Rev* 2006;CD003793.
18 Carone M, Patessio A, Ambrosino N, et al. Efficacy of pulmonary rehabilitation in chronic respiratory failure (CRF) due to chronic obstructive pulmonary disease (COPD): Tthe Maugeri Study. *Respir Med* 2007;101:2447-53.
19 Higginson IJ, Bausewein C, Reilly CC, et al. An integrated palliative and respiratory care service for patients with advanced disease and refractory breathlessness: a randomised controlled trial. *Lancet Resp Med* 2014, published online 29 Oct.
20 Nava S, Ferrer M, Esquinas A, et al. Palliative use of non-invasive ventilation in end-of-life patients with solid tumours: a randomised feasibility trial. *Lancet Oncol* 2013;14:219-27.
21 Struik FM, Lacasse Y, Goldstein R, et al. Nocturnal non-invasive positive pressure ventilation for stable chronic obstructive pulmonary disease. *Cochrane Database Syst Rev* 2013;6:CD002878.
22 Bausewein C, Booth S, Gysels M, et al. Effectiveness of a hand-held fan for breathlessness: a randomised phase II trial. *BMC Palliat Care* 2010;9:22.
23 Mahler DA, Gifford AH, Waterman LA, et al. Effect of increased blood levels of beta-endorphin on perception of breathlessness. *Chest* 2013;143:1378-85.
24 Johnson MJ, Bland JM, Oxberry SG, et al. Opioids for chronic refractory breathlessness: patient predictors of beneficial response. *Eur Respir J* 2013;42:758-66.
25 Oxberry SG, Torgerson DJ, Bland JM, et al. Short-term opioids for breathlessness in stable chronic heart failure: a randomized controlled trial. *Eur J Heart Fail* 2011;13:1006-12.
26 Johnson MJ, McDonagh TA, Harkness A, et al. Morphine for the relief of breathlessness in patients with chronic heart failure—a pilot study. *Eur J Heart Fail* 2002;4:753-6.
27 Currow DC, McDonald C, Oaten S, et al. Once-daily opioids for chronic dyspnea: a dose increment and pharmacovigilance study. *J Pain Symptom Manage* 2011;42:388-99.
28 Ekstrom MP, Bornefalk-Hermansson A, Abernethy AP, et al. Safety of benzodiazepines and opioids in very severe respiratory disease: national prospective study. *BMJ* 2014;348:g445.
29 Uronis H, McCrory DC, Samsa G, et al. Symptomatic oxygen for non-hypoxaemic chronic obstructive pulmonary disease. *Cochrane Database Syst Rev* 2011;6:CD006429.
30 SY, O'Driscoll BR. Is nebulized saline a placebo in COPD? *BMC Pulm Med* 2004;4:9.

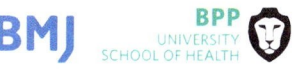

An introduction to advance care planning in practice

Anjali Mullick, consultant in palliative medicine[1][2], Jonathan Martin, consultant in palliative medicine and visiting fellow[1][3], Libby Sallnow, specialty registrar in palliative medicine and research fellow[1]

[1]St Joseph's Hospice, London E8 4SA, UK

[2]Newham University Hospital, London, UK

[3]Harris Manchester College, University of Oxford, Oxford, UK

Correspondence to: A Mullick
a.mullick@stjh.org.uk

Cite this as: *BMJ* 2013;347:f6064

DOI: 10.1136/bmj.f6064

http://www.bmj.com/content/347/bmj.f6064

Advance care planning has been defined as a process of formal decision making that aims to help patients establish decisions about future care that take effect when they lose capacity.[1] It recently gained increased importance in the United Kingdom, after being recommended by the end of life care strategy.[2] The first national guidance for health and social care staff in the UK was produced in 2007 and revised in 2011.[3] Before this, terms and concepts used in the UK had included "living wills" and "advance directives," which have been replaced by terminology outlined in the national guidance and the Mental Capacity Act 2005.[4]

Advance care planning differs from general care planning in that it is usually used in the context of progressive illness and anticipated deterioration. This has implications for its acceptability to patients. It is a voluntary process and may result in a written record of a patient's wishes, which can be referred to by carers and health professionals in the future. If a patient loses capacity, health and social care professionals should make use of information gleaned from the advance care planning process to guide them in decision making when needed.

The Royal College of Physicians and other national organisations stress the need to avoid a document driven or "tick box" approach to this process,[5] and many authors advise focusing on communication rather than on specific interventions or outcomes.[6][7][8] The success of advance care planning should therefore not be defined on the basis of completed paperwork alone.[9]

This review aims to provide an overview of the potential benefits and risks of advance care planning, to summarise barriers to taking part in it, and to give practical guidance to health professionals on how to approach the process, with reference to the Mental Capacity Act 2005. Although this article is based on UK law and practice, we believe that the concepts and approaches discussed could be applied more widely. For example, both the Australian and American Medical Associations endorse similar concepts to those used in the UK.[10][11]

SUMMARY POINTS

- Advance care planning aims to help patients establish decisions about future care that take effect when they lose capacity

- Evidence for the benefit of advance care planning is mixed; more recent evidence suggests that it can facilitate the delivery of care more in keeping with patient wishes and increase patient and family satisfaction with care

- Advance care planning discussions should be centred around the beliefs, goals, and values of patients, rather than on specific outcomes or interventions

- A sound working knowledge of the Mental Capacity Act 2005 is important when facilitating advance care plan discussions

What are the benefits of advance care planning?

Theoretically, the process can facilitate patient autonomy so that patients' future wishes can be carried out once they can no longer decide for themselves,[1] but evidence regarding real benefit is mixed. A controlled trial of the impact of combining improved communication about resuscitation preferences with information on prognosis found no improvement in the quality of end of life care.[12] Other authors have suggested that the wider advance care planning process may also be ineffective in achieving positive outcomes.[13][14][15][16]

Conversely, some evidence, including that from a recent small systematic review in patients with dementia and cognitive impairment,[17] points to several possible benefits. These include less aggressive medical care and better quality of life near death, decreased rates of hospital admission, especially of care home residents, and increased rates of hospice admission,[18][19][20] with those having completed an advance care plan being more likely to receive care that is aligned with their wishes.[21][22] A UK retrospective study of 969 deceased hospice patients found that those who had completed such a plan (57%) spent less time in hospital in their last year of life. It also found that those who died outside of hospital had a lower mean hospital treatment cost than those who died in hospital.[23]

Advance care planning is also thought to help families prepare for the death of a loved one, to resolve family conflict, and to help with bereavement.[24][25] For example, a randomised controlled trial of facilitated advance care planning versus usual care in elderly patients in Australia showed that 86% of patients in the intervention arm had their end of life wishes known and respected compared with 30% in the control arm. The same study highlighted a greater level of satisfaction among patients and relatives in the intervention group. Family members of patients in the intervention group who died had lower levels of psychological morbidity.[25]

A systematic review published in 2008 examined evidence for improving palliative care at the end of life. It included 41 articles relating to advance care planning and found moderate evidence supporting multicomponent interventions to increase patient uptake of advance directives; however, these studies seldom measured clinically important outcomes. The paper also concluded that recent research supports an approach to care planning that engages values, involves skilled facilitators, and focuses on key decision makers (for example, patients, care givers, and providers).[26]

Patients can find the process itself helpful, particularly when discussion focuses on their goals, values, and beliefs, rather than on particular treatments or interventions.[25][27][28]

Patients report several reasons for wishing to make advance decisions, including not wanting to be a burden on others and concern for self,[27][29] with underlying specific issues relating to their personal experiences and fears.[29][30]

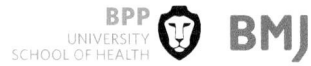

What are the risks and barriers to advance care planning?

Some patients will not wish to engage in discussions about future care because this involves thinking about a deterioration in their condition.[6] [30] [31] [32] There may also be cultural sensitivities to such conversations. Self identified barriers to the process in one qualitative study of older medical patients included perceiving advance care planning as irrelevant, having insufficient information to engage in the discussions, and the time constraints of health professionals.[33] A further challenge is that the process asks patients to predict their future experience of illness, which some may find difficult.[34] [35] However, a person's willingness to engage in the conversation may change over time, so it may be appropriate to re-offer discussions at a later stage.

Equally, barriers may exist for professionals[31] [36] [37]; in particular, doctors may be unwilling to initiate such discussions, because this may "bring death into full view."[6] Some may fear that honesty about prognosis will cause patients undue distress or destroy their hope.[6] [38] However, although caution in discussion is obviously needed, a longitudinal qualitative study found that patients have a variety of responses to, on the one hand, wanting support for hope and, on the other, wanting honest prognostic information; responses included being able to hope for things other than cure.[38] This accords with our experience—some degree of emotional upset may occur, but it is usually appropriate to the situation, and most patients who accept the offer of a discussion for advance care planning find such conversations empowering.

Some patients think that professionals should raise the matter,[39] so if we do not do this their needs may remain unmet. Being in a trusting relationship with patients,[24] or being able to develop such a relationship,[40] is helpful in this context.

How can we initiate discussions?

Advance care planning can apply to patients with a wide range of diagnoses, but particularly those with long term conditions or receiving end of life care.[5] It should be offered when the patient is still well enough to participate in the discussions and before any relevant loss of mental capacity.[5] [41] This can mean that for certain conditions, such as dementia, discussions may have to be offered early in the course of disease. One UK systematic review found that a maximum of 36% of patients with cognitive impairment and dementia being admitted to a nursing home had capacity to participate in advance care planning.[17] However, data on the best timing of advance care planning discussions in patients with dementia are conflicting. One recent qualitative study suggested that patients with mild dementia find such discussions acceptable,[42] but another found that people with dementia had difficulty considering their future selves.[35]

More generally, some studies have identified particular triggers for initiating these conversations, such as recurrence of cancer.[6] The timing of conversations with patients with non-cancer conditions, such as chronic obstructive pulmonary disease, may also prove challenging. This disease is often not perceived to be terminal and therefore not relevant to the principles of advance care planning.[36] This reflects the nature of chronic conditions in which disease can be stable and well managed for many years, before moving on to the terminal phase. However, because sudden changes in condition can occur, the opportunity to take part in advance care planning could be missed if the subject is not broached early on.

Another crucial factor is the communication skills of health professionals. A number of authors recognise the potentially challenging, sensitive, and complex nature of conversations about advance care planning,[13] [43] with others recommending that practitioners need specific training.[5] [39] [44] One component of such highly skilled communication is knowing when not to proceed with discussions—for example, when doing so might cause disproportionate levels of distress[5]—and how to "titrate" information over time.

Box 1 includes a list of suggested triggers for initiating or reviewing such discussions.

Practical approaches to communication

When preparing to offer discussions it may be useful to consider the following:

- Patients may need time to think and reflect, so the initial advance care planning process may extend over several conversations.[5] [6] One study found that the process took a median of 60 minutes over one to three conversations[25]
- Ensure that any outcomes of these discussions are appropriately shared among relevant teams and organisations,[26] [45] and updated if decisions change
- Avoid giving the impression that it is possible to anticipate and plan for every eventuality[13]
- Do not assume that other health or social care professionals have offered opportunities for such discussions[36] [37]
- Discussions that take place in the patient's wider family or social network may give rise to conflict, which is best dealt with early, to avoid conflict coming to light when the patient has lost capacity or died.[24]

Mahon suggests two questions that may be useful for initiating an advance care planning discussion that focuses on the patient's goals:

1) If you cannot, or choose not to, participate in healthcare decisions with whom should we speak?

2) If you cannot, or choose not to, participate in decision making what should we consider when making decisions about your care?[8]

For some patients answering question 1 may be as far as they wish to take such a discussion, and hopefully this question can be asked without causing patients undue anxiety. Box 2 outlines our communication suggestions.

How does advance care planning fit with the Mental Capacity Act 2005?

As well as knowing about a patient's disease and its likely consequences,[5] an adequate understanding of the law (including capacity assessment), the advance care planning process, and the related documentation is necessary.[9] [48] However, two UK studies have shown that some professionals have a limited understanding of advance care planning,[44] [49] with the authors of one suggesting that those with specialist skills in particular diseases may be better placed to undertake more complex aspects of the process.[44] This section serves as a brief introduction to some of the key legal problems.

The Mental Capacity Act 2005 legislates for England and Wales on the way in which decisions are made by, and on behalf of, people with impaired mental capacity.[4] It sets out five principles and a legal framework designed to protect patients with impaired capacity and their carers, who have to make decisions about their care and treatment. It is accompanied by the Mental Capacity Act 2005 code of practice, and practitioners have a legal duty

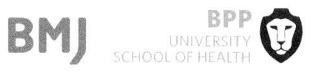

BOX 1 TRIGGERS FOR INITIATING OR REVIEWING ADVANCE CARE PLANNING DISCUSSIONS

There is no agreed standard frequency with which to review these discussions, so the interval should be based on patients' wishes, taking into account their clinical condition.

Triggers include:

- Patient initiates the conversation
- Diagnosis of a progressive life limiting illness
- The diagnosis of a condition with a predictable trajectory, which is likely to result in a loss of capacity, such as dementia or motor neurone disease
- A change or deterioration in condition
- Change in a patient's personal circumstances, such as moving into a care home or loss of a family member
- Routine clinical review of the patient, such as clinic appointments or home visits
- When the previously agreed review interval elapses

BOX 2 COMMUNICATION TIPS

Initiating the conversation

Start with general open questions, then be guided by the patient's cues and responses to know whether to explore further

Examples:

- How have you been coping with your illness recently?
- Do you like to think about or plan for the future?
- When you think of the future, what do you hope for?[46]
- When you think about the future, what worries you the most?[46]
- Have you given any thought to what kinds of treatment you would want (and not want) if you became unable to speak for yourself?[47]
- What do you consider your quality of life to be like now?[47]

During the conversation

- Use language that patients can understand and any other communication aids you might need
- Give patients enough information to make informed choices without overloading them
- Clarify any ambiguous statements that patients make—for example:
- Patient: "I don't want heroics"
- Professional: "What do you mean by heroics?"

Ending the conversation

- Summarise what has been discussed to check mutual understanding, or ask the patient to do so
- Screen for any other problems—for example: "Is there anything else you would like to discuss?"
- Arrange another time to continue, complete, or review the discussion if necessary—for example, if the patient would like help completing an advance decision to refuse treatment
- Document the contents of the discussion in the patient record
- Share the contents (with the patient's permission) with anyone else who needs to know, such as family, carers, the community team, and the general practitioner or specialists

to have regard to this.[50] Abiding by a person's wishes about a health related advance decision comes into effect only once the person has lost capacity to make that particular decision.

Mental capacity

People are assumed to have capacity unless it is established that they lack capacity despite all practicable steps taken to help them make the decision in question (see box 3 for the mental capacity assessment).

Best interests

Section 4 of the act deals with making decisions in accordance with the best interests of the person lacking capacity and specifies an initial checklist of common factors that must always be considered. It states that whoever determines what is in someone's best interests must consider, so far as is reasonably ascertainable, the person's past and present wishes and feelings, particularly any relevant written statement made when he or she had capacity,[4] thus giving "weight" to the advance care planning process.

What are the potential outcomes of an advance care planning discussion?

In addition to documents recording a person's preferred place of care or death, advance care planning has three main tools—advance statements, advance decisions to refuse treatment, and lasting powers of attorney.

Advance statements

These are statements about what the patient would or would not want to happen in the future, their goals of care, or their personal values; they are sometimes known as a statement of preferences and wishes. They can be about medical treatment ("I would wish to be ventilated if I stop breathing") or about social aspects of care ("I prefer coffee in the morning"). They are not legally binding but must be taken into account when best interest decisions are made about the person after capacity has been lost. They can be written by the patient or be verbal statements. It is useful to record verbal statements in the patient record, and it is important that they are accessible for those making decisions in the future.

Advance decision to refuse treatment

Valid and applicable advance decisions to refuse treatment (box 4) are legally binding statements (usually written documents) that allow patients to refuse specific medical treatments if they lose capacity in the future. Patients can refuse only medical and nursing treatments in advance and not basic care (such as the offer of food and drink by mouth and repositioning in bed).

It is best, but not a requirement, if the specific circumstances in which patients wish to refuse treatments are made clear, because this information will be used by clinicians in the future to determine if the refusal is applicable. The wording of these statements can be difficult, because potential future situations must be anticipated and described unambiguously. If more than one circumstance is specified for a given refusal of treatment, all have to be present at the same time for the advance decision to apply. Verbal wishes to refuse treatments that do not sustain life can be recorded in the patient's notes.

If you are satisfied that the advance decision to refuse treatment is valid and applicable then you will have to abide by it (best interests do not apply). The only circumstance in which an advance decision is not binding is when the person is detained under the Mental Health Act 1983.[51] Such patients can be treated for their mental disorder without their consent, even if they have a valid and applicable

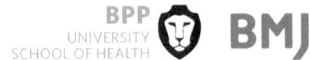

SOURCES AND SELECTION CRITERIA

We searched Medline, Embase, and the *Cochrane Database of Systematic Reviews* using the search terms "advance care planning" and "advance directives", focusing on publications in the past five years, but including older papers that seemed relevant. Where possible we prioritised systematic reviews and controlled trials. We did not carry out a systematic review of the literature and studies are of variable quality, with many being small.

BOX 3 ASSESSING MENTAL CAPACITY

Mental capacity is decision specific and time specific—it is specific to the decision in question and may be of time limited relevance.

The test for mental capacity has two parts:

- The diagnostic test. This is positive if the person has "an impairment of, or disturbance in the functioning of, the mind or brain" (Mental Capacity Act 2005 section 2). Otherwise, by definition, the person has capacity
- The functional test (Mental Capacity Act 2005 section 3) applies only if the diagnostic test is positive. People who can understand, retain, and use or weigh information relating to a decision, as well as be able to communicate their decision, have not lost capacity, even if the diagnostic test is positive. Loss of one or more of these four elements confirms loss of capacity for the specific decision

Mental capacity for a particular decision may fluctuate over time and may need to be reviewed frequently. For example, a patient may be temporarily incapacitated by an episode of sepsis, or through the use of alcohol.

BOX 4 DETERMINING WHETHER AN ADVANCE DECISION TO REFUSE TREATMENT IS VALID AND APPLICABLE

Such decisions come into effect only if the person has lost mental capacity to make the decision in question. The person must have had relevant capacity at the time the advance decision was made and it must be about the decision in question.

Validity

For such a decision to be valid, it should not have been withdrawn by the person, and the person should not have later behaved in a way that is inconsistent with it. In addition, if the person has subsequently made a lasting power of attorney regarding the same decision the advance decision is rendered invalid.

Applicability

For the refusal to be applicable it must be about the treatment currently in question and relate to the circumstances in which the patient now finds himself or herself, if these have also been specified. For example, a person specifically refusing antibiotics for treatment of a chest infection might receive antibiotics for a urinary tract infection if clinically appropriate. However, if the advance decision covers all antibiotics under the specified circumstances then health professionals would be bound not to administer them.

An advance decision may not be applicable if circumstances have changed (for example, an unanticipated advance in medical treatment) and there are reasonable grounds to believe that these changes would have affected the advance decision if the person had known about them when making the decision.

Life sustaining treatment

When the treatment to be refused is potentially life sustaining, such as cardiopulmonary resuscitation, as well as being valid and applicable, the decision must be written, signed by the patient in the presence of a signed witness, and must state that it applies even if life is at risk.

---

advance decision to refuse the treatment in question (electroconvulsive therapy is an exception to this rule).

Lasting power of attorney

These are legal documents that replace the previous enduring power of attorney. They allow patients (donors) to nominate someone (attorney) to whom they want to give decision making powers (if they lose capacity in the future). There are two types of lasting power of attorney: "property and financial affairs" and "health and welfare." Once made, these documents must be registered with the Office of the Public Guardian (for a fee) before coming into effect. It is possible to nominate more than one person as an attorney, or nominate different people for different decisions.

A health and welfare lasting power of attorney comes into effect only when the donor loses the capacity to make the decisions that are covered by the document. If there are worries that an attorney is not making decisions in the best interests of the donor, the decision should be challenged. It can then be adjudicated on by the Court of Protection (which might appoint a court appointed deputy, usually someone close to the patient, who would be able to take best interests decisions for the patient).

What are electronic palliative care coordination systems?

Appropriate dissemination of advance care planning decisions is a challenge; other than for lasting powers of attorney, the UK has no central register of advance care plans. Electronic palliative care coordination systems are designed to improve communication and facilitate health professionals' access to this information. Electronic registers, or urgent care records, such as Coordinate my Care in London (www.coordinatemycare.co.uk/index.html), hold immediately accessible information about patients' advance care plans and other information, such as treatment escalation plans, and are available to a wide range of relevant professionals. In some areas, this has led to an increase in patients dying in their preferred place of care.[52]

When should advance care planning decisions be reviewed? (see box 1)

Although no specific evidence or recommendations are available on when to review these decisions, on the basis of personal experience, several factors may be relevant and should prompt review. For example, if the personal circumstances of patients change, such as place of residence or perception of quality of life, they may wish to reconsider their decisions. New therapeutic options may become available or, as the condition progresses, the patient's values and goals may change, and this may affect earlier decisions. Advance care planning must be reconsidered regularly, either to confirm or amend the content, while the person has mental capacity to do so. This will allow the document to reflect the patient's current wishes and increase the likelihood that it will be judged as valid and applicable at the relevant time.

Contributors: All authors conceived, planned, and helped write this review. JM did the literature search and both AM and JM reviewed the literature. All authors reviewed the article before submission. AM is guarantor. Michael Ball and Claire Kerlin, both trust solicitors, Barts Health NHS Trust, reviewed the draft article in its earlier stages, but made no important changes to content.

Funding: No special funding received.

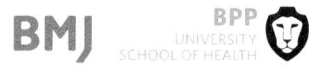

ADDITIONAL EDUCATIONAL RESOURCES

Resources for patients

- National End of Life Care Programme (www.endoflifecare. nhs.uk/search-resources/resources-search/publications/ planning-for-your-future-care.aspx)—Outlines the different options available to people when planning for their end of life care and comes in a range of languages
- Aging with Dignity (www.agingwithdignity.org/ forms/5wishes.pdf)—US based website that aims to help people take control of how they are treated if they are seriously ill
- Regents of the University of California (www. prepareforyourcare.org)—Aims to help patients make medical decisions for themselves and get the right medical care

Resources for professionals

- Thomas K, Lobo B, eds. Advance care planning in end of life care. Oxford University Press, 2011
- National End of Life Care Programme. Capacity, care planning and advance care planning in life limiting illness. A guide for health and social care staff. 2011. www.endoflifecare.nhs.uk/ assets/downloads/ACP_booklet_2011_Final_1.pdf
- Office of the Public Guardian. A guide for people working in health and social care. OPG603. 2009. www.justice.gov.uk/ downloads/protecting-the-vulnerable/mca/opg-603-0409.pdf
- Macmillan Cancer Support/NHS. Tips for advance care planning for GPs. 2012. www.endoflifecare.nhs.uk/search-resources/resources-search/publications/acp-tips-for-gps. aspx

Competing interests: We have read and understood the BMJ Group policy on declaration of interests and declare the following interests: None.

Provenance and peer review: Not commissioned; externally peer reviewed.

1 Hayhoe B, Howe A. Advance care planning under the Mental Capacity Act 2005 in primary care. *Br J Gen Pract* 2011;61:e537-41.
2 Department of Health. End of life care strategy: promoting high quality care for adults at the end of their life. 2008. https://www.gov. uk/government/publications/end-of-life-care-strategy-promoting-high-quality-care-for-adults-at-the-end-of-their-life.
3 NHS National End of Life Care Programme. Capacity, care planning and advance care planning in life limiting illness. A guide for health and social care staff. Department of Health, 2011. www.endoflifecare.nhs. uk/assets/downloads/ACP_booklet_2011_Final_1.pdf.
4 National Archives. The Mental Capacity Act 2005. www.legislation.gov. uk/ukpga/2005/9/contents.
5 Royal College of Physicians. Advance care planning. Concise Guidance to Good Practice series. No 12. 2009. www.rcplondon.ac.uk/sites/ default/files/concise-advance-care-planning-2009.pdf.
6 Barnes K, Jones L, Tookman A, King M. Acceptability of an advance care planning interview schedule: a focus group study. *Palliat Med* 2007;21:23-8.
7 Billings JA. The need for safeguards in advance care planning. *J Gen Intern Med* 2012;27:595-600.
8 Mahon MM. An advance directive in two questions. *J Pain Symptom Manage* 2011;41:801-7.
9 Fried TR, O'Leary JR. Using the experiences of bereaved caregivers to inform patient- and caregiver-centered advance care planning. *J Gen Intern Med* 2008;23:1602-7.
10 Australian Medical Association. The role of the medical practitioner in advance care planning. 2006. https://ama.com.au/position-statement/ role-medical-practitioner-advance-care-planning-2006.
11 American Medical Association. Opinion 2.191—advance care planning. 2011. www.ama-assn.org/ama/pub/physician-resources/medical-ethics/code-medical-ethics/opinion2191.page.
12 The SUPPORT Principal Investigators. A controlled trial to improve care for seriously ill hospitalized patients. The study to understand prognoses and preferences for outcomes and risks of treatments (SUPPORT). *JAMA* 1995;274:1591-8.
13 Perkins HS. Controlling death: the false promise of advance directives. *Ann Intern Med* 2007;147:51-7.
14 Tonelli MR. Pulling the plug on living wills. A critical analysis of advance directives. *Chest* 1996;110:816-22.
15 Schneiderman LJ, Kronick R, Kaplan RM, Anderson JP, Langer RD. Effects of offering advance directives on medical treatments and costs. *Ann Intern Med* 1992;117:599-606.
16 Goodman MD, Tarnoff M, Slotman GJ. Effect of advance directives on the management of elderly critically ill patients. *Crit Care Med* 1998;26:701-4.
17 Robinson L, Dickinson C, Rousseau N, Beyer F, Clark A, Hughes J, et al. A systematic review of the effectiveness of advance care planning interventions for people with cognitive impairment and dementia. *Age Ageing* 2012;41:263-9.
18 Wright AA, Zhang B, Ray A, Mack JW, Trice E, Balboni T, et al. Associations between end-of-life discussions, patient mental health, medical care near death, and caregiver bereavement adjustment. *JAMA* 2008;300:1665-73.
19 O'Malley AJ, Caudry DJ, Grabowski DC. Predictors of nursing home residents' time to hospitalisation. *Health Serv Res* 2011;46:82-104.
20 Molloy DW, Guyatt GH, Russo R, Goeree R, O'Brien BJ, Bédard M, et al. Systematic implementation of an advance directive program in nursing homes: a randomized controlled trial. *JAMA* 2000;283:1437-44.
21 Silveira MJ, Kim SY, Langa KM. Advance directives and outcomes of surrogate decision making before death. *N Engl J Med* 2010;362:1211-8.
22 Mack JW, Weeks JC, Wright AA, Block SD, Prigerson HG. End-of-life discussions, goal attainment, and distress at the end of life: predictors and outcomes of receipt of care consistent with preferences. *J Clin Oncol* 2010;28:1203-8.
23 Abel J, Pring A, Rich A, Malik T, Verne J. The impact of advance care planning of place of death, a hospice retrospective cohort study. *BMJ Support Palliat Care* 2013;3:168-73.
24 Rhee JJ, Zwar NA, Kemp LA. Advance care planning and interpersonal relationships: a two-way street. *Fam Pract* 2013;30:219-26.
25 Detering KM, Hancock AD, Reade MC, Silvester W. The impact of advance care planning on end of life care in elderly patients: randomised controlled trial. *BMJ* 2010;340:c1345.
26 Lorenz KA, Lynn J, Dy SM, Shugarman LR, Wilkinson A, Mularski RA, et al. Evidence for improving palliative care at the end of life: a systematic review. *Ann Intern Med* 2008;148:147-59.
27 Pautex S, Hermann FR, Zulian GB. Role of advance directives in palliative care units: a prospective study. *Palliat Med* 2008;22:835-41.
28 Kaldjian LC, Curtis AE, Shinkunas LA, Cannon KT. Goals of care toward the end of life: a structured literature review. *Am J Hosp Palliat Care* 2008-2009;25:501-11.
29 Levi BH, Dellasega C, Whitehead M, Green MJ. What influences individuals to engage in advance care planning? *Am J Hosp Palliat Care* 2010;27:306-12.
30 Piers RD, van Eechoud IJ, Van Camp S, Grypdonck M, Deveugele M, Verbeke N, et al. Advance care planning in terminally ill and frail older persons. *Patient Educ Couns* 2013;90:323-9.
31 Rhee JJ, Zwar NA, Kemp LA. Uptake and implementation of advance care planning in Australia: findings of key informant interviews. *Aust Health Rev* 2012;36:98-104.
32 Knauft E, Nielsen EL, Engelberg RA, Patrick DL, Curtis JR. Barriers and facilitators to end-of-life care communication for patients with COPD. *Chest* 2005;127:2188-96.
33 Schickedanz AD, Schillinger D, Landefeld CS, Knight SJ, Williams BA, Sudore RL. A clinical framework for improving the advance care planning process: start with patients' self-identified barriers. *J Am Geriatr Soc* 2009;57:31-9.
34 Halpern S. Shaping end-of-life care: behavioral economics and advance directives. *Semin Respir Crit Care Med* 2012;33:393-400.
35 Dening KH, Jones L. Sampson EL. Preferences for end-of-life care: a nominal group study of people with dementia and their family carers. *Palliat Med* 2013;27:409-17.
36 Gott M, Gardiner C, Small N, Payne S, Seamark D, Barnes S, et al. Barriers to advance care planning in chronic obstructive pulmonary disease. *Palliat Med* 2009;23:642-8.
37 Spence A, Hasson F, Waldron M, Kernohan WG, McLaughlin D, Watson B, et al. Professionals delivering palliative care to people with COPD: qualitative study. *Palliat Med* 2009;23:126-31.
38 Curtis JR, Engelberg R, Young JP, Vig LK, Reinke LF, Wenrich MD, et al. An approach to understanding the interaction of hope and desire for explicit prognostic information among individuals with severe chronic obstructive pulmonary disease or advanced cancer. *J Palliat Med* 2008;11:610-20.
39 Barnes KA, Barlow CA, Harrington J, Ornadel K, Tookman A, King M, et al. Advance care planning discussions in advanced cancer: analysis of dialogues between patients and care planning mediators. *Palliat Support Care* 2011;9:73-9.
40 Prendergast TJ. Advance care planning: pitfalls, progress, promise. *Crit Care Med* 2001;29:N34-9.
41 National Institute for Health and Care Excellence. Dementia: supporting people with dementia and their carers in health and social care. CG42. 2006. http://guidance.nice.org.uk/CG42.
42 Poppe M, Burleigh S, Banerjee S. Qualitative evaluation of advanced care planning in early dementia (ACP-ED). *PLoS One* 2013;8:e60412.
43 Callaghan D. Once again, reality: now where do we go? *Hastings Cent Rep* 995;25:S33-6.
44 Robinson L, Dickinson C, Bamford C, Clark A, Hughes J, Exley C. A qualitative study: professionals' experiences of advance care planning in dementia and palliative care, "a good idea in theory but . . ." *Palliat Med* 2013;27:401-8.
45 Randall F. Advance care planning: ethical and clinical implications for hospital medicine. *Br J Hosp Med* 2011;72:437-40.
46 Pantilat S, Steimle A. Palliative care for patients with heart failure. *JAMA* 2004;291:2476-83.

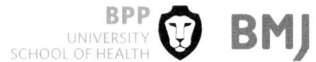

47   Quill T. Initiating end-of-life discussions with seriously ill patients—addressing the elephant in the room. *JAMA* 2000;284:2503-7.

48   Boddy J, Chenoweth L, McLennan V, Daly M. It's just too hard! Australian health care practitioner perspectives on barriers to advance care planning. *Aust J Prim Health* 2013;19:38-45.

49   Boyd K, Mason B, Kendall M, Barclay S, Chinn D, Thomas K, et al. Advance care planning for cancer patients in primary care: a feasibility study. *Br J Gen Pract* 2010;60:e449-58.

50   Department for Constitutional Affairs. Mental Capacity Act 2005. Code of practice. 2007. www.justice.gov.uk/downloads/protecting-the-vulnerable/mca/mca-code-practice-0509.pdf.

51   National Archives. The Mental Health Act 1983. www.legislation.gov.uk/ukpga/1983/20/contents.

52   Smith CF, Riley J. Coordinate My Care: a clinical service for end-of-life care underpinned by an IT solution [electronic response to: There IT goes again. Cross M]. www.bmj.com/rapid-response/2011/11/03/coordinate-my-care-clinical-service-end-life-care-underpinned-it-solution.

Related links

bmj.com/archive
Previous articles in this series
- Post-mastectomy breast reconstruction (BMJ 2013;347:f5903)
- Identifying brain tumours in children and young adults (BMJ 2013;347:f5844)
- Gout (BMJ 2013;347:f5648)
- Testicular germ cell tumours (BMJ 2013;347:f5526)
- Managing cows' milk allergy in children (BMJ 2013;347:f5424)

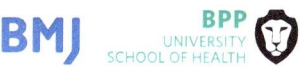

Cognitive assessment of older people

John Young, head[1], David Meagher, professor of psychiatry[2], consultant psychiatrist[3], Alasdair MacLullich, professor of geriatric medicine[4]

[1]Academic Unit of Elderly Care and Rehabilitation, Leeds Institute for Health Sciences, University of Leeds, Leeds LS2 9LJ, UK

[2]University of Limerick Medical School, Castletroy, Limerick, Ireland

[3]Midwestern Regional Hospital, Dooradoyle, Limerick, Ireland

[4]Edinburgh Delirium Research Group, Geriatric Medicine, University of Edinburgh, Royal Infirmary of Edinburgh, Edinburgh EH16 4TJ, UK

Correspondence to: Professor J Young, Academic Unit of Elderly Care and Rehabilitation, Bradford Institute for Health Research, Bradford Teaching Hospitals NHS Foundation Trust, Bradford BD9 6RJ john.young@bradfordhospitals.nhs.uk

Cite this as: BMJ 2011;343:d5042

DOI: 10.1136/bmj.d5042

http://www.bmj.com/content/343/bmj.d5042

This is the second in a series of four articles about assessing older people

Cognitive assessment involves examination of higher cortical functions, particularly memory, attention, orientation, language, executive function (planning activities), and praxis (sequencing of activities). This article will focus on cognitive assessment of older people (those aged over about 65 years) in the context of possible dementia, delirium, and depression. These are common and serious clinical syndromes affecting older people, and accurate cognitive assessment is an essential component for diagnosis. Dementia affects 20% of people aged over 80 years,[1] and delirium may affect 30-50% of older people in hospitals and an estimated 16% in long term care facilities.[2] The annual incidence of major depression in the general older population is about 15% a year and doubles after age 70.[3]

Why does cognitive assessment matter?

Cognitive assessment helps to clarify the presence of one or more of the clinical syndromes of dementia, delirium, and depression. The case scenario box (part 1) describes a patient presenting with a gradual deterioration of cognitive function and a recent, abrupt deterioration. The abrupt change in mental state with reported sleepiness is highly suggestive of delirium, with a urinary tract infection (new onset incontinence) as a possible trigger. Dementia or depressive illness (loss of interest, poor concentration, forgetfulness), or both, are also possible so need consideration, but the immediate priority is to assess for delirium.

Patients with dementia have a very high risk of developing delirium (often triggered by an infection, surgery, or drugs), and delirium is often associated with progression of dementia.[4] Conversely, patients without baseline dementia who present with delirium may develop persisting cognitive deficits and effectively a new onset of dementia.[5] Depression in older people often presents with complaints of memory impairment, and people with dementia may have an associated depression.[3]

Cognitive assessment helps to clarify the presence of these syndromes. Currently many older people presenting with dementia, delirium, and depression do not receive a diagnosis, or they receive a misdiagnosis. In a 2010

observational study, only 25% of patients with delirium presenting to a medical assessment unit received a correct diagnosis.[6] Failure to detect delirium may mean missing a treatable condition (such as a chest or urinary infection, or a drug side effect), which may be life threatening as every 48 hours spent with delirium is associated with an 11% increase in mortality.[7] Hence, patients presenting with rapid (hours, days) onset of cognitive symptoms or a worsening of established symptoms should be assessed urgently for delirium. The timely recognition of dementia when symptoms are causing anxiety to the patient or carer brings the possibility of better support, anticipatory care, initiation of drug treatment, and reduced distress for the patient and their carers.[1] Failure to detect depression denies the opportunity for identifying a potentially treatable and debilitating illness. Depression in older people is just as treatable as in younger people.[3]

What is the best way to assess cognition?

The key to the reliable identification of cognitive impairment is to integrate three components: observation of the patient; a collateral account from a carer; and the results of standardised tests. These components should consider key questions for immediate and ongoing management (box 1).

Observation of the patient

The clues to the presence of cognitive impairment may be subtle and are often overlooked, particularly in dementia, where the onset may be insidious, with the family adapting to the impairments, r egarding them as "normal" behaviour. The discussion with the patient can be sensitively directed to inquiries about intrusions into everyday life, such as forgetting appointments, problems with finances, mislaying objects, and kitchen mishaps. There may be indicators of personal neglect—sometimes obvious (such as a dishevelled appearance), sometimes less so (a mis-buttoned jacket in a previously fastidious man, or a usually immaculate lady who has left off her lipstick). The primary care practitioner, who may have known the person for some years, is particularly well placed to notice these. Close attention to the content, organisation, and presentation of the patient's narrative is critical. Points to look out for:

- Dementia—Features include impaired fluency of language, vagueness with dates and sequence of events, a tendency to repeat phrases, or a predilection to dwell excessively on distant events
- Delirium—Features include poor attention (such as seemingly not following questions; distractibility; or inability to focus), incoherent speech (hard to fully understand what the patient is trying to say), and altered level of alertness (sleepiness or agitation). The key is substantial change or fluctuation in mental status over hours or days: this is the cardinal feature of delirium
- Depression—Features include low mood, loss of interest and diminished capacity for enjoyment, poor self care, and a negative outlook with feelings of hopelessness that can include suicidal thoughts. However, it is important to be aware that these features are less prominent in older

SUMMARY POINTS

- Dementia, depression, and delirium are common and serious clinical syndromes in older people that are underdiagnosed in routine care
- Formal detection of these syndromes may enable identification of treatable conditions, is associated with better outcomes for patients, and requires routine cognitive assessment
- Cognitive assessment requires integration of information acquired from observing the patient and talking with carers, and from the results of an assessment instrument
- Cognitive assessment instruments are brief, easy to use, and sensitive to cognitive impairment, but an overall clinical assessment is needed to establish the underlying cause
- The character and time frame of cognitive problems are key considerations in establishing an accurate diagnosis and a coherent management plan

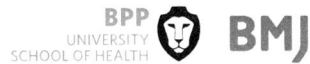

CASE SCENARIO: PART 1

A woman aged 89 years attends your clinic accompanied by her daughter. The daughter explains that her mother has not been herself over the past few months, that she is less interested in her usual activities, has poor concentration during conversation, and forgets day to day events. Two days ago she became incontinent of urine, which was unusual for her, and was noted to be confused and sleepy.

---

patients, in whom somatic symptoms (reduced energy, poor appetite, insomnia) are more typical.

Drugs are a common cause of delirium in older people, and a medication review is therefore essential. A systematic review of 14 randomised controlled trials and observational studies showed that opioids, benzodiazepines, and dihydropyridines (such as amlodipine)—and possibly antihistamines (H1 antagonists)—confer an increased risk of delirium. Digoxin and antipsychotics confer no increased risk, and uncertainty remains for other drug classes.[8]

Examination

Examination should specifically assess for nutritional status (evidence of self neglect) and for uncorrected visual and hearing problems (easy to resolve and risk factors for delirium and depression). Examination should also assess for new physical illness (such as anaemia and cardiac or respiratory failure) or deterioration in a pre-existing chronic disease, as these are possible aggravating factors for dementia or depression or precipitants for delirium. For suspected delirium, focus the examination on detecting chest, urinary, and skin infections; heart failure and new or fast atrial fibrillation; urinary retention; and rectal examination if impaction is suspected. In suspected dementia perform a neurological examination to assess for abnormalities in the pyramidal pathway (brisk reflexes and extensor plantar responses may indicate vascular dementia) and the extrapyramidal system (expressionless face, bradykinesia, and cogwheel rigidity may indicate dementia with Lewy bodies).

Investigations

The investigations for suspected dementia, depression, and delirium are similar (box 2) but have different rationale. For dementia the aim is to detect potentially reversible causes for the cognitive impairment; for depression to identify physical problems that might be contributing to the low mood; and for delirium, to identify possible precipitants. Brain imaging is recommended for suspected dementia to identify the very few people with intracerebral tumours or normal pressure hydrocephalus, and to contribute to the diagnosis of the specific dementia type.[1]

Collateral account from carer

A collateral account from a carer is essential for clarifying what the symptoms are, their timescale (weeks or months for dementia and depression, and hours or days for delirium), and their relation to baseline mental function. Again, a primary care practitioner who is familiar with the person is often better placed than a practitioner in secondary care, who must purposefully seek collateral information. Failure to undertake this straightforward task may result in misdiagnosis. Informant based questionnaires such as the AD8 (ascertain dementia 8) (box 3)[9] or the short form of the informant questionnaire on cognitive decline in the elderly[10] may be used to structure the conversation. They are both simple and quick to complete (three and five minutes respectively), either face to face or over the telephone.

BOX 1 KEY ASPECTS OF COGNITIVE ASSESSMENT TO GUIDE ONGOING MANAGEMENT

- Does this patient have substantial cognitive impairment now, and what was his or her baseline function?
- What is the time frame over which this has developed?
- What is the character of this impairment? (For example, short term memory difficulties might point to dementia, and prominent inattention to delirium)
- Are there associated disturbances of behaviour? (For example, a day-night sleep reversal pattern is common in delirium; restlessness and wandering in dementia; and lethargy indicates possible depression)
- Do the problems follow a pattern indicative of delirium, depression, or dementia?
- Could the patient have a serious underlying physical cause for this presentation (typically "yes" for suspected delirium), and is immediate intervention or urgent investigation needed? (Immediate intervention is warranted, for example, if the patient's safety is at risk (such as high risk of falls or dehydration), and urgent investigation is warranted if delirium is suspected or cognitive decline is marked or sudden)
- Is specialist input needed to clarify diagnosis, conduct more detailed assessment, or advise on management?

BOX 2 INVESTIGATIONS FOR SUSPECTED DEMENTIA, DEPRESSION, AND DELIRIUM*

- Full blood count
- Electrolytes
- Renal function tests
- Liver function tests
- Thyroid function tests
- Calcium
- Glucose
- C reactive protein
- Serum folate
- Serum vitamin B12

Additional investigations for suspected dementia

- Brain imaging (computed tomography or magnetic resonance imaging)

Additional investigations for suspected delirium

- Chest radiography
- Urine microscopy and culture
- Blood cultures (if bacteraemia is suspected)

*Adapted from NICE guidance[2]

The questionnaires focus on long term changes in aspects of cognitive function and behaviour rather than current function and are thus less influenced by a person's cultural and educational background and can reliably contribute to the diagnosis of early, mild, or more severe dementia. Reports of recent changes in usual behaviour (box 4) as an indication of delirium should also be specifically sought in any older person who is unwell. Indeed, the question, "Do you think [patient's name] has been more confused lately?" had 80% sensitivity for delirium.[11]

Standardised assessments

Although the routine use of standardised assessment instruments is recommended, they are not diagnostic instruments—the diagnosis of dementia, delirium, and depression is eventually a clinical one that synthesises all available evidence. Indeed, the testing process can sometimes be more diagnostically informative than the actual test score achieved because it provides insights

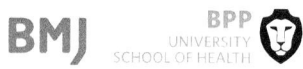

BOX 3 INFORMANT BASED AD8 (ASCERTAIN DEMENTIA 8) QUESTIONNAIRE

An informant who knows the patient well is asked to respond yes or no to the eight questions of the AD8 questionnaire (below). The instructions are given to the informant either in person or over the phone: "Remember, 'yes, a change' indicates that you think there has been a change in the last several years caused by cognitive (thinking and memory) problems." Two positive responses indicate possible dementia (sensitivity 92%, specificity 46%).[10]

1 Has problems with judgment (such as falling for scams, bad financial decisions, buying gifts inappropriate for recipients)?

2 Shows reduced interest in hobbies and activities?

3 Repeats questions, stories, or statements?

4 Has trouble learning how to use a tool, appliance, or gadget (such as computer, microwave, remote control)?

5 Forgets correct month or year?

6 Has difficulty handling complicated financial affairs (such as balancing a bank account, dealing with income tax, paying bills)?

7 Has difficulty remembering appointments?

8 Has consistent problems with thinking and/or memory?

BOX 4 COMMON PRESENTING SYMPTOMS OF DELIRIUM*

- *Cognitive function*—for example, worsened concentration, slow responses, confusion
- *Perception*—for example, visual or auditory hallucinations
- *Physical function*—for example, reduced mobility, reduced movement, restlessness, agitation, changes in appetite, sleep disturbance
- *Social behaviour*—for example, lack of cooperation with reasonable requests, withdrawal, or alterations in communication, mood, and/or attitude

*From NICE guidance[2]

BOX 5 ABBREVIATED MENTAL TEST SCORE

Score 1 for each correct answer. A score of ≤7 out of a possible 10 suggests cognitive impairment.

- 1 How old are you?
- 2 What is the time (to the nearest hour)?
- 3 Give the patient an address (such as "42 West Street") for recall at the end of the test
- 4 What year is it?
- 5 What is the name of this place?
- 6 Can the patient recognise two relevant people (such as a nurse and a doctor)
- 7 What was the date of your birth?
- 8 When was the second world war?
- 9 Who is the present prime minister?
- 10 Count down from 20 to 1. (Allow no errors, and give no cues)

---

ceiling, so people with mild cognitive impairment may score in the "normal" range of 25-30 points, particularly if they have high educational attainment. Scores of 21-24, 10-20, and 9 or less indicate mild, moderate, and severe cognitive impairment respectively. However, copyright protection is now enforced, and the mini-mental state examination must be purchased from the publishers (www.parinc.com/).

Abbreviated mental test score

This 10 item assessment (box 5) is commonly used in hospitals, although it has lower sensitivity and specificity to detect cognitive impairment than the mini-mental state examination. A four item version of the 10 item test (known as the four item abbreviated mental test score) is used in emergency departments or acute assessment units, and its performance seems broadly equivalent to the full version;[13] completion of this shorter abbreviated version takes less than one minute, and failure on any of the four items (age, date of birth, place, and year) implies cognitive impairment.

The general practitioner assessment of cognition (GPCOG)

This simple, two step assessment was developed for use in primary care and is particularly suited to multicultural populations. It is available as a web based tool (www.gpcog.com.au/index.php) and takes less than four minutes to administer. Step 1 comprises an assessment of orientation and memory, and requires the completion of the clock drawing test (figure). A score of ≤4 (out of 9) indicates cognitive impairment. A score of 5-8 is indeterminate and triggers an informant based assessment (step 2) with six questions. A negative response to three of these items suggests cognitive impairment (sensitivity 85%, specificity 86%).[14]

Brief assessment for depression

A quick, validated example is the patient health questionnaire 2 (PHQ2), a two item screening test that focuses on two key symptoms of depression: depressed mood and lack of interest or pleasure in activities (anhedonia).[15] The stem question is, "Over the last two weeks, how often have you been bothered by any of the following problems: (1) Little interest or pleasure in doing things; (2) Feeling down, depressed, or hopeless?" For each option the respondent chooses from "not at all" (score 0), "several days" (1), "more than half the days" (2), and "nearly every day" (3). A score of ≥3 suggests depression. A large study of over 8000 community dwelling older people showed a sensitivity of 100% and specificity of 77%.[15]

into cognitive processes such as attentiveness and disorganised thinking. "Untestability" is itself an important sign of severe disturbance of the mental status and often indicates delirium. No consensus has been reached on which standardised assessments to use, but by becoming thoroughly familiar with and competent in the use of a few core instruments and basing this selection on local use, practitioners can maximise communication between teams. The reliability of responses on brief standardised assessments of depression can be reduced in people with moderate to severe cognitive impairment. However, coexisting depression is common, and if any uncertainty remains, consider referral for specialist assessment.

Brief cognitive tests

Many brief, standardised tests of cognitive function have been developed, mostly assessing memory and orientation.[12] The test scores may help to gauge dementia severity and progression, and repeated scores (such as preoperatively and postoperatively) can also help with the diagnosis of delirium, especially if superimposed on dementia. Falsely low scores may arise in people with a low educational background, deafness (through mishearing questions), or depression (no interest in questions). The tests need to be conducted with sensitivity to prevent undue distress. Some commonly used tests are described below.

Mini-mental state examination

The mini-mental state examination is a widely used, well validated, 30 point cognitive test that comprises 11 items and takes about eight minutes to complete. It has a low

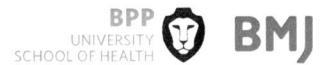

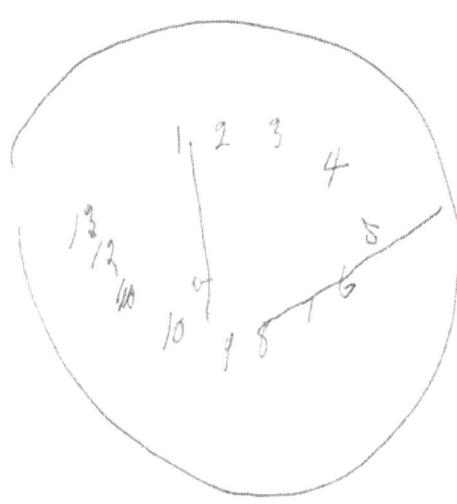

An example of the clock drawing test. The patient is asked to draw a circle, add the clock numbers, and set the hands (one small, one long) to "10 past 11," with a potential total score of 3 (1 for each element). This patient has drawn an incomplete circle (score 0); used uneven spacing of clock numbers (0); but has drawn reasonably correct clock hands (1). Total score is 1 out of 3, interpreted as evidence of cognitive impairment. Although the clock test is part of the general practitioner assessment of cognition (GPCOG) test, it can be used separately to test for visuospatial, constructional praxis and for executive (planning) impairments, which are common in dementia

Brief assessment for delirium

The confusion assessment method (box 6) is a tool for screening for delirium.[16] Training in its use is recommended to ensure adequate sensitivity and reliability.[17] A cognitive test such as the mini-mental state examination must be done before completion of the confusion assessment method, and the total time for completion (of the two combined) is typically 10-12 minutes.

What are the challenges?

The unenlightened but entrenched view that memory loss is a normal consequence of old age limits clinical thinking, as does the intellectually lazy use of the term "confusion" as a diagnosis. Becoming more open to the possibility of the three inter-related syndromes of dementia, depression, and delirium in day to day practice is a critical first step, and healthcare professionals could overcome the idea that cognitive assessment is too complicated or time consuming by becoming familiar with selected core instruments. Better training in how to diagnose dementia, depression, and delirium is also needed.[18 19] Embedding brief cognitive assessment tests and prompts to seek information from carers within patient documentation systems could also improve accuracy and speed of diagnosis. The reliable diagnosis of dementia and depression in older people may emerge only over time (box, Case scenario: part 2), and regular reviews over several weeks are usually needed.

Contributors: JY planned and wrote the first draft. All authors helped to develop and revise the paper. JY is the guarantor.

Competing interests: All authors have completed the ICMJE uniform disclosure form at www.icmje.org/coi_disclosure.pdf (available on request from the corresponding author) and declare: no support from any organisation for the submitted work; no financial relationships with any organisations that might have an interest in the submitted work in the previous three years, no other relationships or activities that could appear to have influenced the submitted work.

CASE SCENARIO: PART 2

Your patient has a score on the mini-mental state examination of 15 out of 30, indicating moderate cognitive impairment. During testing, you observe that her attention is poor. Questions to her daughter confirm a recent change in mental status. You review your patient's drugs and do not find any that might be responsible. You diagnose delirium, probably triggered by a urinary tract infection on a background of dementia and/or depression. You request blood and urine tests (box 2) and initiate antibiotics.

A week later, your patient is now alert and attentive, but her daughter is still worried that she remains "quiet," withdrawn, and lacking in spontaneity. She continues to struggle to recall recent events. Her score on the mini-mental state examination has improved to 21. Both questions of the patient health questionnaire 2 are answered positively, supporting the clinical suspicion of depression. Antidepressant treatment is started, and regular review over the coming weeks confirms improvement in her depressive symptoms, with a brighter mood, greater spontaneity, and more interest in usual activities and self care. However, she remains forgetful and struggles to perform day to day tasks. Her score on the mini-mental state examination (23) has still not reached a "normal" level (25-30). You therefore refer her to the local memory clinic, where Alzheimer's dementia is diagnosed and she is started on a cholinesterase inhibitor.

BOX 6 CONFUSION ASSESSMENT METHOD TO DIAGNOSE DELIRIUM*

The diagnosis of delirium requires a present or abnormal rating for criteria 1 and 2, plus a present or abnormal rating for either criterion 3 or criterion 4.

1 Acute onset and fluctuating course
- Is there evidence of an acute change in mental status from the patient's baseline? Has this behaviour fluctuated during the past day—that is, tended to come and go, or increase and decrease in severity?

2 Inattention
- Does the patient have difficulty in focusing attention (for example, is he or she easily distracted) or in keeping track of what is being said?

3 Disorganised thinking
- Is the patient's speech disorganised or incoherent, such as rambling or irrelevant conversation, unclear or illogical flow of ideas, or unpredictable switching from subject to subject?

4 Altered level of consciousness
- Overall, how would you rate this patient's level of consciousness? Alert (normal), vigilant (hyperalert), lethargic (drowsy, easily aroused), stupor (difficult to arouse), coma (unarousable). Any rating other than "alert" is scored as abnormal

Rating the four items

The four items of this assessment method provide prompts for the cardinal features of delirium. To establish an acute onset and/or fluctuating course usually requires information from a family member or carers. Inattention can be detected by the digit span test or reciting days of the week backwards. Disorganised thinking and sleepiness (altered level of consciousness) can be detected during conversation with the patient—this implies spending some time with the patient. The features of delirium typically fluctuate with deceptively lucid moments; this further emphasises the importance of information from family members and carers.

*Adapted from: Inouye et al[16] and Inouye[17]

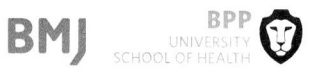

SOURCES AND SELECTION CRITERIA

We have used personal archives of references and our own experience. We also examined the guidelines on dementia, delirium, and depression published by the National Institute for Health and Clinical Excellence (NICE) and a systematic review of cognitive assessment instruments.

HOW CAN I CHANGE MY PRACTICE?

General resources

- Depression: http://guidance.nice.org.uk/CG90/SlideSet/ppt/ English)

- Dementia: http://guidance.nice.org.uk/CG42/SlideSet/ppt/ English

- Delirium: http://guidance.nice.org.uk/CG103/SlideSet/ppt/ English

- Management of patients with dementia. SIGN guideline 86. www.sign.ac.uk/pdf/sign86.pdf. (Highly practical dementia guideline)

- Woodford HJ, George J. Cognitive assessment in the elderly: a review of clinical methods. *Q J Med* 2007;100:469-84. http://qjmed.oxfordjournals.org/content/100/8/469.full. (Thorough review of the role of cognitive assessment and the instruments that can be used)

BMJ Group resources

BMJ Learning modules

- Dementia: diagnosis and assessment. http://learning.bmj. com/learning/search-result.html?moduleId=5004452

- Alzheimer's disease: diagnosis and management http://learning.bmj.com/learning/search-result. html?moduleId=5004421

Best Practice

- Assessment of memory deficit: http://bestpractice.bmj.com/ best-practice/monograph/710.html

- Assessment of dementia: http://bestpractice.bmj.com/best-practice/monograph/242.html

Provenance and peer review: Commissioned; externally peer reviewed.

Patient consent not required (patient anonymised, dead, or hypothetical).

1   National Institute for Health and Clinical Excellence. Dementia: supporting people with dementia and their carers in health and social care. (Clinical guideline 42.) 2006. http://guidance.nice.org.uk/CG42.

2   National Institute for Health and Clinical Excellence. Delirium: diagnosis, prevention and management. (Clinical guideline 103.) 2010. http://guidance.nice.org.uk/CG103.

3   Alexopoulos GS. Depression in the elderly. *Lancet* 2005;365:1961-70.

4   Fong TG, Jones RN, Shi P, Marcantonio ER, Yap L, Rudolph JL, et al. Delirium accelerates cognitive decline in Alzheimer disease. *Neurology* 2009;72:1570-5.

5   MacLullich AMJ, Beaglehole A, Hall RJ, Meagher DJ. Delirium and long-term cognitive impairment. *Int Rev Psychiatry* 2009;21:30-42.

6   Collins N, Blanchard MR, Tookman A, Sampson EL. Detection of delirium in the acute hospital. *Age Ageing* 2010;39:131-5.

7   González M, Martínez G, Calderón J, Villarroel L, Yuri F, Rojas C, et al. Impact of delirium on short-term mortality in elderly inpatients: a prospective cohort study. *Psychosomatics* 2009;50:234-8.

8   Clegg A, Young J. Which medications to stop in people at risk of delirium: a systematic review. *Age Ageing* 2011;40:23-9.

9   Galvin JE, Roe CM, Xiong C, Morris JC. Validity and reliability of the AD8 informant interview in dementia. *Neurology* 2006;67:1942-8.

10   Jorm AF. The informant questionnaire on cognitive decline in the elderly (IQCODE): a review. *International Psychogeriatrics* 2004;16:1-19.

11   Sans MB, Dantoc BP, Hartshorn A, Ryan CJ, Lujic S. Single question in delirium (SQiD): testing its efficacy against psychiatrist interview, the confusion assessment method and the memorial delirium assessment scale. *Palliat Med* 2010;24:561-5.

12   Woodford HJ, George J. Cognitive assessment in the elderly: a review of clinical methods. *Q J Med* 2007;100:469-84. (Systematic review.)

13   Schofield I, Stott DJ, Tolson D, McFadyen A, Monaghan J, Nelson D. Screening for cognitive impairment in older people attending accident and emergency using the 4-item abbreviated mental test. *European J Emerg Med* 2010;17:340-2.

14   Brodaty H, Pond D, Kemp N, Luscomb G, Harding L, Berman K, et al. The GPCOG: a new screening test for dementia designed for general practice. *JAGS* 2002;50:530-4.

15   Li C, Friedman B, Conwell Y, Fiscella K. Validity of the patient health questionnaire 2 (PHQ-2) in identifying major depression in older people. *JAGS* 2007;55:596-602.

16   Inouye SK, van Dyck CH, Alessi CA, Balkin S, Siegal AP, Horwitz RI. Clarifying confusion: the confusion assessment method. A new method for detection of delirium. *Ann Intern Med* 1990;113:941-8.

17   Inouye SK. Confusion assessment method: training manual and coding guide. 2003. www.hospitalelderlifeprogram.org/private/cam-disclaimer.php?pageid=01.08.00.

18   Davis D, MacLullich AMJ. Understanding barriers to delirium care: a multicentre survey of knowledge and attitudes amongst UK junior doctors. *Age Ageing* 2009;38:559-63.

19   Royal College of Psychiatrists' Centre for Quality Improvement. National audit of dementia (care in general hospitals). 2010. www. rcpsych.ac.uk/pdf/The%20Interim%20Report.pdf.

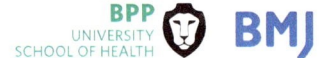

Dementia

Alistair Burns, professor of old age psychiatry[1], honorary consultant psychiatrist[2], Steve Iliffe, professor of primary care for older people[3]

[1]University of Manchester Psychiatry Research Group, Manchester M13 9PL

[2]Manchester Mental Health and Social Care Trust, Manchester

[3]Department of Primary Care & Population Health, University College London, London NW3 2PF

Correspondence to: A Burns alistair. burns@manchester.ac.uk

Cite this as: BMJ 2009;338:b75

DOI: 10.1136/bmj.b75

http://www.bmj.com/content/338/bmj.b75

Dementia is a clinical syndrome characterised by a cluster of symptoms and signs manifested by difficulties in memory, disturbances in language, psychological and psychiatric changes, and impairments in activities of daily living. Alzheimer's disease is a specific disease entity and is the commonest cause of dementia. In this, the first of two articles, we will review the clinical and service implications of dementia syndrome; the second will concentrate on Alzheimer's disease.

What is the burden of disease?

About 12 million people worldwide have dementia, and this total is likely to increase to 25 million by 2040.[1] The Dementia UK report[2] estimated that about 637 000 people in the UK have dementia syndrome and the annual cost of their care is £17bn (€18.7bn; $24.7bn), which is more than heart disease (£4bn), stroke (£3bn), and cancer (£2bn). Annual costs per patient have been estimated at $57 000 in the United States and $64 000 in Italy (including estimates for informal care) and $24 000 in Sweden and $14 000 in Canada (excluding informal care).[w1] Dementia is one of the main causes of disability in later life; in terms of global burden of disease, it contributes 11.2% of all years lived with disability—higher than stroke (9.5%), musculoskeletal disorders (8.9%), heart disease (5%), and cancer (2.4%).[w2] The scale of the problem of dementia, and the under-response to it that is evident world wide, has prompted governments to review their policies. One example of the political pressure facing industrial societies can be seen in the arguments of the UK's Alzheimer's Society (box 1), which has been influential in developing the dementia strategy for England.

What are the barriers to making a diagnosis early?

The benefits of early investigation and diagnosis include identification of treatable physical and psychiatric causes, treatment of comorbid conditions, initiation of psychosocial support, and instigation of pharmacological symptomatic treatments. However, early recognition is not easy because of the insidious and variable onset of the syndrome, which emerges through the personality of the individual, sometimes without a clear demarcation until late in the disease process. Patients, families, and general practitioners may all be reluctant to diagnose dementia because it is such a serious and largely unmodifiable disease that still carries a huge burden of stigma. Physicians may unconsciously hesitate to label a patient as such,[3] and family members may gradually take over social roles from the patient, protecting him or her from difficulties in daily life, but also delaying the conscious recognition of the disorder by offsetting impairments.[4]

How can clinicians recognise dementia?

Recognition of an emerging dementia syndrome depends on the triad of patient report, informant history, and assessment of cognitive function.

Awareness that memory problems in old age, particularly when deteriorating and interfering with daily activities, may be the harbinger of dementia is the most important factor in recognition. The most commonly used cognitive assessment tool is the mini-mental state examination,[5] which is scored out of 30: a score of <24 suggests dementia. However, performance requires intact language and is dependent on educational attainment and cultural background. It can take up to 20 minutes to complete and so may be practical for use only in secondary care. The general practitioner assessment of cognition test,[6] and two other cognitive screening tests (the mini-cog assessment instrument[w3] and the memory impairment screen[w4]) are as clinically and psychometrically robust as and more appropriate for use in primary care than the mini-mental state examination.[7] The six item cognitive impairment test (box 2) was designed for use in general practice and produces more reliable results than the mini-mental state examination.[8]

How is dementia usually diagnosed?

Current UK guidance recommends that the general practitioner perform some routine investigations (standard blood screening and possibly chest radiography if the patient has a history of chest disease and electrocardiography if heart disease is suspected) before referring the patient for a specialist secondary care assessment, preferably by an old age psychiatrist.[9] The second step comprises the exclusion of potentially reversible conditions (such as normal pressure hydrocephalus) and the confirmation of the dementia pathology via detailed neurocognitive assessment and, if available, computed tomography. This allows the subtyping of dementia that is important for prognosis and treatment, particularly given that some physicians are reluctant to diagnose Alzheimer's disease, the only one of the dementias in which symptom modification with drug treatment is possible. Box 3 summarises the investigations that should be considered.

The diagnostic process may be iterative and extended.[w5] From first symptom to presentation to the general practitioner takes about 18 months, with a similar time to diagnosis thereafter. This time period can be shortened by using a structured educational intervention based on adult learning principles and conducted as a workshop in general practice. This educational package can improve diagnostic rates of dementia syndromes, as can decision support software designed to help diagnostic and management thinking.[10] The curriculum for the educational intervention has been distributed as an electronic tutorial on CD to all

---

SUMMARY POINTS

- Dementia is a global health and social care crisis
- In the United Kingdom 700 000 people have dementia, and the annual cost of care is £17bn a year; these values are set to rise
- People with mild cognitive impairment are up to 15 times more likely to develop Alzheimer's disease than those with normal cognition
- Complaints of memory loss often indicates the presence of depression
- Trazodone, clomethiazole, and selective serotonin reuptake inhibitors are suitable alternatives to antipsychotic drugs in people with dementia who are agitated
- Interventions by carers can be as powerful as drug treatment in terms of outcome
- Apathy and withdrawal in people with dementia can be as distressing to carers as agitation and aggression

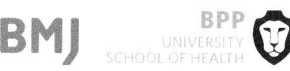

BOX 1 SEVEN RECOMMENDATIONS FROM THE *DEMENTIA UK* REPORT[2]

- Make dementia a national priority
- Increase funding for dementia research
- Improve skills in dementia care
- Develop community support
- Guarantee support packages for carers
- Hold a national debate on who pays for care
- Develop comprehensive dementia care models

BOX 2 THE 6 ITEM COGNITIVE IMPAIRMENT TEST*

Six questions

- What year is it?
- What month is it?
- Give the patient an address phrase to remember with five components (such as John, Smith, 42, High Street, Bedford)
- About what time is it (within one hour)
- Count backwards from 20-1
- Say the months of the year in reverse

Repetition

- Ask the patient to repeat the address phrase requested earlier

See Brooke et al[8] for the scoring system

BOX 3 INVESTIGATIONS FOR DEMENTIA*

In primary care

- Blood tests: full blood count, erythrocyte sedimentation rate, urea and electrolytes, thyroid function tests (to detect comorbid conditions such as anaemia resulting from vitamin B-12 deficiency or renal disease and to exclude reversible causes such as hypothyroidism).
- Syphilis serology is not recommended as a routine test but can be justified if the apparent course of the syndrome or the presentation is atypical.

In secondary care

- Computed tomography (to exclude intracranial lesions; cerebral infarction and haemorrhage; extradural and subdural haematomas; normal pressure hydrocephalus)
- Magnetic resonance imaging (sensitive indicator of cerebrovascular disease, higher resolution to detect focal atrophy—for example, in hippocampal area)
- Single photon emission tomography (to assess regional blood flow and dopamine scan to detect Lewy body disease)
- Carotid ultrasonography (if large vessel atherosclerosis is suspected)
- Electroencephalography is not part of routine investigations but can be useful if epilepsy or an encephalopathy is suspected

General medical investigations

- Chest radiography
- Mid-stream specimen urine if clinical symptoms indicate
- Lumbar puncture (but not to be carried out routinely)
- Electrocardiography (especially if treatment with a cholinesterase drug is being considered)

Informed by the guideline of the National Institute for Clinical Excellence and the Social Care Institute for Excellence[5]

---

practices in England by the Alzheimer's Society, and the decision support software has been incorporated into the EMIS clinical software system for general practice.

How can clinicians distinguish dementia and depression?

To diagnose someone with dementia when in fact they are depressed is traditionally taught as one of the great errors of clinical practice. This rule was based largely on the fact that depression is potentially treatable and dementia largely untreatable. What is now known is that the comorbidity of depressive dementia symptoms is high. People with dementia syndrome have high rates of depression and people with depression often have prominent complaints of memory loss, neuropsychological deficits, and often organic brain changes.

In addition, the fear of triggering a depressive response, denial, or withdrawal from contact with services is one factor that inhibits practitioners from discussing dementia as a diagnosis.[11] As treatments for specific causes of dementia emerge, the traditional dichotomy of a treatable versus a non-treatable condition is less relevant to clinical practice, but nevertheless awareness of the overlap between these disorders is clinically important because clinical trials have shown that antidepressant treatment can be beneficial.[9]

Why is it important to determine the cause of dementia?

Box 4 outlines the different causes (sometimes referred to as subtyping) of dementia syndrome. The causes are important because different types of dementia can have different courses, with different patterns of symptoms, and can respond differently to treatment. For example, the symptoms of Alzheimer's disease can be modified with cholinesterase inhibitors (discussed in detail in our second article). Lewy body dementia differs from the other types because of the dominance of motor symptoms (like Parkinson's disease) and the salience of visual hallucinations. People with Lewy body dementia who take antipsychotic drugs may have adverse effects.[9] The identification of vascular disease means that comorbidities can be treated.

It is important to differentiate between different types of dementia because patients (and with their permission their carers) have the right to a definitive diagnosis (for example, saying someone has jaundice is not a diagnosis in itself) and specific treatments are available for Alzheimer's disease. None the less, the different subtypes have much in common, and there are some generic approaches to dementia that should inform clinical practice.

What is the evidence for managing patients with dementia?

The most comprehensive review of the evidence for different approaches to long term care for people with dementia was carried out jointly by the National Institute for Health and Clinical Excellence (NICE) and the Social Care Institute for Excellence in 2006.[9] This review identified key priorities for service development and the implementation of the guidelines (box 5).

How can clinicians judge mental capacity?

The Mental Capacity Act 2005[12] is complex, and all those working with older people need to be aware of its principles, which include the following propositions:

- Adults are assumed to have capacity unless proved otherwise
- Individuals must be given all available support before concluding that they cannot make decisions for themselves
- People must retain the right to make what may be seen as eccentric and unwise decisions
- Anything done for a person without capacity must be in their best interests and should restrict their rights and basic freedoms as little as possible.

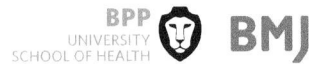

BOX 4 CAUSES OF DEMENTIA

- Alzheimer's disease (about 50% of cases)
- Vascular dementia (about 25%)
- Mixed Alzheimer's disease and vascular dementia (included in the above, 25%)
- Lewy body dementia (15%)
- All others (about 5% combined) including frontotemporal dementia, focal dementias (such as progressive aphasia), subcortical dementias (such as Parkinson's disease dementia), and secondary causes of dementia syndrome (such as intracranial lesions)

BOX 5 KEY PRIORITIES FOR IMPLEMENTATION OF THE GUIDELINE ON DEMENTIA PRODUCED JOINTLY BY NICE AND THE SOCIAL CARE INSTITUTE FOR EXCELLENCE[9]

- Memory services need further development
- Structural imaging is essential for diagnosis
- No discrimination should exist in provision of medical and surgical services for people with dementia
- Capacity to make decisions must be assessed according to the rules of the Mental Capacity Act 2005
- Carers' needs must be recognised and met
- Coordination and integration of health and social care are likely to improve the quality of life of people with dementia
- Challenging behaviour can be managed without necessarily using drug treatment
- Training for professionals should have high priority
- The needs of people with dementia in acute hospitals requires attention

---

Doctors are increasingly being asked to assess capacity in people with cognitive impairment. The medical assessment is based on a person's ability to understand what is being asked, retain the information long enough to make a judgment, and be able to express that judgment. The important issues of capacity are that they may vary over time and are specific to a decision—for example, giving consent to a medical procedure, to a move to a nursing home, or to making a will.

What psychosocial interventions are helpful in dementia?
Cognitive behavioural therapy in patients with mild to moderate dementia seems useful for overcoming "catastrophic thinking" (experiencing all adversity as a disaster) and depressive withdrawal.[13] "Cognitive reframing" (see box 6) can play a role in developing positive coping strategies in carers and may be more effective than problem solving approaches or support group interventions for carers.[w6] Case studies of cognitive behavioural therapy involving people with dementia[14] have shown how a person centred approach can help to alleviate fears of other people "finding out" the diagnosis, to reduce rapid deterioration in abilities, to avoid socially embarrassing behaviour, and to avoid losing any influence over care planning. The techniques used include combinations of reality orientation, memory strategies, and reframing (box 6). Psychotherapeutic approaches to dementia are successful.[15]

What information do people with dementia and their families need?
For people with newly diagnosed dementia and members of their family accurate information about local support should be available in primary and secondary care, social care, and voluntary and community settings.[16] Information for patients with dementia is most useful if people with dementia have been involved in its compilation and presentation, and

---

BOX 6 PSYCHOSOCIAL INTERVENTIONS

- Reality orientation focuses on the likely slow progression in early dementia and offsets "catastrophic" fears that may be triggered by mild memory lapses
- Memory enhancement strategies include setting shorter term goals and maintaining a social circle and useful family roles that reinforce memory
- Reframing dementia means presenting dementia to the patient as a disability that can be accommodated and emphasising the persistent abilities

---

examples of good practice should be adapted for local circumstances and services.[17] [w7] Family members may have concerns that differ from those anticipated by clinicians and so should have access to information and advice from sources that are able to resolve these differences.[18]

How should carers be supported?
Carers of people with dementia are more likely to experience depressed mood, report a higher burden, and have worse general health than carers of patients with other chronic diseases,[6] [19] but some evidence also exists that carers feel reluctant to ask for professional help.[18] [w8] Depressed mood in the carer is one of the factors that determine transfer of the person with dementia to residential care.[3]

The experience of burden is related to the type of coping strategies used by the carer, the experience of loneliness, and the lack of accessible support rather than to "objective" measures of tasks and responsibilities.[w9] Supporting positive coping strategies and promoting problem solving behaviour seem effective in reducing depression,[20] but interventions for people with dementia living at home do not reduce perceived burden.[21]

How should behavioural and psychological symptoms in dementia be managed?
Non-cognitive symptoms (also called "behavioural and psychological symptoms in dementia" or "challenging behaviour") are particularly distressing for families. Non-cognitive symptoms encompass a range of symptoms from agitation and pacing around through to wandering and getting lost, and up to 90% of people with dementia will experience such symptoms to some degree at some time, particularly in the middle and later stages of the illness.[22] While the risks of the behaviours may not be high, they can lead to high levels of stress in carers and may be one of the crucial factors leading to care home admission.[23]

Little high quality evidence exists for the clinical and cost effectiveness of non-drug treatments,[22] although research findings are starting to show the potential of exercise, aromatherapy, and behavioural interventions such as the ABC (antecedents, behaviour, consequences) approach.[9] Management of non-cognitive symptoms in dementia requires a thorough clinical assessment to exclude treatable causes such as infection or pain. Non-drug approaches should be used where possible and specialist advice sought. In the current situation of limited resources it is all too easy to prescribe drug treatment for such symptoms, and 20-50% of people with dementia in institutional care receive antipsychotic drugs,[24] despite widespread concerns over the hazards of these drugs in people with dementia.[25] Box 7 outlines potential alternative drugs.

Conclusion
The ageing of populations in industrialised and developing countries makes dementia syndrome everybody's business. It requires all practitioners working with older patients to understand the insidious onset, main features, and impact

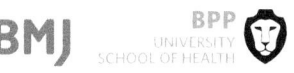

BOX 7 DRUG TREATMENTS (DAILY DOSES) FOR BEHAVIOURAL PROBLEMS IN DEMENTIA

For mild agitation

- Trazodone 50-300 mg
- Benzodiazepines, such as lorazepam 0.5-4 mg
- Clomethiazole up to three capsules (5-15 ml liquid)
- Selective serotonin reuptake inhibitors, such as citalopram 10-20 mg, sertraline 50-100 mg
- Also consider sodium valproate 250 mg to 1 g, carbamazepine (50-300 mg), cholinesterase inhibitors (particularly rivastigmine 1.5-6 mg in Lewy body dementia), promazine 25-100 mg

For severe agitation or if psychosis is present

- Quetiapine 25-200 mg
- Risperidone 0.5-2 mg
- Olanzapine 2.5-10 mg
- Aripiprazole 5-15 mg

If depressive symptoms are present

- Selective serotonin reuptake inhibitors such as citalopram 10-20 mg, sertraline 50-100 mg
- Mirtazapine 15-45 mg

If severe behavioural problems are present

- Consider haloperidol in small doses (0.5-4 mg) and time limited

BOX 8 CURRENT PRIORITIES IN DEMENTIA*

- Raise the national profile of dementia (both in professionals and the public)
- Gain wider acceptance of the need for early diagnosis and investigation
- Improve care for people with dementia in general hospitals (for example, by raising awareness among medical and nursing staff)
- Improve care for people with dementia in institutional settings (such as in the management of behavioural problems)
- Focus on the benefits of non-drug interventions (alone and in combination with drug treatment)
- Develop a research agenda to investigate the potential for preventive strategies

*Based on the Department of Health's proposed national dementia strategy[26]; the joint guideline from NICE and the Social Care Institute for Excellence[9]; and the Dementia UK report[2]

of dementia and to be aware of the range of responses available. Box 8 outlines a wider agenda for professional and service development that is likely to have an impact on most primary and secondary care clinicians.

Both authors are associate directors of the Dementia and Neurodegenerative Diseases Research Network (DeNDRoN).

Contributors: Both authors contributed equally to the preparation of this manuscript. AB is the guarantor of the paper.

Competing interests: AB is editor in chief of the International Journal of Geriatric Psychiatry and receives research funding and consultancy fees from pharmaceutical companies involved in the manufacture and marketing of drugs for Alzheimer's disease including Eisai, Pfizer, Shire, Novartis, Janssen-Cilag, Lundbeck, and Wyeth. SI was a member of the guidelines development group (2004-6) for the joint NICE and Social Care Institute for Excellence guidelines and of the Dementia Strategy External Reference Group (2008).

Provenance and peer review: Commissioned; externally peer reviewed.

SOURCES AND SELECTION CRITERIA

We searched Medline and Pubmed from 2006 to September 2008, previous work having been summarised in the joint dementia guideline published by NICE and the Social Care Institute for Excellence in 2006. We searched the Cochrane database (2008 version) for randomised controlled trials for drug treatment and psychosocial interventions and used our own knowledge of the literature and selected authoritative reviews to supplement these sources.

TIPS FOR NON-SPECIALIST

- Occasional lapses of memory are common, especially in the presence of physical illness or stress—if in doubt, offer to see someone again in three months
- If you ask a patient a simple question and they immediately turn their head to the spouse, suspect dementia
- If you suspect dementia, take a history from an informant
- Have a low threshold for referring someone to a memory clinic if you suspect he or she may have dementia
- Always consider dementia when seeing a patient, especially an older patient, who complains of memory problems
- Generally, memory problems developing over days are due to vascular disease, over weeks are due to depression, and over months are due to dementia

ADDITIONAL EDUCATIONAL RESOURCES

- Alzheimer's Australia. Mind your mind: a user's guide to dementia risk reduction. www.alzheimers.org.au/upload/MYM_book_lowres.pdf
- National Institute for Health and Clinical Excellence, Social Care Institute for Excellence. Dementia: supporting people with dementia and their carers in health and social care. 2006. www.nice.org.uk/Guidance/CG42
- Iliffe S, Drennan V. Primary care and dementia. London: Jessica Kingsley, 2001.
- Alzheimer's Society. Dementia in the community: management strategies for primary care. London: AS, 2006
- Burns A, O'Brien J, Ames D. Dementia. 3rd ed. London: Hodder Arnold, 2005.

1 Ferri CP, Prince M, Brayne C, Brodaty H, Fratiglioni L, Ganguli M, et al. Global prevalence of dementia: a Delphi consensus study. Lancet 2005;366:2112-7.

2 Alzheimer's Society. Dementia UK: the full report. London: AS, 2007.

3 Downs M, Bowers B. Caring for people with dementia. BMJ 2008;336:225-6.

4 De Lepeleire J, Heyrman J, Buntinx F. The early diagnosis of dementia: triggers, early signs and luxating events. Fam Pract 1998;15:431-6.

5 Folstein MF, Folstein SE, McHugh PR. Mini-mental state: a practical method for grading the cognitive state of patients for the clinician. J Psychiatr Res 1975;12:189-98.

6 Brodaty H, Pond D, Kemp NM, Luscombe G, Harding L, Berman K, et al. The primary care physician COG: a new screening test for dementia designed for general practice. J Am Geriatr Soc 2002;50:530-4.

7 Milne A, Culverwell R, Guss R, Tuppen J, Whelton R. Screening for dementia in primary care: a review of the use, efficacy and quality of measures. Int Psychogeriatr 2008;3:431-58.

8 Brooke P, Bullock R. Validation of the 6 item cognitive impairment test. Int J Geriatr Psychiatr 1999;14:936-40.

9 National Institute for Health and Clinical Excellence, Social Care Institute for Excellence. Dementia: supporting people with dementia and their carers in health and social care . 2006. www.nice.org.uk/Guidance/CG42

10 Downs M, Turner S, Bryans M, Wilcock J, Keady J, Levin E, et al. Effectiveness of educational interventions in improving detection and management of dementia in primary care: a cluster randomised controlled study. BMJ 2006;332:692-5.

11 Iliffe S, Wilcock J. The identification of barriers to the recognition of and response to dementia in primary care using a modified focus group method. Dementia 2005;4:12-23.

12 Office of the Public Guardian. Mental Capacity Act 2005. www.publicguardian.gov.uk/mca/mca.htm.

13 Thompson LW, Wenger G, Zeuss JD and Gallagher D. CBT with early stages Alzheimer's disease patients: an exploratory view of the utility of this approach. In: Light E, Lebowitz BD, eds. Alzheimer's disease—treatment and family stress. New York: Hemisphere, 1990.

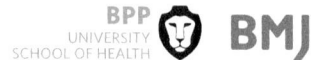

14   Husband HJ. The psychological consequences of learning a diagnosis of dementia: three case examples. *Aging and Mental Health* 1999;3:179-83.

15   Burns A, Guthrie E, Marino-Francis F, Busby C, Morris J, Russell E, et al. Brief psychotherapy in Alzheimer's disease. *Br J Psychiatry* 2005;187:143-7.

16   Audit Commission. *Forget me not.* London: AC, 2000.

17   Gely-Nargeot M, Derousene C, Selmes J, Groupe ODAL. European survey on current practice and disclosure of the diagnosis of Alzheimer's disease. A study based on caregivers report. *Psychol Neuropsychtr Vieil* 2003;1:45-55.

18   Brodaty H, Thompson C, Fine M. Why caregivers of people with dementia and memory loss don't use services. *Int J Geriatr Psychiatry* 2005;20:537-46.

19   Grasel E. When home care ends—changes n the physical health of informal caregivers caring for dementia patients: a longitudinal study. *JAGS* 2002;50:843-9.

20   Zanetti O, Frisoni G, Bianchetti A, Tamanza G, Cigoli V, Trabucchi M. Depressive symptoms of Alzheimer's caregivers are mainly due to personal rather than patient factors. *Int J Geriatr Psychiatry* 1998;13:358-67.

21   Gitlin L, Belle S, Burgio L, Czaja S, Mahoney D, Gallagher-Thompson D, et al. Effects of multicomponent interventions on caregiver burden and depression: the REACH multisite initiative at 6 month follow-up. *Psychology Ageing* 2003;18:361-74.

22   Robinson L, Hutchings D, Corner L, Beyer F, Dickinson H, Vanoli A, et al. Wandering in dementia: a systematic literature review of the effectiveness of non-pharmacological interventions to prevent wandering in dementia and evaluation of the ethical implications and acceptability of their use. *Health Technology Assessment* 2006;10(26).

23   Balestreri L, Grossberg A, Grossberg GT. Behavioural and psychological symptoms of dementia as a risk factor for nursing home placement. *Int Psychogeriatr* 2000;12:59-62.

24   Fossey J, Ballard C, Juszczak E, James I, Alder N, Jacoby R, et al. Effect of enhanced psychosocial care on antipsychotic use in nursing home residents with severe dementia: cluster randomised trial. *BMJ* 2006;332:756-61.

25   Schneider LS, Dagerman KS, Insel P. Risk of death with atypical antipsychotic drug treatment for dementia: meta-analysis of randomized placebo-controlled trials. *JAMA* 2005;294:1934-43.

26   Department of Health. *National dementia strategy* . (In press.) www.dh.gov.uk/en/socialcare/deliveringadultsocialcare/olderpeople/nationaldementiastrategy/index.htm

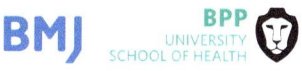

Dementia: timely diagnosis and early intervention

Louise Robinson, general practitioner and professor of primary care[1], Eugene Tang, NIHR academic clinical fellow in general practice[1], John-Paul Taylor, senior clinical lecturer and honorary consultant in old age psychiatry[2]

[1]Institute of Health and Society, Newcastle University, Newcastle upon Tyne, NE2 4AX, UK

[2]Institute of Neuroscience, Newcastle University, Newcastle upon Tyne, UK

Correspondence to L Robinson
a.l.robinson@ncl.ac.uk

Cite this as: BMJ 2015;350:h3029

DOI: 10.1136/bmj.h3029

http://www.bmj.com/content/350/bmj.h3029

Dementia describes a clinical syndrome that encompasses difficulties in memory, language, and behaviour that leads to impairments in activities of daily living. Alzheimer's disease is the most common subtype of dementia, followed by vascular dementia, mixed dementia, and dementia with Lewy bodies. Because the global population is rapidly ageing, dementia has become a concern worldwide[1]; the illness places considerable burden on individuals and their families and also on health and social care provision.

By 2050 an estimated 135 million people worldwide will have dementia. In 2010 the global cost of dementia care was estimated at $604bn (£396bn; €548bn) and estimated to increase to $1tr by 2030.[1] Of all chronic diseases, dementia is one of the most important contributors to dependence and disability.[23] In the absence of a cure, a professional belief that nothing can be done has contributed to delays in diagnosis.[4] However, increasing evidence showing that dementia may be preventable[15] has led to an international focus on earlier diagnosis and intervention.[6] This review aims to summarise current evidence and best practice in the diagnosis and early intervention in dementia care.

Why is timely diagnosis important?

In some countries the introduction of a national dementia strategy has led to greater emphasis on earlier diagnosis, although population based screening is not recommended as dementia does not fulfil the criteria of a condition suitable for screening.[7] With evidence from large longitudinal cohort studies showing that the prevalence of dementia is declining globally, there is now greater emphasis on prevention and risk reduction.[15] In England, policy has rightly or wrongly influenced the introduction of case finding in high risk groups—including people over 75 years of age, as age is the strongest risk factor for dementia—and those with high vascular risk, Parkinson's disease, and learning disabilities.[8] The policy comprises proactive memory assessment of people in both primary care and acute hospital settings who may not have symptoms; however, there is little evidence that such initiatives, which inevitably lead to increased referrals to specialist services, are cost effective and whether they are distressing to patients.[46]

How can clinicians recognise dementia?

Diagnosing dementia can be difficult owing to its insidious onset, symptoms resembling "normal ageing" memory loss, and a diversity of other presenting symptoms—for example, difficulty in finding words or making decisions.[10] An individual's ability to accommodate, compensate, or even deny his or her symptoms in the early stages should also be considered. The individual's family may also have noticed difficulties in communication and personality or mood changes; family concern is of particular importance.[9] Increasing frequency of patients' visits to their general practice, missed appointments, or confusion over drugs may also be warning signs.[8]

Diagnosis of subtype is important given differences in management, disease course, and outcomes for different dementias; awareness of early symptoms in less common dementias can assist generalists in deciding to which specialist services patients are referred (box 1). Duration over which symptoms have developed is also important, with Alzheimer's disease tending to have a more insidious onset than vascular dementia.

How is dementia diagnosed?

The role of primary care

General practitioners are often the first point of contact for patients who are worried that they may have dementia. The role of primary care is to exclude a potentially treatable illness or reversible cause of the "dementia"—for example, depression, vitamin B12 deficiency, or thyroid disturbance; refer for specialist assessment, especially those with unusual symptoms (neurological, psychiatric, or behavioural changes) or those with major risk factors (for example, important medical comorbidities, psychosocial problems, harm to self); and ensure patients who have mild cognitive impairment (objective cognitive loss not affecting function and daily living activities) are followed up in primary care, and, if their symptoms become more severe, re-referred for specialist assessment.

Initial assessment should include a careful history from both the patient and the main carer, with particular emphasis on disturbance of cognitive function and activities of daily living. A physical examination should be undertaken to look for any focal neurological signs and exclude any visual or auditory problems. Baseline investigations and a brief cognitive assessment, using one of the many tools available (box 2), should also be carried out before referral to secondary care.[9]

The mini-mental state examination[16] has traditionally been recommended as the brief cognitive assessment tool of choice, although copyright restrictions are influencing its use in practice. The tools listed in box 2 have been found to be as clinically and psychometrically robust as the mini-mental state examination[17]; a clock drawing

THE BOTTOM LINE

- Dementia is a major global health problem; in the absence of a cure there is increasing focus on risk reduction, timely diagnosis, and early intervention
- Primary and secondary care doctors play complementary roles in dementia diagnosis; differential diagnoses include cognitive impairment due to normal ageing and depression
- Cost effective drug (acetylcholinesterase inhibitors) and non-drug interventions such as cognitive stimulation therapy exist that help to delay cognitive deterioration and improve quality of life; information provision and practical support are also important
- Discussions about a person's wishes for future care should occur at an early stage of illness while the person has mental capacity
- Family carers of people with dementia are at high risk of physical and mental illness as a consequence of caring and they require equal attention and support

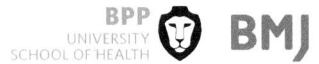

PATIENT AND PUBLIC INVOLVEMENT

Patient and public involvement in this clinical review has been achieved through several processes: the inclusion of patients and the public in the groups responsible for developing the national guidelines referenced in this review; liaising with patient and public representatives from the National Institute of Health Research Dementia and Neurodegenerative Diseases Research Network who contributed to systematic reviews included in this review[49]; and asking the UK Alzheimer's Society to comment on the final draft of the paper and provide up to date information resources for patients and carers.

test may be added to the assessment if it is not already incorporated into the tool.[18] The Addenbrooke's cognitive examination,[19] especially the revised version, has superior diagnostic accuracy to the mini-mental state examination but takes about 25 minutes to complete and has better accuracy in moderate to high prevalence settings.[20] No one brief cognitive assessment tool is more accurate than another and all are inadequate for assessing early or subtle changes, with scores affected by factors such as education. Mini-mental state examination scores are used to indicate the severity of Alzheimer's disease: mild, scores 21-26; moderate, scores 10-20; moderately severe, scores 10-14; severe, scores less than 10.

Depression masquerading as dementia is probably the most common differential diagnosis and should always be considered; however, they can coexist and depression may precede dementia. If suspected, a trial of antidepressants may be indicated, with reassessment of the individual's capabilities and cognitive function 6-8 weeks later.

The role of secondary care
Primary care is increasingly taking on a greater role in both the assessment and the long term care of people with dementia; one multicentre randomised controlled trial found no evidence that specialist memory clinics were more effective than general practice services in providing post-diagnostic support.[21] Secondary services have an important role in defining the dementia subtype, dealing with more complex cases, and stratifying which patients with mild cognitive impairment are at greatest risk of developing dementia and most in need of follow-up.

What are the roles of imaging and other investigations?

Imaging, in particular structural scanning (computed tomography or magnetic resonance imaging), is recommended as part of the investigations of people with suspected dementia in UK,[9] European,[22] and US guidelines.[23] Imaging is now also embedded in several modern diagnostic criteria for different dementias, including Alzheimer's disease and dementia with Lewy bodies.[24] [25] [26] In modern dementia imaging there is now less focus on "excluding" reversible causes of dementia (for example, tumours) and more on determination of subtype. Structural imaging, particularly magnetic resonance imaging, can also help clarify whether a vascular disease is contributing to the cognitive impairment and thus whether strict adherence to treatment guidance for vascular risks is warranted.

BOX 1 EXAMPLES OF LESS COMMON DEMENTIAS AND THEIR EARLY PRESENTING SYMPTOMS

Vascular dementia

- Wide range of signs and symptoms depending on extent, location, and severity of the cerebrovascular disease
- Symptoms can develop abruptly after a stroke or more insidiously with small vessel disease
- Memory loss can be a feature but typically is less noticeable than in Alzheimer's disease. Language, information processing, decision making, and visuospatial deficits can also be found
- Mood changes and apathy are common symptoms; can co-occur with Alzheimer's disease and this is termed mixed dementia

Frontotemporal dementias

- More common in younger age groups (50-60 years)
- The most common clinical type is behavioural variant frontotemporal dementia, with changes in personality and behaviour. Disinhibition and impulsiveness can be features. Memory function is typically intact early on

Dementia with Lewy bodies

- Complex visual hallucinations are a key feature. In the early stages they may only occur during periods of physical stress (for example, infections) or at night time and may be followed by more subtle visuoperceptual symptoms—for example, illusions
- Parkinsonism (tremor, slowed movements, postural instability, shuffling gait) is also a feature. Tremor may be less evident, but people with early dementia with Lewy bodies may be slower in movements and more prone to falls
- Fluctuations or noticeable variations in cognitive function can occur and can be difficult to separate from delirium
- Autonomic symptoms may occur—for example, postural hypotension
- Sleep disturbances such as rapid eye movement sleep behaviour disorder (shouting out or moving while asleep) can occur many years before the onset of dementia

Parkinson's disease with dementia

- As many as 80% of patients with Parkinson's develop dementia
- Symptoms are similar to those of dementia with Lewy bodies, although motor Parkinson's symptoms typically predate cognitive and psychiatric symptoms by more than a year

Posterior cortical atrophy

- A less common form of Alzheimer's disease, which tends to affect younger people (50s and 60s)
- Visual agnosias (difficulties with recognising faces, objects, or perceiving more than one object at a time), apraxias (motor planning difficulties), acalculia (difficulty with calculation), and alexia (difficulty reading) are symptoms
- Memory typically preserved early on

Other uncommon to rare causes of dementia

- Alcohol related dementia, Creutzfeldt-Jakob disease, HIV related cognitive impairment, Huntington's chorea, corticobasal syndrome, movement related dementias (for example, progressive supranuclear palsy), multiple sclerosis, Niemann-Pick disease type C, normal pressure hydrocephalus

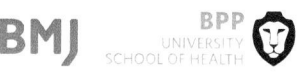

BOX 2 INVESTIGATIONS AND BRIEF COGNITIVE ASSESSMENT TOOLS FOR DEMENTIA IN PRIMARY CARE

Blood tests

- Blood tests that should be ordered are: full blood count, erythrocyte sedimentation rate, urea and electrolytes, thyroid function, vitamin B12, and folate. Midstream specimen of urine, chest radiography, and electrocardiography may also be needed where clinically appropriate

Brief cognitive assessment tools

General practitioner assessment of cognition[11]

- Takes no longer than five minutes to administer and comprises two components: a six item cognitive assessment with the patient and an informant questionnaire (if the cognitive assessment score is equivocal: 5-8 inclusive). Scores >8 are deemed to represent cognitive impairment and <5 intact cognition. Sensitivity 82-85%; specificity 83-86%[12]

6 item cognitive impairment test[13]

- Takes 3-4 minutes to perform and consists of six questions on orientation and memory, although the test may be susceptible to influences of language and education. Scores of 0-7 are considered normal and >8 suggest cognitive impairment. Sensitivity 78.5-83%; specificity 77-100%[12]

Mini-cog assessment instrument[14]

- Takes 2-4 minutes to complete and consists of two components, a three item recall and the clock drawing test. Cognitive impairment is considered to be present if people are unable to recall any of the three items or if they recall only one or two items and draw an abnormal clock. Sensitivity 76-99%; specificity 89-96%[12]

Memory impairment screen[15]

- Takes around four minutes to complete and is a brief four item delayed free recall and cued recall memory impairment test. A score of <4 indicates possible dementia. Sensitivity 74-86%; specificity 96-97%[12]

In the United Kingdom, functional neuroimaging, including hexamethylpropyleneamine oxime (HMPAO) single photon emission computed tomography (SPECT) and [18F] fluoro-2-deoxy-D-glucose positron emission tomography (FDG-PET), is available but usually used as a second line approach to assist with subtype diagnoses, particularly where the diagnosis is in doubt. Dopaminergic iodine-123-radiolabelled 2β-carbomethoxy-3β-(4-iodophenyl)-N-(3-fluoropropyl) nortropane (FP-CIT) SPECT imaging is licensed in Europe and in a number of other countries for the diagnosis of dementia with Lewy bodies and may also be helpful where the clinical diagnosis of dementia with Lewy bodies is not clear.[27]

What new investigations are emerging in the diagnosis of dementia?

Cerebrospinal fluid sampling is used to exclude inflammatory, infective, and malignancy related causes of dementia and is typically recommended in individuals with rapid cognitive decline, unusual or neurological presentations, or cognitive impairment at less than 55 years of age.[28] More recently there has been a focus on developing cerebrospinal fluid based markers, such as β amyloid and tau, for changes in Alzheimer's disease that can predate the onset of the dementia, the so called prodromal phase of Alzheimer's disease. Although such markers have been incorporated into recent diagnostic criteria for Alzheimer's disease,[25] [26] whether they are effective at predicting those who will

develop dementia[29] and, more importantly, practically acceptable, makes their widespread clinical use challenging at present.

It is now possible to directly image amyloid in the brain using several positron emission tomography radiotracers, and this imaging technique may have a future role clinically in predicting which people with mild cognitive impairment will develop Alzheimer's disease. However there is still major heterogeneity in how these scans are interpreted. For example, a recent meta-analysis found that although amyloid imaging has high sensitivity (83-100%) in detecting people with mild cognitive impairment who convert to Alzheimer's disease related dementia, diagnostic specificities varied considerably between studies (46-88%).[30]

What constitutes best practice in early intervention?

Discussing the diagnosis: saying the "D" word

Health professionals can be reluctant to speak openly and honestly with patients and their families about dementia, with some refraining from using the "D" word.[28] Although initially discussing the diagnosis may be distressing, evidence suggests most people prefer to know if they have dementia in order to access appropriate support and treatment and to plan for the future.[4] [31]

What options are available after diagnosis?

Drug interventions

Clinically and cost effective drugs for dementia are available; the emphasis is to improve or maintain function after neuronal damage rather than to alter the underlying pathogenesis leading to the dementia syndrome. Two classes of drugs are currently recommended for symptomatic (Alzheimer's disease and mixed) dementia[6][32]: acetylcholinesterase inhibitors donepezil, galantamine, and rivastigmine, and N-methyl-D-aspartic acid receptor antagonists such as memantine. At present, acetylcholinesterase inhibitors are the only recommended options to manage mild to moderate Alzheimer's disease and there is no evidence that one is more efficacious than another[33]; notwithstanding, a large randomised controlled trial has recently shown that continued treatment with donepezil is associated with cognitive benefits in moderate to severe dementia.[34] Memantine has been approved for people with moderate to severe Alzheimer's disease or those with intolerance to acetylcholinesterase inhibitors; it has also been used in mild Alzheimer's disease but the evidence for this is currently lacking despite its frequent off-label use.[35]

Non-drug approaches

The evidence base is steadily increasing for non-drug interventions in dementia care, although further research in many areas is still needed.[6] In a large systematic review evaluating both drug and non-drug interventions in dementia care, cognitive stimulation therapy was found to be as clinically and cost effective as the acetylcholinesterase inhibitors[36]; reminiscence therapy is also recommended in national guidelines.[9] However, the evidence base for innovative service provision such as case management, whereby a case manager, usually a nurse or social worker acts as the main care coordinator between key stakeholders, including primary and secondary care, is mixed.[6] [36] Although the evidence base for cost effectiveness is low,[37] specially developed assistive technology—any device or system that

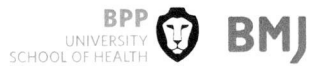

SOURCES AND SELECTION CRITERIA

We searched for articles through Medline, PubMed, and the Cochrane database of systematic reviews from January 2006 to December 2014—the period after publication of the current UK national dementia guidance[9]—using the search terms "dementia", "Alzheimer's", "carer", and "caregiver". Additional searches were carried out for specific subsections—for example, "pharmacologic treatment" and "non-pharmacologic interventions/strategies/treatment". Where possible, we focused on systematic reviews, meta-analyses, and high quality randomised controlled trials. We included only articles in English and excluded those published in non-peer reviewed journals. Recommendations in this review are derived from the most recent international and UK national guidance[9] on evidence based practice in dementia care and the authors' interpretation of the included evidence.

allows an individual to perform tasks that they would otherwise be unable to do, or increases the ease and safety with which the task can be performed—to help people with dementia is available and can be useful in relieving carer anxiety and helping people with dementia to remain living at home (www.atdementia.org.uk/).

Information provision

People with dementia and their families require emotional and practical support to help them live as good a quality of life as they can; the family doctor is in a key position to provide ongoing support and advice once the diagnosis is confirmed.[46] Voluntary organisations such as Alzheimer's International provide a wide range of information resources and practical support for people living with all types of dementia (www.alz.co.uk/). Signposting to local sources of support as well as social services and respite care are integral to the consultation. Listening to an individual patient's difficulties and concerns and providing simple cognitive and emotional strategies in the primary care consultation are beneficial to both patients and their families.

Discussing the future

One important area to be discussed in the earlier stages of dementia, while people still have mental capacity, is personal wishes for future care and also who should make decisions when the patients are no longer able to do so. In dementia, such discussions—termed advance care planning—have been shown to reduce inappropriate hospital admissions towards the end of life, but the evidence base is weak.[38] [39] Discussions about advance care planning require both sensitivity and honesty; general practitioners or hospital specialists are well placed to undertake these discussions if they have an established relationship with the patient. After such conversations, patients can formally record their wishes in several ways, including the completion of an advance directive, or "living will" as it was previously known (box 3).

Primary care doctors may find it difficult to assess the mental capacity of an individual with dementia; mental capacity may fluctuate with time and also with acute illness. In England, the introduction of the Mental Capacity Act in 2005 provided much needed guidance for health and social care professionals on how to undertake an assessment of capacity and to make decisions in the best interests of adults who lack the mental capacity to do so for themselves (box 4).

BOX 3 OUTCOMES OF ADVANCE CARE PLANNING DISCUSSIONS: INTERNATIONAL AND NATIONAL TERMINOLOGY

- *Statement of wishes and preferences*—this documents an individual's wishes for future care and is not legally binding; in the UK this is known as an advance statement
- *An advance directive for refusal of treatment (or "living will")*—this is a statement of an individual's refusal to receive specific medical treatment in a predefined future situation. It is legally binding and comes into effect when a person loses mental capacity. In the UK, this is known as an advance decision to refuse treatment
- *A proxy decision maker or power of attorney*—This is a legally binding document whereby an individual ("donor") nominates another ("attorney") to make decisions on his or her behalf should he or she lose capacity. In England, following the Mental Capacity Act, this is now known as a lasting power of attorney and there are two separate aspects to lasting power of attorney, one for an individual's health and welfare and a second for property and financial affairs

---

BOX 4 ASSESSMENT OF MENTAL CAPACITY (AS DERIVED FROM UK MENTAL CAPACITY ACT 2005)

Two stage test for determining whether an individual has mental capacity to make a specific decision

1. Does the patient have an impairment or disturbance of function of the brain?
2. Regarding a specific decision, can the patient:
- understand the decision to be made?
- retain sufficient information to make an informed decision?
- use information appropriately?
- communicate their decision?

Practical tips for assessment of capacity:
- Information may need to be provided in different forms
- General practitioners may need to assess patients on several occasions—that is, if morning is the best time for them
- Record information and the two stages described above accurately in patient notes
- Refer to experts (old age psychiatry) if in doubt

Caring for family carers

In the UK, two thirds of people with dementia live independently in the community, with most of their care and support provided by family and friends. Such informal carers are more likely to experience depressed mood, to report a higher care "burden," and to have worse physical health than carers of people with other long term conditions.[40] They may grieve as their family member loses functional and cognitive abilities, and as companionship, affection, and intimacy are affected; this is termed a living bereavement. Notwithstanding the satisfaction carers experience from caring, the support they receive and their ability to seek help when needed influence how they cope. Supporting informal carers, monitoring their health and wellbeing, and providing or referring them for additional practical and psychological support is another crucial role for general practitioners and community care services.[41]

We thank Tim Beanland, knowledge services manager at the Alzheimer's Society, London for advice. LR is supported by a National Institute for Health Research professorship (NIHR-RP-011-043).

Contributors: LR drafted the outline and overview of the article; all authors contributed equally to the content. LR is the guarantor of the paper.

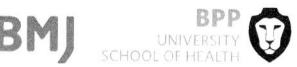

TIPS FOR NON-SPECIALISTS

- Occasional memory lapses are common as people get older, especially in the presence of stress, depression, and acute physical illness; review the patient after appropriate treatment has been given or a reasonable length of time has elapsed
- If you suspect dementia, take a history from both the patient and the main family carer; the latter's suspicions are often correct
- Be aware that certain groups of people are at greater risk of developing dementia—for example, those who have had a stroke and those with Parkinson's disease
- Early identification of modifiable risk factors for dementia may reduce the numbers of people developing dementia in later life
- Effective and useful treatments exist for people with dementia; have a low threshold for referring someone with suspicious symptoms for a specialist memory assessment
- Assess both the physical and the mental health of the main family carer; supporting informal carers is an important part of dementia care

Competing interests: We have read and understood the BMJ policy on declaration of interests and declare the following interests: none.

Provenance and peer review: Commissioned; externally peer reviewed.

1   Prince M, Albanese E, Guerchet M, et al. World Alzheimer report 2014. Dementia and risk reduction: an analysis of protective and modifiable risk factors. Alzheimer's Disease International, 2014.
2   Prince M, Knapp M, Guerchet M, et al. Dementia UK. 2nd ed. Alzheimer's Society, 2014.
3   Prince M, Prina M, Guerchet M. World Alzheimer report 2013. An analysis of long term care for dementia. Alzheimer's Disease International, 2013.
4   Iliffe S, Robinson L, Brayne C, et al. Primary care and dementia: 1. diagnosis, screening and disclosure. Int J Geriatr Psychiatry 2009;24:895-901.
5   Matthews FE, Arthur A, Barnes LE, et al. A two-decade comparison of prevalence of dementia in individuals aged 65 years and older from three geographical areas of England: results of the Cognitive Function and Ageing Study I and II. Lancet 2013;382:1405-12.
6   Prince M, Bryce R, Ferri C. World Alzheimer report 2011: the benefits of early diagnosis and intervention. Alzheimer's Disease International, 2011
7   Alzheimer Europe. National Dementia Strategies (diagnosis, treatment and research): country comparisons. 2013. www.alzheimer-europe.org/Policy-in-Practice2/Country-comparisons/National-Dementia-Strategies-diagnosis-treatment-and-research.
8   Bamford C, Eccles M, Steen N, et al. Can primary care record review facilitate earlier diagnosis of dementia? Fam Pract 2007;24:108-16.
9   National Institute for Health and Care Excellence/Social Care Institute of Excellence (NICE/SCIE). Dementia: supporting people with dementia and their carers in health and social care. (Clinical guideline CG42) 2006. http://guidance.nice.org.uk/CG42.
10 Kostopoulou O, Delaney BC, Munro CW. Diagnostic difficulty and error in primary care—a systematic review. Fam Pract 2008;25:400-13.
11 Brodaty H, Pond D, Kemp NM, et al. The GPCOG: a new screening test for dementia designed for general practice. J Am Geriatr Soc 2002;50:530-4.
12 Yokomizo JE, Simon SS, Bottino CM. Cognitive screening for dementia in primary care: a systematic review. Int Psychogeriatr 2014;26:1783-804.
13 Brooke P, Bullock R. Validation of a 6 item cognitive impairment test with a view to primary care usage. Int J Geriatr Psychiatry 1999;14:936-40.
14 Borson S, Scanlan J, Brush M, et al. The mini-cog: a cognitive 'vital signs' measure for dementia screening in multi-lingual elderly. Int J Geriat Psychiatry 2000;15:1021-7.
15 Buschke H, Kuslansky G, Katz M, et al. Screening for dementia with the memory impairment screen. Neurology 1999;52:231-8.
16 Folstein MF, Folstein SE, McHugh PR. "Mini-mental state". A practical method for grading the cognitive state of patients for the clinician. J Psychiatr Res 1975;12:189-98.
17 Milne A, Culverwell A, Guss R, et al. Screening for dementia in primary care: a review of the use, efficacy and quality of measures. Int Psychogeriatr 2008;20:911-26.
18 Shulman KI. Clock-drawing: is it the ideal cognitive screening test? Int J Geriatr Psychiatry 2000;15:548-61.
19 Mioshi E, Dawson K, Mitchell J, et al. The Addenbrooke's Cognitive Examination Revised (ACE-R): a brief cognitive test battery for dementia screening. Int J Geriat Psychiatry 2006;21:1078-85.

ADDITIONAL EDUCATIONAL RESOURCES

Resources for healthcare professionals

- Alzheimer's Society. Assessing cognition in older people (www.alzheimers.org.uk/cognitiveassessment)—a practical toolkit for health professionals
- BMJ Group resources: BMJ Learning modules. (http://learning.bmj.com/learning/module-intro/dementia-primary-care)—describes the management of dementia in primary care
- BMJ Quality (http://quality.bmj.com)—four e-projects to improve quality of care in the areas of support for carers, antipsychotic drug prescribing, timely diagnosis, and palliative care

Resources for patients and carers

- Social Care Institute for Excellence. Dementia gateway (www/scie/org.uk/dementia)—web based information and e-learning resources written by experts mainly for professional carers and supporters
- Alzheimer's Society. The dementia guide: living well after diagnosis (www.alzheimers.org.uk/dementiaguide or request copies at publications@alzheimers.org.uk)—comprehensive practical information for people with dementia and families with a recent diagnosis. Includes a free booklet, video case studies, and downloadable translations
- Lewy body Society (http://lewybody.org/aboutdlb)—website of the only charity in Europe exclusively concerned with dementia with Lewy bodies
- FTD Talk (www.ftd.org)—accessible updates and web information for people with frontotemporal dementia from researchers
- Alzheimer's Disease International. Help for caregivers (www.alz.co.uk/ADI-publications)—a downloadable booklet produced in collaboration with the World Health Organization: practical tips on caring for someone with dementia
- Carers UK Factsheets (http://carersuk.org)—practical information for carers about topics such as benefits and getting help and support
- at dementia (www.atdementia.org.uk)—a website providing information on assistive technology for people with dementia

20 Larner AJM. A meta-analysis of the accuracy of the Addenbrooke's Cognitive Examination (ACE) and the Addenbrooke's Cognitive Examination-Revised (ACE-R) in the detection of dementia. Int Psychogeriatr 2014:26:555-63.
21 Meeuwsen EJ, Melis RJ, Van der Aa GC, et al. Effectiveness of dementia follow-up care by memory clinics or general practitioners: randomised controlled trial. BMJ 2012;344:e3086.
22 Hort J, O'Brien JT, Gainotti G, et al. EFNS guidelines for the diagnosis and management of Alzheimer's disease. Eur J Neurol 2010;17:1236-48.
23 .Jack CR Jr, Albert MS, Knopman DS, et al. Introduction to the recommendations from the National Institute on Aging-Alzheimer's Association workgroups on diagnostic guidelines for Alzheimer's disease. Alzheimers Dement 2011;7:257-62.
24 McKeith IG, Dickson DW, Lowe J, et al. Diagnosis and management of dementia with Lewy bodies: third report of the DLB Consortium. Neurology 2005;65:1863-72.
25 McKhann GM, Knopman DS, Chertkow H, et al. The diagnosis of dementia due to Alzheimer's disease: recommendations from the National Institute on Aging-Alzheimer's Association workgroups on diagnostic guidelines for Alzheimer's disease. Alzheimers Dement 2011;7:263-9.
26 Dubois B, Feldman HH, Jacova C, et al. Advancing research diagnostic criteria for Alzheimer's disease: the IWG-2 criteria. Lancet Neurol 2014;13:614-29.
27 Walker Z, Moreno E, Thomas A, et al. Clinical usefulness of dopamine transporter SPECT imaging with 123I-FP-CIT in patients with possible dementia with Lewy bodies: randomised study. Br J Psychiatry 2015;206:145-52.
28 Rossor MN, Fox NC, Mummery CJ, et al. The diagnosis of young-onset dementia. Lancet Neurol 2010;9:793-806.
29 Ritchie C, Smailagic N, Noel-Storr AH, et al. Plasma and cerebrospinal fluid amyloid beta for the diagnosis of Alzheimer's disease dementia

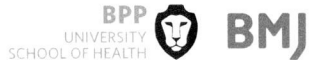

and other dementias in people with mild cognitive impairment (MCI). *Cochrane Database Syst Rev* 2014;6:CD008782.

30 Zhang S, Smailagic N, Hyde C, et al. (11)C-PIB-PET for the early diagnosis of Alzheimer's disease dementia and other dementias in people with mild cognitive impairment (MCI). *Cochrane Database Syst Rev* 2014;7:CD010386.

31 Robinson L, Gemski A, Abley C, et al. The transition to dementia: individual and family experiences of receiving a diagnosis: a review. *Int Psychogeriatr* 2011;23:1026-43.

32 National Institute for Health and Care Excellence. Donepezil, galantamine, rivastigmine and mementine for the treatment of Alzheimer's disease. (Technology appraisal guidance TA217) 2011. http://guidance.nice.org.uk/guidanceTA217.

33 Birks J. Cholinesterase inhibitors for Alzheimer's disease. *Cochrane Database Syst Rev* 2006;1:CD005593.

34 Howard R, McShane R, Lindesay J, et al. Donepezil and memantine for moderate-to-severe Alzheimer's disease. *N Engl J Med* 2012;366:893-903.

35 Schneider LS, Dagerman KS, Higgins JP, et al. Lack of evidence for the efficacy of memantine in mild Alzheimer disease. *Arch Neurol* 2011;68:991-8.

36 Knapp M, Iemmi V, Romeo R. Dementia care costs and outcomes: a systematic review. *Int J Geriatr Psychiatry* 2013;28:551-61.

37 Gibson G, Newton L, Pritchard G, et al. The provision of assistive technology products and services for people with dementia in the United Kingdom. Dementia (London) 2014; published online 5 May.

38 Robinson L, Dickinson C, Rousseau N, et al. A systematic review of the effectiveness of advance care planning interventions for people with cognitive impairment and dementia. *Age Ageing* 2012;41:263-9.

39 Van der Steen JT. Dying with dementia: what we know after more than a decade of research. *J Alzheimers Dis* 2010;22:37-55.

40 Brodaty H, Green A, Koschera A. Meta-analysis of psychosocial interventions for caregivers of people with dementia. *J Am Geriatr Soc* 2003;51:657-64.

41 Cameron ID, Aggar C, Robinson AL, et al. Assessing and helping carers of older people. *BMJ* 2011;343:d5202.

Related links

thebmj.com
previous articles in this series

- The diagnosis and management of hypocalcaemia (BMJ 2015;350:h2723)
- Management of the unstable shoulder (BMJ 2015;350:h2537)
- Childhood attention-deficit/hyperactivity disorder (BMJ 2015;350:h2168)
- Identifying and managing common childhood language and speech impairments (BMJ 2015;350:h2318)
- The diagnosis and management of interstitial lung diseases (BMJ 2015;350:h2072)
- Sudden infant death syndrome and advice for safe sleeping (BMJ 2015;350:h1989)

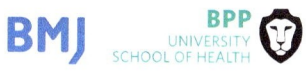

Alzheimer's disease

Alistair Burns, professor of old age psychiatry[1], honorary consultant psychiatrist[2], Steve Iliffe, professor of primary care for older people[3]

[1]University of Manchester Psychiatry Research Group, Manchester M13 9PL

[2]Manchester Mental Health and Social Care Trust, Manchester

[3]Department of Primary Care & Population Health, University College London, London NW3 2PF

Correspondence to: A Burns alistair. burns@manchester.ac.uk

Cite this as: BMJ 2009;338:b158

DOI: 10.1136/bmj.b158

http://www.bmj.com/content/338/bmj.b158

In this, the second of two review articles about dementia, we focus on Alzheimer's disease, which is the most common cause of dementia. Dementia is a clinical syndrome characterised by a cluster of symptoms and signs manifested by difficulties in memory, disturbances in language, psychological and psychiatric changes, and impairments in activities of daily living. Alzheimer's disease is a specific disease that affects about 6% of the population aged over 65 and increases in incidence with age.[1]

Patients with Alzheimer's disease are often identified and managed in primary care, where they may present diagnostic and management challenges. The benefits of early investigation and diagnosis of Alzheimer's disease include instigation of pharmacological symptomatic treatments and initiation of psychosocial support, plus treatment of comorbid conditions. Here we review the diagnosis and medical management of Alzheimer's disease, relying where possible on evidence from randomised controlled trials.

What is Alzheimer's disease?
Alzheimer's disease is a chronic progressive neurodegenerative disorder characterised by three primary groups of symptoms. The first group (cognitive dysfunction) includes memory loss, language difficulties, and executive dysfunction (that is, loss of higher level planning and intellectual coordination skills). The second group comprises psychiatric symptoms and behavioural disturbances—for example, depression, hallucinations, delusions, agitation—collectively termed non-cognitive symptoms.[2] The third group comprises difficulties with performing activities of daily living (deemed "instrumental" for more complex activities such as driving and shopping and "basic" for dressing and eating unaided). The symptoms of Alzheimer's disease progress from mild symptoms of memory loss to very severe dementia (figure). Increasingly, the coexistence of vascular disease and Alzheimer's disease is being recognised clinically, pathologically, and epidemiologically.[4]

What is the relation between normal ageing and Alzheimer's disease?
Population studies of ageing and cognition suggest that impairment in multiple cognitive domains is observable several years before a clinical diagnosis of Alzheimer's disease is made.[5] This observed cognitive dysfunction is not qualitatively different from that seen in normal ageing, suggesting continuity rather than discontinuity in the shift from normal ageing to preclinical dementia.[6]

Global cognitive deterioration, affecting memory and other aspects of cognitive functioning (verbal ability, visuospatial skills, attention, and perceptual speed), is almost always a presenting symptom.[w1] There is considerable overlap in cognitive performance between normal ageing and this stable phase,[w2] and little evidence exists as yet that these changes are detectable in clinical encounters. A person with symptoms of Alzheimer's disease is about 30% more likely to display the clinical features of dementia if they have coexisting symptoms of vascular disease.[4]

What is the benefit of identifying mild cognitive impairment?
Longitudinal studies suggest that cognitive impairments in this early stage may remain relatively constant for several years.[w3] This phase corresponds to the clinical concept of mild cognitive impairment, in which the individual has subjective symptoms (predominantly of memory loss) and measurable cognitive deficits but without notable impairment in defined activities of everyday life (box 1). Controversy surrounds the concept of mild cognitive impairment: is it really an identifiable precursor ripe for preventive interventions, or is it merely medicalising normal ageing? The debate continues, but prospective studies have shown that people with amnestic mild cognitive impairment (the form characterised by memory loss) are up to 15 times more likely to have developed dementia at follow-up,[w4] suggesting it may be a precursor to Alzheimer's disease.

Currently, stringent tests of episodic memory are the best neuropsychological predictors of subsequent conversion from mild cognitive impairment to Alzheimer's disease at group level. Imaging techniques can identify early brain changes, both structural and metabolic, but no single technique if used as a screening test can accurately identify individuals with mild cognitive impairment who will subsequently develop Alzheimer's disease or other dementias.[7] A combination of neuropsychological testing and neuroimaging improves the diagnostic accuracy of predicting cognitive decline in people in this phase compared with that achieved with either modality alone.[8] However, the tools for identifying the early changes of Alzheimer's disease are outpacing the therapeutic options, so the usefulness of such early "preclinical" diagnosis remains uncertain.[w5]

The stable phase of mild cognitive impairment ends with a detectable decline in cognitive function, lasting two to five years, in which semantic memory (the store of facts and general knowledge) and implicit memory (the non-conscious influence of past experience on subsequent performance) also becomes degraded.[9] Trial evidence shows that early recognition of cognitive impairment and clinical assessment and management at this point delays the subsequent need for nursing home care and reduces the risk of misdiagnosis and inappropriate management.[w5]

How does Alzheimer's disease present?
Memory loss is universal and is the first symptom in the vast majority of cases. The gradual onset of memory loss means that it may (understandably) be misattributed to normal ageing and is often recognised only in retrospect

SUMMARY POINTS

- People with mild cognitive impairment are up to 15 times more likely to develop Alzheimer's disease than those with normal cognition
- Memory loss is a presenting symptom in most people who develop Alzheimer's disease
- The cause of Alzheimer's disease is unknown, but genetic and environmental risk factors have been implicated
- Cholinesterase inhibitors are safe and effective and can be prescribed for people in the moderate stages of Alzheimer's disease
- Antipsychotic drugs reduce agitation but are linked with an increased risk of mortality and impair cognition
- Evidence is growing that some strategies are successful at preventing Alzheimer's disease

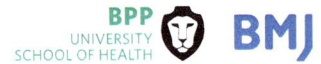

as the onset of Alzheimer's disease. The onset is insidious, emerging with mild loss of memory and difficulty with word finding, symptoms that are common in everyday life to varying degrees. It is only when the symptoms interfere significantly with social and work activities, or are recognised by others, who sense they are progressing, that suspicion of a dementia is justified. Emotional changes are common, major depression occurs in 24-32% of cases, anxiety in 17-27%, apathy in up to 41%, and delusions in 23%.[10]

How do we diagnose and assess Alzheimer's disease?
The clinical diagnosis of Alzheimer's disease follows a logical sequence: the history should include information from an informant; a mental state assessment should include a validated cognitive function test; and the physical examination should focus on vascular and neurological signs supplemented by investigations. Assessment of dementia involves a two step process. Firstly, it is important to distinguish dementia syndromes from other conditions that can mimic them, such as depression, delirium, and mild cognitive impairment. Secondly, once dementia syndrome is recognised, the diagnosis of a subtype is important because it may determine the kind of treatment possible. Current criteria for the main causes of dementia (Alzheimer's disease,[11] [12] vascular dementia,[13] [14] and Lewy body dementia[15]) are well summarised by Dubois.[12]

For cognitive screening in general practice, the clock test is popular because of its non-confrontational nature and because the normal drawing of a clock more or less excludes the presence of important cognitive impairment. However, the rules for scoring the tests can be quite complex and using a solitary cognitive test to screen for the presence of a dementia syndrome does not do justice to the wide variety of symptoms that make up the clinical syndrome of dementia. Activities of daily living are assessed alongside cognition, but there is less consistency in the assessment instruments used.

What is the cause of Alzheimer's disease?
The cause of Alzheimer's disease is unknown, but case-control studies have linked several risk factors with the disease including age, family history, apolipoprotein (Apo) E4 status, head injury, depression, hypertension, diabetes,

high cholesterol, atrial fibrillation, presence of cerebral emboli, and low physical and cognitive activity (box 2). Some risk factors are potentially modifiable.

Neuritic (or senile) plaques and neurofibrillary tangles are the primary histological features of Alzheimer's disease; the presence of phosphorylated tau is the hallmark of the former, and the deposition of the insoluble protein amyloid denotes the latter. Both have been correlated with the severity of the clinical features of the dementia syndrome (as has synaptic density, a measure of neuronal loss).[w12] [w13]

What is the genetic contribution to Alzheimer's disease?
Familial aggregation of Alzheimer's disease has been known for some 75 years, and the risk for first degree relatives of people with the disease is estimated at 10-40% higher than in unrelated people.[w14] Twin studies have found that concordance is higher in monozygotic twins than in dizygotic twins, indicating the presence of a genetic component, although the modest concordance levels in monozygotic twins (who share 100% genetic material) would suggest that environmental factors are at play as well.[w15]

Mutations have been described in three genes: the amyloid precursor protein, presenilin 1, and presenilin 2, on chromosomes 21, 14, and 1 respectively. For late onset Alzheimer's disease, the only known genetic risk factor is ApoE, located on chromosome 19. Three gene forms exist (ApoE e2, ApoE e3, and ApoE e4), with possession of one e4 allele being associated with a threefold risk for the development of Alzheimer's disease, whereas those with the homozygous condition have an eightfold risk.[w16] The importance of environmental factors is confirmed by the fact that the strongest association is not true across all races and 50% of white patients with Alzheimer's disease do not carry an e4 allele.

What treatments work for Alzheimer's disease?
Although we focus here on treatments for Alzheimer's disease, many psychosocial interventions are appropriate for the clinical syndrome of dementia regardless of its cause. As most psychosocial interventions and some drug treatments are for symptomatic benefit they do not rely for their efficacy on modifying the underlying pathophysiology. For example, the treatment of depression in dementia is essentially the same whether the dementia results from Alzheimer's disease or vascular dementia, alone or in combination.

In clinical practice, non-drug interventions should be tried first[w17] especially when symptoms are neither causing distress nor placing a person at risk to themselves or others.[16] Therapeutic interventions that are tailored to the individual and establish a good rapport with the person with dementia and their carers are essential. Continuity of clinical care may also be important because it permits a complex appreciation of individuals. For example, a person's own awareness of changes in their cognitive function is associated with better treatment outcomes after cognitive rehabilitation, but awareness can be difficult to assess as individuals with Alzheimer's disease may deny problems in one context but report awareness of them in another.[w18] General practitioners are well placed to have this understanding of their patients, and collaboration between specialists and general practitioners in the care of people with Alzheimer's disease is essential.

Pharmacotherapy
Cholinesterase inhibitors are the mainstay of drug treatment for Alzheimer's disease (box 3).[17] They inhibit cholinesterase, which breaks down acetylcholine, raising

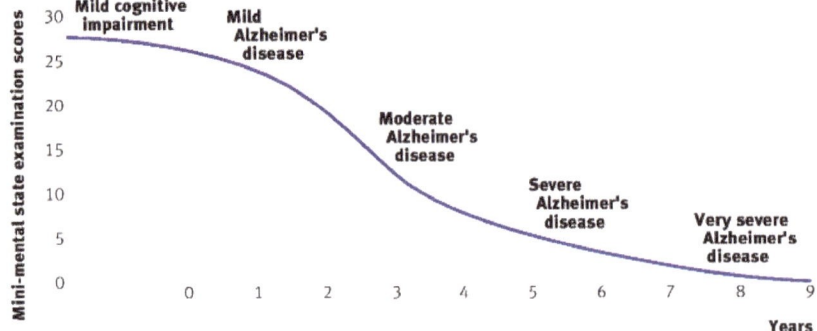

Mild cognitive impairment: Complaints of memory loss, intact activities of daily living, no evidence of Alzheimer's disease
Mild Alzheimer's disease: Forgetfulness, short term memory loss, repetitive questions, hobbies, interests lost, impaired activities of daily living
Moderate Alzheimer's disease: Progression of cognitive deficits, dysexecutive syndrome, further impaired activities of daily living, transitions in care, emergence of behavioural and psychological symptoms of dementia
Severe Alzheimer's disease: Agitation, altered sleep patterns, assistance required in dressing, feeding, bathing, established behavioural and psychological symptoms of dementia
Very severe Alzheimer's disease: Bedbound, no speech, incontinent, basic psychomotor skills lost

Symptom progression in Alzheimer's disease. Adapted from Feldman et al[3]

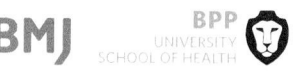

BOX 1 CRITERIA FOR DIAGNOSING MILD COGNITIVE IMPAIRMENT[W4]

- Memory complaints, preferably corroborated by an informant
- Impaired memory function for age and education
- Preserved general cognitive function
- Intact activities of daily living
- No evidence of dementia

BOX 2 RISK FACTORS FOR ALZHEIMER'S DISEASE[W6]

Sociodemographic[W7]

- Age: increasing age
- Sex: no consistent evidence
- National and ethnic profile: some evidence of regional variations

Familial and genetic factors[W8] [W9]

- Family history: 3.5-fold increase in risk when a first degree relative is affected
- Diseases causing mutations: on chromosomes 1, 14, and 21 (see later in the article)
- ApoE genotype
- Down's syndrome: everyone eventually develops the neuropathological features of Alzheimer's disease
- Premorbid cognitive reserves: longer education and higher intelligence are protective

Medical history and treatments[W10]

- Head injuries: anti-inflammatory drugs are associated with a reduction in risk
- Oestrogen replacement: no consistent evidence
- Vascular risk factors: hypertension, diabetes, homocysteine, and cholesterol are all implicated
- Depression: associated with Alzheimer's disease
- Herpes simplex: a risk factor, possibly mediated by the presence of ApoE e4

HABITS[W11]

- Alcohol: drinking wine is protective
- Smoking: no consistent evidence
- Diet: no consistent evidence (including for aluminium)
- Occupational and recreation factors: no consistent evidence

---

BOX 3 DRUG TREATMENTS FOR ALZHEIMER'S DISEASE

Cholinesterase inhibitors (for moderate disease)

- Donepezil 5-10 mg
- Rivastigmine 6-12 mg
- Galantamine 8-24 mg

Glutamatergic partial antagonist* (for moderately severe disease)

- Memantine 10-20 mg

*Not recommended by the National Institute for Health and Clinical Excellence

---

people taking the active drug responded compared with those taking the placebo. Core efficacy is essentially the same for the drugs, with choice determined on the basis of familiarity by the clinician, "once daily" dosing (rivastigmine is available in patch form), and ability to manipulate the dose (rivastigmine). Since April 2004 all English primary care trusts have been required by the national service framework for older people (2001) to have a shared-care protocol in place for prescribing and monitoring use of cholinesterase inhibitors in general practice and specialist settings.

Memantine is a glutamatergic partial antagonist that some trials have found effective in people with more severe dementia, but its use in the UK National Health Service is restricted to those involved in clinical trials of this drug (see NICE's technology appraisal at www.nice.org.uk/TA111).

Amnesia and activities of daily living

Non-drug approaches are not effective in modifying memory loss, although memory retraining techniques can offer support and improve wellbeing in people with mild dementia.[W21] Both cholinesterase inhibitors and memantine produce modest but identifiable improvements in activities of daily living.[17] Patients and their carers often report that improvements in activities of daily living make the biggest positive impact on their lives.[W20]

How can behavioural and psychological difficulties be managed?

General assessment

If a person with dementia develops distressing symptoms or challenging behaviour, an assessment to identify modifiable factors that may influence behaviour (such as depression, adverse effects of drugs, individual biography, and psychosocial or physical environmental factors) is important. A physical examination may, for example, discover a source of pain that underlies challenging behaviour. Environmental and psychosocial factors that may increase the likelihood of challenging behaviour include overcrowding, poor communication between the person and staff, lack of privacy, lack of activities, conflicts between staff and carers, and inadequate attention from staff.[W17]

The sequence of events is often more important than phenomenology in determining causation. For example, did a change happen after an alteration in medication, moving rooms in a nursing home, or even a change in staffing? The management of behavioural disturbance is closely linked to the underlying cause and is generally independent of the type of dementia.

Agitation

Environmental factors play a role in the genesis and maintenance of agitation, and non-drug approaches are important first line treatments. Advice on behavioural management and support for carers is essential, and when symptoms are mild and the environment supportive this

---

the level of the neurotransmitter and resulting in symptom modification. Controversy emerged after guidance from the National Institute for Health and Clinical Excellence (NICE) recommended that cholinesterase inhibitors should be used only to treat moderate Alzheimer's disease and not mild or severe disease.[W17] Underpinning this guideline is a cost effectiveness analyses by NICE that suggested that cholinesterase inhibitors are beneficial only for people with dementia whose scores on the (30 point) mini-mental state examination are between 10 and 20.[W17] The NICE dementia guidelines point out the unreliability of the mini-mental state examination and advocate treatment based on clinical assessment of "significant impairment."[W17] This latter criterion is the one that clinicians will find more useful. Uptake of dementia drugs in the United Kingdom is lower than in other European countries.[18] [W19]

Cochrane reviews show that cholinesterase inhibitors have a moderate but worthwhile symptom modifying effect in a substantial minority of people with Alzheimer's disease and are generally well tolerated.[W20] The difference between active treatment and placebo on core measures of cognitive function is about three points on a 70 point scale over six months. This equates approximately to the decline expected over the same period. About 10% more

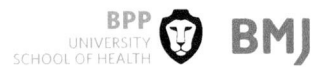

is usually sufficient to manage the situation. Non-drug approaches that have been used with benefit include aromatherapy, bright light therapy, music or dance, massage, pet therapy, and multisensory stimulation.[w17]

Although antipsychotic drugs consistently reduce agitated behaviour, concerns have been expressed recently over the safety of both the older (such as haloperidol) and second generation (such as risperidone, olanzapine, and quetiapine) antipsychotics[19] in terms of an increased risk of stroke and mortality[20] and a detrimental effect on cognition.[w22] Antipsychotic drugs have long been used to treat problem behaviours such as sexual disinhibition, wandering (often associated with agitation), swearing, and shouting. Other sedatives may be effective, as may β blockers, benzodiazepines, and carbamazepine.[w23] The evidence for efficacy is patchy, with few well described methodologically sound randomised controlled trials.

Drug treatment should be used with great caution, if at all, and general practitioners caring for patients with dementia should seek specialist advice about the management of behaviour and psychological symptoms in dementia. Recent trials using the cholinesterase inhibitor donepezil have shown conflicting results in its ability to improve behavioural problems[21] [w24] while rivastigmine may be beneficial in reducing behavioural symptoms in Lewy body dementia.[15]

Depression
Exercise may help reduce the symptoms of depression, and randomised controlled trials support the use of antidepressants. Newer selective serotonin reuptake inhibitors are the preferred class, rather than the older tricyclic agents, which have troublesome side effects.[w24]

Psychosis
Second generation antipsychotic drugs have been more extensively studied in prospective randomised controlled trials than the older tricyclics, but evidence has accumulated to show they have the same side effect profile and increased mortality rate as first generation antipsychotics, and both have been shown to be associated with more rapid cognitive decline.[22] Although the second generation antipsychotics reduce agitation, probably independently of a sedative effect, they seem to have little specific benefit on psychosis. Concerns over the safety of second generation antipsychotics led to a warning about their use for people with agitation in dementia, but their licence still allows for the treatment of psychosis. The NICE dementia guidelines recommend that if drug treatment is used, it should be at the lowest effective dose. The guidelines advise caution if using drugs to control behaviour, particularly if the person has been restrained, because of the risks of loss of consciousness instead of sedation, over-sedation with loss

of alertness, and damage to the relationship between the person with dementia, their carers, and the care team.

Carers' needs
Loss of function and psychological and behavioural symptoms in people with Alzheimer's disease are sources of stress and a burden for carers. Some interventions reduce psychological morbidity in carers and help people with dementia stay at home longer; programmes that involve both the patients and their families and are more intensive and modified to carers' needs may be more successful.[23]

The PREVENT trial found significant improvements in care processes and outcomes for both people with dementia (increased prescribing of cholinesterase inhibitors and antidepressant drugs and fewer behavioural and psychological symptoms) and family carers (improved depression scores and higher carer satisfaction ratings).[24] Multicomponent interventions that included, for example, educational sessions, group support, and practical training were the most successful interventions for both people with dementia and their family carers.[23] [w25]

Is prevention of Alzheimer's disease possible?
Evidence is growing that some interventions may delay the onset of Alzheimer's disease. Predicting the onset of dementia is possible (table). Prevention is a complex area: interventions with single agents (such as antihypertensive drugs or statins) are unlikely to result in a large scale reduction because many risk factors are involved and intervention studies would therefore be complex to design and execute. Whether interventions affect the core biological mechanisms of Alzheimer's disease or are mediated through reduction of vascular risk factors is unclear. For example, statins not only reduce cholesterol but also have, for example, antithrombotic and anti-inflammatory actions. Ageing and family history (genetic) factors are traditionally regarded as non-modifiable risk factors, but that view may be challenged by the avoidance of the effects of chronological ageing by lifestyle interventions and perhaps ultimately by gene therapy. Public interest in the possibility of preventing Alzheimer's disease is high (box 4).

Conclusion
The ageing of populations in industrialised and developing countries makes Alzheimer's disease everybody's business. It requires all practitioners working with older patients to understand the insidious onset, main features, and impact of dementia and to be aware of the range of responses available.

Both authors are associate directors of the Dementia and Neurodegenerative Diseases Research Network (DeNDRoN).

Contributors: Both authors contributed equally to the preparation of this manuscript. AB is the guarantor of the paper.

Newly developed scoring system based on mid-life vascular and non-vascular characteristics that predicts risk of dementia over 20 years. Adapted from Kivipelto et al[w26]

Characteristic	Low risk profile (risk 0.1%*)	High risk profile (risk 48.9%*)
Age (years)	<47	>53
Sex	Female	Male
Education (no of years)	≥10	≤6
Systolic blood pressure (mm Hg)	≤140	>140
Total cholesterol (mmol/l)	≤6.5	>6.5
Body mass index (kg/m²)	≤30	>30
Physical activity	Active	Inactive
Presence of apolipoprotein E e4	No	Yes

*The risk of dementia if all characteristics apply.

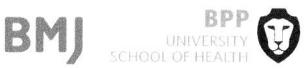

BOX 4 SEVEN SIGNPOSTS FOR A "BRAIN HEALTHY" LIFESTYLE [W27]

- Keep your brain active
- Eat healthily
- Be physically active
- Manage your blood pressure, blood cholesterol, blood sugar, and weight
- Participate in social activities
- Avoid tobacco smoke and drink alcohol only in moderation
- Protect your head from injury

SOURCES AND SELECTION CRITERIA

We searched Medline and Pubmed from 2006 to September 2008, previous work having been summarised in the joint dementia guideline published by NICE and the Social Care Institute for Excellence in 2006. We searched the Cochrane database (2008 version) for randomised controlled trials for drug treatment and psychosocial interventions and used our own knowledge of the literature and selected authoritative reviews to supplement these sources.

TIPS FOR THE NON-SPECIALIST

- History from a knowledgeable informant is as useful in the diagnosis of Alzheimer's disease as a direct interview with the patient
- Take care when discussing Alzheimer's disease or dementia—many people have seen a relative with a disease and will have their own preconception, often profoundly negative, of what the disease is
- It is always worth doing a physical assessment and routine blood tests in people with Alzheimer's disease—coexisting, easily treatable illness may be found

ADDITIONAL EDUCATIONAL RESOURCES

- Burns A, O'Brien J. Clinical practice with anti-dementia drugs: a consensus statement from British Association for Psychopharmacology. *J Psychopharmacol* 2006;20:732-55.
- Alzheimer's Society. *Dementia in the community: management strategies for primary care.* London: AS, 2006.
- Alzheimer's Australia. *Mind your mind: a user's guide to dementia risk reduction.* www.alzheimers.org.au/upload/MYM_book_lowres.pdf

Competing interests: AB is editor in chief of the *International Journal of Geriatric Psychiatry* and receives research funding and consultancy fees from pharmaceutical companies involved in the manufacture and marketing of drugs for Alzheimer's disease including Eisai, Pfizer, Shire, Novartis, Janssen-Cilag, Lundbeck, and Wyeth. SI was a member of the guidelines development group (2004-6) for the joint NICE and Social Care Institute for Excellence guidelines and of the Dementia Strategy External Reference Group (2008).

Provenance and peer review: Commissioned; externally peer reviewed.

1 Ferri CP, Prince M, Brayne C, Brodaty H, Fratiglioni L, Ganguli M, et al. Global prevalence of dementia: a Delphi consensus study. *Lancet* 2005;366:2112-7.
2 Burns A, Jacoby R, Levy R. Psychiatric phenomena in Alzheimer's disease. *Br J Psychiatry* 1990;157:72-94.
3 Feldman H, Woodward M. The staging and assessment of moderate to severe Alzheimer disease. *Neurology* 2005;65:S10-7.
4 Snowdon DA, Greiner LH, Mortimer JA, Riley KP, Greiner PA, Markesbery WR. Brain infarction and the clinical expression of Alzheimer disease. The Nun Study. *JAMA* 1997;277:813-7.
5 Matthews FE, McKeith I, Bond J, Brayne C; MRC CFAS. Reaching the population with dementia drugs: what are the challenges? *Int J Geriatr Psychiatry* 2007;7:627-31.
6 Brayne C. The elephant in the room—healthy brains in later life, epidemiology and public health. *Nat Rev Neurosci* 2007;8:233-9.
7 Nestor PJ, Scheltens P, Hodges JR. Advances in the early detection of Alzheimer's disease. *Nat Rev Neurosci* 2004;5:S34-41.
8 Chong MS, Sahadevan S. An evidence-based clinical approach to the diagnosis of dementia. *Ann Acad Med Singapore* 2003;32:740-8

9 Spaan PE, Raaijmakers JG, Jonker C. Alzheimer's disease versus normal ageing: a review of the efficiency of clinical and experimental memory measures. *J Clin Exp Neuropsychol* 2003;25:216-33.
10 Leroi I, Lyketsos C. Neuropsychiatric aspects of dementia. In: Burns A, O'Brien J, Ames D, eds. *Dementia* . 3rd ed. London:Hodder Arnold, 2005:55-64.
11 McKhann G, Drachman D, Folstein M, Katzman R, Price D, Stadlan EM. Clinical diagnosis of Alzheimer's disease: report of the NINCDS-ADRDA Work Group under the auspices of Department of Health and Human Services Task Force on Alzheimer's Disease. *Neurology* 1984;34:939-44.
12 Dubois. Research criteria for the diagnosis of Alzheimer's disease: revising the NINCDS–ADRDA criteria. *Lancet* 2007;6:734-46.
13 Chui HC, Victoroff JI, Margolin D, Jagust W, Shankle R, Katzman R. Criteria for the diagnosis of ischemic vascular dementia proposed by the State of California Alzheimer's Disease Diagnostic and Treatment Centers. *Neurology* 1992;42:473-80.
14 Román GC, Tatemichi TK, Erkinjuntti T, Cummings JL, Masdeu JC, Garcia JH, et al. Vascular dementia: diagnostic criteria for research studies: report of the NINDS-AIREN International Workshop. *Neurology* 1993;43:250-60.
15 McKeith IG, Dickson DW, Lowe J, Emre M, O'Brien JT, Feldman H, et al. Diagnosis and management of dementia with Lewy bodies: third report of the DLB consortium. *Neurology* 2005;65:1863-72.
16 Burns A, Byrne J, Ballard C, Holmes C. Sensory stimulation in dementia: an effective option for managing behavioural problems. *BMJ* 2002;325:1312-3.
17 Burns A, O'Brien J. Clinical practice with anti-dementia drugs: a consensus statement from British Association for Psychopharmacology. *J Psychopharmacol* 2006;20:732-55.
18 Waldemar G, Phung KTT, Burns A, Georges J, Hansen FR, Iliffe S, et al. Access to diagnostic evaluation and treatment for dementia in Europe. *Int J Geriatr Psychiatry* 2007;22:47-54.
19 Wang PS, Schneeweiss S, Avorn J, Fischer MA, Mogun H, Solomon DH, et al. Risk of death in elderly users of conventional vs. atypical antipsychotic medications. *N Engl J Med* 2005;353:2335-41.
20 Schneider LS, Dagerman KS, Insel P. Risk of death with atypical antipsychotic drug treatment for dementia: meta-analysis of randomized placebo-controlled trials. *JAMA* 2005;294:1934-43.
21 Holmes. The efficacy of donepezil in the treatment of neuropsychiatric symptoms in Alzheimer disease. *Neurology* 2004;63:214 -9
22 O'Brien J. Antipsychotics for people with dementia. *BMJ* 2008;337:a602.
23 Brodaty H, Green A, Koschera A. Meta-analysis of psychosocial interventions for caregivers of people with dementia. *J Am Geriatr Soc* 2003;51:657-64.
24 Callahan C, Boustani M, Unverzagt F, Austrom M, Damush T, Perkins A, et al. Effectiveness of collaborative care for older adults with Alzheimer's disease in primary care: a randomized controlled trial. *JAMA* 2006;295:2148-57.

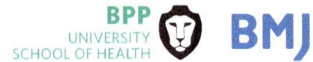

Depression in older adults

Joanne Rodda, clinical training fellow in old age psychiatry, Zuzana Walker, reader in old age psychiatry, Janet Carter, senior lecturer in old age psychiatry

Department of Mental Health Sciences, University College London, London W1W 7EJ, UK

Correspondence to: J Carter j.carter@ucl.ac.uk

Cite this as: BMJ 2011;343:d5219

DOI: 10.1136/bmj.d5219

http://www.bmj.com/content/343/bmj.d5219

Depression is a major contributor to healthcare costs and is projected to be the leading cause of disease burden in middle and higher income countries by the year 2030.[w1] Depression in later life, traditionally defined as age older than 65, is associated with disability, increased mortality, and poorer outcomes from physical illness. Most clinicians will encounter older patients with depression in their day to day practice, but although treatment is as effective for older patients as for younger adults, the condition is often under-recognised and under-treated. According to WHO data, proportionately more people aged over 65 commit suicide than any other age group, and most have major depression. Older people who attempt suicide are more likely to die than younger people, while in those who survive, prognosis is worse for older adults.[1]

With a progressively ageing population worldwide, identification and treatment of depression in older adults becomes increasingly important, especially as older patients may have different presentations and needs than younger ones. We consider recent systematic reviews, meta-analyses, and randomised controlled trials to provide generalists with an understanding of current approaches to the diagnosis and management of patients who develop late life depression.

What is late life depression and who gets it?

Traditionally, the age of 65 has been used to differentiate between "older" and "younger" adults, although there is no set point at which an individual becomes "older" and assessment and care must be based on individual need. Arbitrary definitions of "late life" and differences between studies in terms of diagnostic criteria and populations sampled have produced varying reports of prevalence. Individuals with late life depression represent a heterogeneous group with symptoms that may fall anywhere on a spectrum ranging from sub-threshold mood disorder to major depression. A recent comprehensive meta-analysis using studies with moderate to high methodological quality showed that the point prevalence of major depression in over 75s ranged from 4.6% to 9.3%[2] whereas rates for sub-threshold depressive symptoms (those failing to reach diagnostic criteria) ranged from 4.5% to 37.4%. A related meta-analysis in people aged over 55 found that sub-threshold depressive symptomatology was two to three times more prevalent than major depression.[2] Most depressive episodes in late life will be a recurrence rather than a first ever episode[w2] and the increased female to male ratio is in line with that in younger adults.

Prevalence rates of depression are increased in brain disorders including dementia, Parkinson's disease, and stroke, and also in systemic disease, for example diabetes mellitus and cardiovascular disease (box 1). Prevalence estimates for depression in Alzheimer's disease cluster around 30% but range from 0% to 86%,[w3] reflecting the difficulty associated with definition and diagnosis of depression in dementia.

How is depression diagnosed in older patients?

Box 2 lists the Diagnostic and Statistical Manual of Mental Disorders (DSM-IV) criteria for diagnosis of a major depressive episode. Ideally diagnosis is based on clinical interview, observation of the patient's behaviour, and a collateral history from relatives and care givers. When taking a background history it is important to identify factors that may precipitate and maintain depression. The main risk factors for late life depression are comorbid physical illness, cognitive impairment, functional impairment, lack or loss of close social contacts, and a previous history of depression (box 1), according to the findings of large community based studies.

The risk assessment is important in any psychiatric presentation, and in patients with depression the main area of risk is suicide. Methodologically sound controlled studies have identified some key risk factors for suicide, listed in box 3.

Older patients often have symptoms of depression that do not meet the criteria for a major depressive episode (box 2) but are nonetheless clinically important. Identification of the psychological and functional effects of these symptoms determines whether or not treatment is indicated and who may benefit from interventions.

Current guidance for the assessment and management of depression from the UK National Institute for Health and Clinical Excellence (NICE) (http://guidance.nice.org.uk/CG90/QuickRefGuide/pdf/English) recommends the use of rating scales to determine severity, although many are weighted towards the presence of somatic symptoms and may therefore overestimate depression in older people, in whom such symptoms are common.

A recent comparison of several assessment scales (patient health questionnaire, Beck depression inventory, hospital anxiety and depression scale) in a primary care population found that treatment and referral rates were identical even though each tool identified differing numbers of patients with moderate to severe depression. However, regardless of the tool used, rates for treatment in older people still remained lower than for younger adults.[w4] Many rating scales are in common use to assess depression but

SUMMARY POINTS

- Depression in older adults is associated with an increased risk of death and disability
- Cognitive and functional impairment and anxiety are more common in older than in younger adults with depression
- Older adults with depression are at increased risk of suicide and are more likely than younger adults to complete suicide
- Depression is associated with cognitive impairment and an increased risk of dementia
- A selective serotonin reuptake inhibitor should be the first line pharmacological treatment for depression for most older adults, including those with chronic physical illness
- Psychological and drug treatment is as effective in older as in younger adults
- Subthreshold depressive symptoms that substantially affect older patients' lives are common and management with psychosocial and drug strategies may be effective and prevent further deterioration

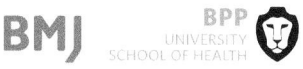

BOX 1 RISK FACTORS FOR DEPRESSION IN ELDERLY PEOPLE[30]

Physical factors

- Chronic disease, such as diabetes, ischaemic heart disease, heart failure, chronic obstructive pulmonary disease
- Acute myocardial infarction
- Organic brain disease: dementia, stroke, Parkinson's disease, cerebrovascular disease
- Endocrine/metabolic disorders: thyroid disease, hypercalcaemia, B12 and folate deficiency
- Malignancy
- Chronic pain and disability

Psychosocial factors

- Social isolation
- Change in financial circumstances
- Being a carer
- Change of role and loss of social status
- Bereavement and loss
- Difficulty in adapting to illness/pain/disability
- Poor defences against anxiety about death
- History of depression
- Being in institutional care

BOX 2 DSM-IV CRITERIA FOR MAJOR DEPRESSIVE EPISODE

- Nearly every day for the preceding two weeks the patient has experienced five or more of:
- Depressed mood for most of the day*
- Decreased interest or pleasure in nearly all activities for most of the day*
- Marked loss or gain of weight or markedly increased or decreased appetite
- Excessive sleep or not enough sleep
- Observable psychomotor agitation or retardation
- Tiredness or loss of energy
- Feelings of guilt or worthlessness
- Poor concentration or indecisiveness
- Thoughts of dying or suicide, suicide attempt

*One of these features must be present. Depressed mood for .2 weeks not meeting these criteria is defined as a minor depressive episode. Diagnostic and statistical manual of mental disorders (DSMIV), American Psychiatric Association, 1994

BOX 3 RISK FACTORS FOR SUICIDE IN OLDER PEOPLE[1]

- Older age, male sex
- Social isolation
- Bereavement
- History of attempts
- Evidence of planning
- Chronic painful illness or disability
- Drug or alcohol use
- Sleep disorders

BOX 4 USEFUL SCALES FOR DEPRESSION

Geriatric depression scale (GDS-15)*

- Specifically developed for use in geriatric patients; contains fewer somatic items; suitable only for patients with no, mild, or moderate cognitive impairment (>15/30 on mini-mental state examination)
- Well validated in older people. Cut-off score in population over 60 of ≥5 indicates a case of depression: sensitivity 92%, specificity 54%[w12 w13]

Cornell scale for depression in dementia (CSDD)*

- Suitable for patients with cognitive deficit, not diagnostic for depression but higher scores indicate greater need for further evaluation[w14]

Patient health questionnaire (PHQ-9)*

- Self reported depression assessment tool scoring each of the nine DSM-IV criteria as 0 (not at all) to 3 (nearly every day)
- Validated in adults over 60 in primary care in the United States and Netherlands. With cut-off score of >9 has sensitivity 88%, specificity 80%[w15 w16]

Beck depression inventory (BDI)

- Self reported seven item scale
- Not recommended for use in older people owing to focus on somatic symptoms[w17]

Hospital anxiety and depression scale (HADS)*

- Self-rating scale containing two subscales measuring symptoms of depression (HADS-D) and anxiety (HADS-A) during previous week. Scores >8 for both HADS-A and HADS-D have sensitivity and specificity of 80% and predictive validity of 70%
- HADS identifies equal numbers of patients with depression regardless of age[w18]

Montgomery and Åsberg depression rating scale (MADRS)

- Clinician rated 10 item scale, measures severity of depressive symptoms; sensitive to change; mainly used to assess response to treatment but no agreement on cut-off score for remission (between ≤4 and ≤10), popular in Europe

*Validated in older adults

few are well validated in older people, with the exception of the patient health questionnaire, geriatric depression scale, hospital anxiety and depression scale, and the Cornell scale for depression in dementia (box 4).

Is depression more difficult to diagnose in older adults?

Several studies have shown that older adults are significantly less likely than younger ones to recognise depressive symptoms, which they attribute to normal ageing or physical illness, and that both patients and their doctors tend to view depression as a problem that can be explained away, rather than as an objective illness that warrants treatment.[w5] These findings suggest that older adults might be less able to identify, and therefore seek appropriate treatment for, common depressive symptoms.

In our clinical experience, late life depression differs qualitatively from depression in early life. Somatisation, hypochondriasis, psychomotor retardation or agitation, and psychosis more commonly form part of the clinical picture, although this tendency has not been uniformly demonstrated.[3] Furthermore, late life depression has been associated with cognitive impairment, physical disability, and anxiety, with a large community naturalistic study suggesting that clinically important anxiety coexists in around 50% of patients aged 55-85.[4]

Does depression increase the risk of dementia?

Most studies find that depression in late life is accompanied by measurable cognitive impairment, mediated by memory deficits, diminished executive function, and slowed information processing, which may resolve on remission of symptoms, or may persist even after effective treatment of mood. In the past, the term "depressive pseudodementia" was used to describe reversible dementia in depression,

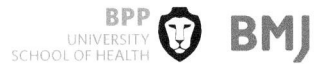

but this oversimplifies the complex spectrum of cognitive impairment.

Two systematic meta-analyses of high quality studies[5][6] report that late onset depression (after age 65) increases the risk of dementia twofold, but as yet no research has ascertained whether depression is a risk factor for dementia or represents a prodromal condition.[7]

Several mechanisms have been proposed to explain the relation between depression and dementia, including hypercortisolaemia, loss of hippocampal volume, neuroinflammatory processes, increased Alzheimer-type pathology, reduced cognitive reserve, and vascular disease. None has yet been conclusively demonstrated, but the link is probably multifactorial and the mechanisms not mutually exclusive.

Of these potential mechanisms, vascular changes in the brain have attracted most attention. The key hypothesis is that disruption of prefrontal-striatal circuitry by cerebrovascular pathology produces a syndrome of mood disorder and executive dysfunction. This syndrome is variously described as "vascular depression" or "depression executive dysfunction syndrome",[8] reflecting fundamental nosological differences. However, the concept is controversial, and a prospective population based postmortem study of over 65s found no association between depression and cerebrovascular pathology.[9] Randomised controlled trials have shown that presence of "vascular depression"/"depression executive dysfunction syndrome" may predict a worse response to antidepressant drug treatment[10] and is associated with increased mortality[11] There is currently no evidence to suggest that treating depression in early or late life reduces the incidence of dementia.

How is late life depression managed?

Given the association between medical morbidity and depression, exclusion of underlying causative or exacerbating factors is an important first step in the management of late life depression (box 1). Baseline investigations, for example routine blood tests, may be indicated (box 5).

In subsyndromal and mild depression, psychosocial interventions may be sufficient to cause an improvement. These include increasing social contact and adding structure to the day; for example, assistance in accessing local community events, day centres, or befriending services. Evidence from randomised trials suggests that depressive symptoms in older adults may improve with structured exercise programmes.[12] A RCT of a stepped care approach to the management of subthreshold depressive symptoms found that the intervention (watchful waiting, bibliotherapy based on cognitive behavioural therapy, problem solving therapy, and medication) was associated with a 50% reduction in depression and anxiety disorders at 12 months[13] compared with treatment as usual and was cost effective[w6].

Current NICE guidance recommends that patients with mild or sub-threshold illness who do not respond well to initial supportive interventions are offered psychological therapy or antidepressant medication, while a combination of both interventions is recommended for those with moderate or severe illness.

When should I refer?

NICE guidance recommends that patients are referred to specialist services if they have not responded adequately to management options available in primary care; in severe depression, psychosis, or complex psychosocial situations; and where the degree of risk warrants specialist input.

> **BOX 5 INVESTIGATIONS TO CONSIDER WHEN DEPRESSION IS SUSPECTED**
>
> - Full blood count
> - Urea and electrolytes
> - Liver function tests
> - Thyroid function tests
> - Vitamin B12
> - Folate
> - Fasting glucose
> - Bone profile
> - Further tests dictated by clinical presentation

We also emphasise the need to refer older people with comorbid cognitive decline.

Services available in the UK vary geographically and are constantly evolving. A randomised controlled trial of home treatment versus conventional outpatient care for patients aged over 64 living independently and recruited from primary and secondary care services in Austria found significantly reduced depressive symptoms, improved global function, fewer admissions and lower costs of care in the home treatment arm at 3 and 12 months' follow-up.[14] Studies of collaborative care interventions, where care is delivered through integrated mental health and primary care providers, have also repeatedly reported improved outcomes compared with usual care[w7] although the effect appeared to be associated with prescription of antidepressant medication rather than better communication between primary care providers and mental health services.

Which medication should be prescribed?

Selective serotonin reuptake inhibitors (SSRIs) are well established as first line treatment for depression in older adults. A Cochrane review included 32 randomised controlled trials of antidepressant treatment in people aged 55 or over and reported that SSRIs and tricyclic antidepressants had similar efficacy, but that tricyclics were associated with more side effects and withdrawal from treatment.[15] It was not possible to compare efficacy for other antidepressant groups. Findings from a 2008 meta-analysis of second generation antidepressants in older adults (SSRIs, selective serotonin and noradrenaline reuptake inhibitors, bupropion, and mirtazapine) found that treatment in studies lasting 10 weeks or longer was associated with an improved response, supporting the long held belief that response to antidepressants is delayed in older adults.[16] A recent meta-analysis showed an advantage of SSRIs or tricyclic antidepressants over placebo in the treatment of patients with depression in the context of chronic physical illness.[17] Furthermore, evidence from randomised controlled trials has shown that antidepressants are efficacious in depression after stroke[18] and myocardial infarction.[19] Interestingly, a 2007 meta-analysis of 10 randomised controlled trials of prophylactic antidepressant treatment after stroke reported a significant reduction in the rate of post-stroke depression in treatment groups.[20] However, a large randomised controlled trial has recently shown that two commonly used antidepressants, sertraline and mirtazapine, were not appreciably different from placebo in treating depression in patients with Alzheimer's disease. This effect was sustained at 10 months' follow-up and side effects were increased in the antidepressant group.[21]

Overall, an SSRI is usually the safest choice in patients with physical illness; the most common drug interactions are mediated via cytochrome p450 enzymes, and citalopram, escitalopram, and sertraline are safest in this regard.

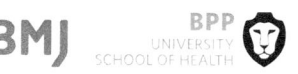

Common side effects of particular concern in the elderly are anticholinergic effects, postural hypotension, and sedation, all of which are more common with tricyclic antidepressants than with SSRIs.[20] The risk can be minimised by starting at a low dose and slowly titrating upward. The risk of hyponatraemia induced by antidepressants increases with age and is associated with female sex, low body weight, renal failure, prescription of other drugs associated with hyponatraemia (such as diuretics), and medical comorbidity.[w8 w9] Older patients prescribed SSRIs are also at increased risk of both upper and lower gastrointestinal bleeding.[w10] Monitoring of serum sodium levels may be necessary, and the risk of gastrointestinal bleeding can be reduced by prescribing proton pump inhibitors.

NICE guidance recommends that antidepressant treatment is continued for at least six months for a single episode and at least two years if patients are thought to be at risk of relapse. A meta-analysis of eight double-blind placebo controlled trials of maintenance antidepressant therapy between 6 and 36 months in people over 55, published in 2011, found that the optimal duration in older adults is uncertain.[22] We suggest that a practical approach is to regularly review depressive symptoms, side effects, comorbidity, and current psychosocial stressors and to involve the patient in the decision making process about ongoing drug treatment.

What if first line drug treatment doesn't work?

A 2011 systematic review and meta-analysis of inadequate response to treatment in older patients included 13 studies, most of which were open label.[23] The overall response rate for active treatment was 52%, and studies reporting positive results for augmentation of treatment with lithium or antipsychotics, and treatment with venlafaxine, duloxetine, selegiline, or phenelzine, were included. Lithium augmentation was the only treatment for which evidence of efficacy was replicated in more than two studies. We suggest that augmentation of treatment with antipsychotic medication should be used with particular caution in view of the susceptibility of older people to adverse drug reactions, and the paucity of data on safety.

Electroconvulsive therapy is sometimes used after inadequate response to drug treatment, although the usual indication is severe depressive illness in which life threatening refusal of food or fluid, risk of suicide, or psychotic features are present. Electroconvulsive therapy is a safe and effective treatment in the elderly despite an absence of methodologically sound evidence from randomised controlled trials.[24]

Can older adults benefit from psychological therapy?

Results from a 2009 meta-regression analysis suggest that psychological therapy—particularly cognitive behavioural therapy, interpersonal therapy, and problem solving therapy—is equally effective in older and younger adults with depression.[25] Combined psychological therapy and pharmacological therapy is more effective than psychological treatment alone for older people with depression.[26]

What is the outlook for older adults with depression?

A 2005 systematic review of studies comparing outcomes in depression in middle life with those in later life found that rates of remission were similar in both groups, but that late life depression was associated with higher rates of relapse.[27] A longitudinal primary care cohort study in the Netherlands reported that the median duration of a major depressive

---

SOURCES AND SELECTION CRITERIA

We based the review on searches of PubMed, EMBASE, and the Cochrane Database of Systematic Reviews using the search terms "depression", "elderly", "aged", and "old age" published between 2006 and 2011 and limited to English language. We focused on well conducted systematic reviews, meta-analyses, and randomised controlled trials.

TIPS FOR THE NON-SPECIALIST

- Exclude physical illness as a cause for apparent depressive symptoms
- Bear in mind that factors associated with ageing and the later stages of life, including physical illness, organic brain disease, pain, disability, losses (such as bereavement), and social isolation, create vulnerability to depression
- Be aware that older people with depression may minimise depressive symptoms and may present with somatic problems
- Discuss options for treatment with the patient
- Consider psychosocial interventions first in subsyndromal depressive states and mild depression
- If medication is needed, use an SSRI at a therapeutic dose as first line treatment unless contraindications are present
- Use the same criteria for referral for psychological therapy as in younger adults; older people are just as able to benefit
- Evaluate risk; more people aged over 65 commit suicide than any other age group and most have major depression
- Refer to specialist care if there is substantial risk of self harm, psychosis, need for complex multiprofessional care, inadequate response to treatment, or cognitive impairment
- If treatment is started, evaluate response and need for ongoing treatment regularly

Points to discuss with the patient

- Depression can affect people in different ways; some people may have strong feelings of sadness, but others may be more aware of feeling tired, slowed down, irritable, indecisive, that everything is an effort, or that they worry unnecessarily about small things and experience various physical problems—all these can be symptoms of depression and are not necessarily just part of "getting old"
- There are many different ways to help people get well, for example taking part in social activities, attending clubs and interest groups; physical exercise; talking therapies, and medication
- The beneficial effects of medication may take two to six weeks to be noticeable, but side effects may occur straight away; medication should ideally be continued for at least six months

---

episode in late life was 18 months, with two thirds of patients taking three years to recover.[28] In the PRISM-E study, a large study of older patients with major depressive disorder, complete remission was attained in only 29% of patients at six month follow-up.[29] Factors associated with prolonged recovery in these studies included severity of depression at baseline, a family history of depression, comorbid anxiety, and general medical comorbidity.

A population based, age stratified, longitudinal study found that adults aged 70-84 years with depression have an increased risk of mortality compared with those who do not have depression, dying on average three years earlier. This risk holds beyond the effects of age, sex, and the presence of dementia, cardiovascular, and other somatic diseases, but did not persist in the oldest old—defined as those aged 85 to 101.[w11]

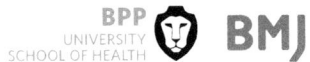

ADDITIONAL EDUCATIONAL RESOURCES

For patients

- Depression (www.ageuk.org.uk/health-wellbeing/conditions-illnesses/depression)—informative web page from Age UK, a charity supporting people in later life
- Depression in older adults—(www.rcpsych.ac.uk/mentalhealthinfoforall/problems/depression/depressioninolderadults.aspx) online information leaflet from the UK Royal College of Psychiatrists
- CG90 Depression in adults: understanding NICE guidance (http://guidance.nice.org.uk/CG90/PublicInfo/pdf/English)—explanation of NICE guidance for those using health services in NHS England and Wales

For healthcare professionals

- Depression: the treatment and management of depression in adults (update) (http://guidance.nice.org.uk/CG90)—guidance from NICE
- Depression (www.cks.nhs.uk/depression/view_whole_topic)—clinical knowledge summary from NHS Evidence
- GPNotebook (www.gpnotebook.co.uk)—online medical encyclopaedia

QUESTIONS FOR FUTURE RESEARCH

- How can we differentiate between depressive syndromes in older adults, for example those overlapping with anxiety and cognitive impairment?
- Does neuroimaging have a role in assessment of depression in older people?
- How can we better identify and manage depression in dementia?
- Are there ways of preventing depression in older adults at a population level?
- What is the optimal period of maintenance treatment for depression in older adults?

Contributors: JR and JC were responsible for the planning, research, writing, and editing of the article. ZW was involved in the planning, writing and editing. JC is the guarantor.

Competing interests: All authors have completed the ICMJE uniform disclosure form at www.icmje.org/coi_disclosure.pdf (available on request from the corresponding author) and declare: no support from any organisation for the submitted work; no financial relationships with any organisations that might have an interest in the submitted work in the previous three years; no other relationships or activities that could appear to have influenced the submitted work.

Provenance and peer review: Commissioned, externally peer reviewed.

1 Manthorpe J, Iliffe S. Suicide in later life: public health and practitioner perspectives. Int J Geriatr Psychiatry 2010;25:1230-8.
2 Meeks TW, Vahia IV, Lavretsky H, Kulkarni G, Jeste DV. A tune in "a minor" can "b major": a review of epidemiology, illness course, and public health implications of subthreshold depression in older adults. J Affect Disord 2011;129:126-42.
3 Alvarez P, Urretavizcaya M, Benlloch L, Vallejo J, Menchon JM. Early- and late-onset depression in the older: no differences found within the melancholic subtype. Int J Geriatr Psychiatry 2011;26:615-21.
4 Beekman AT, de BE, van Balkom AJ, Deeg DJ, van DR, van TW. Anxiety and depression in later life: Co-occurrence and communality of risk factors. Am J Psychiatry 2000;157:89-95.
5 Jorm AF. History of depression as a risk factor for dementia: an updated review. Aust N Z J Psychiatry 2001;35:776-81.
6 Ownby RL, Crocco E, Acevedo A, John V, Loewenstein D. Depression and risk for Alzheimer disease: systematic review, meta-analysis, and metaregression analysis. Arch Gen Psychiatry 2006;63:530-8.
7 Byers AL, Yaffe K. Depression and risk of developing dementia. Nat Rev Neurol 2011;7:323-31.
8 Sneed JR, Culang-Reinlieb ME. The vascular depression hypothesis: an update. Am J Geriatr Psychiatry 2011;19:99-103.
9 Tsopelas C, Stewart R, Savva GM, Brayne C, Ince P, Thomas A, et al. Neuropathological correlates of late-life depression in older people. Br J Psychiatry 2011;198:109-14.
10 Alexopoulos GS, Kiosses DN, Heo M, Murphy CF, Shanmugham B, Gunning-Dixon F. Executive dysfunction and the course of geriatric depression. Biol Psychiatry 2005;58:204-10.
11 Vilalta-Franch J, Planas-Pujol X, Lopez-Pousa S, Llinas-Regla J, Merino-Aguado J, Garre-Olmo J. Depression subtypes and 5-years risk of mortality in aged 70 years: a population-based cohort study. Int J Geriatr Psychiatry 2011, doi:10.1002/gps.2691.
12 Blake H, Mo P, Malik S, Thomas S. How effective are physical activity interventions for alleviating depressive symptoms in older people? A systematic review. Clin Rehabil 2009;23:873-87.
13 Van't Veer-Tazelaar PJ, van Marwijk HW, van Oppen P, van Hout HP, van der Horst HE, Cuijpers P, et al. Stepped-care prevention of anxiety and depression in late life: a randomized controlled trial. Arch Gen Psychiatry 2009;66:297-304.
14 Klug G, Hermann G, Fuchs-Nieder B, Panzer M, Haider-Stipacek A, Zapotoczky HG, et al. Effectiveness of home treatment for elderly people with depression: randomised controlled trial. Br J Psychiatry 2010;197:463-7.
15 Mottram P, Wilson K, Strobl J. Antidepressants for depressed elderly. Cochrane Database Syst Rev 2006;1:CD003491.
16 Nelson JC, Delucchi K, Schneider LS. Efficacy of second generation antidepressants in late-life depression: a meta-analysis of the evidence. Am J Geriatr Psychiatry 2008;16:558-67.
17 Taylor D, Meader N, Bird V, Pilling S, Creed F, Goldberg D. Pharmacological interventions for people with depression and chronic physical health problems: systematic review and meta-analyses of safety and efficacy. Br J Psychiatry 2011;198:179-88.
18 Robinson RG, Spalletta G. Poststroke depression: a review. Can J Psychiatry 2010;55:341-9.
19 Green LA, Dickinson WP, Nease DE, Schellhase KG, Campos-Outcalt D, Schoof BK et al. AAFP guideline for the detection and management of post-myocardial infarction depression. Ann Fam Med 2009;7:71-9.
20 Chen Y, Patel NC, Guo JJ, Zhan S. Antidepressant prophylaxis for poststroke depression: a meta-analysis. Int Clin Psychopharmacol 2007;22:159-66.
21 Banerjee S, Hellier J, Dewey M, Romeo R, Ballard C, Baldwin R, et al. Sertraline or mirtazapine for depression in dementia (HTA-SADD): a randomised, multicentre, double-blind, placebo-controlled trial. Lancet 2011;378:403-11.
22 Kok RM, Heeren TJ, Nolen WA. Continuing treatment of depression in the elderly: a systematic review and meta-analysis of double-blinded randomized controlled trials with antidepressants. Am J Geriatr Psychiatry 2011;19:249-55.
23 Cooper C, Katona C, Lyketsos K, Blazer D, Brodaty H, Rabins P, et al. A systematic review of treatments for refractory depression in older people. Am J Psychiatry 2011.
24 Stek ML, Van der Wurff FB, Hoogendijk WL, Beekman AT. Electroconvulsive therapy for the depressed elderly. Cochrane Database Syst Rev 2006;2:CD003593.
25 Cuijpers P, van SA, Smit F, Andersson G. Is psychotherapy for depression equally effective in younger and older adults? A meta-regression analysis. Int Psychogeriatr 2009;21:16-24.
26 Cuijpers P, van SA, Warmerdam L, Andersson G. Psychotherapy versus the combination of psychotherapy and pharmacotherapy in the treatment of depression: a meta-analysis. Depress Anxiety 2009;26:279-88.
27 Mitchell AJ, Subramaniam H. Prognosis of depression in old age compared to middle age: a systematic review of comparative studies. Am J Psychiatry 2005;162:1588-601.
28 Licht-Strunk E, Van Marwijk HW, Hoekstra T, Twisk JW, De HM, Beekman AT. Outcome of depression in later life in primary care: longitudinal cohort study with three years' follow-up. BMJ 2009;338:a3079.
29 Azar AR, Chopra MP, Cho LY, Coakley E, Rudolph JL. Remission in major depression: results from a geriatric primary care population. Int J Geriatr Psychiatry 2011;26:48-55.
30 Colasanti V, Marianetti M, Micacchi F, Amabile GA, Mina C. Tests for the evaluation of depression in the elderly: a systematic review. Arch Gerontol Geriatr 2010;50:227-30.

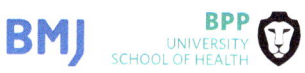

Management of depression in adults

Markku Timonen, professor of general practice[1], Timo Liukkonen, senior consultant[2]

[1]Institute of Health Sciences, University of Oulu, Box 5000, FIN-90014, Finland

[2]Department of Psychiatry, Savonlinna Central Hospital, Finland

Correspondence to: M Timonen markku.timonen@oulu.fi

Cite this as: BMJ 2008;336:435

DOI: 10.1136/bmj.39478.609097.BE

http://www.bmj.com/content/336/7641/435

A study by the World Health Organization ranked depression the fourth global burden of disease and found it to be the largest non-fatal burden of disease, with nearly 12% of total years lived with disability.[1] According to the cross sectional WHO world health survey, carried out in all regions of the world (60 countries), the one year prevalence of a depressive episode (international classification of diseases, 10th revision) was 3.2% (95% confidence interval 3.0% to 3.5%). In patients with several medical conditions the prevalence of depression exceeds that of the general population,[2] with 5-10% of patients affected in primary care and 10-14% of patients under general hospital care.[3] The diagnosis and treatment of depression by general practitioners is not, however, always optimal.[4][5] We review the presentation and assessment of depression and discuss the options for its effective treatment and management.

Why is depression so difficult to diagnose?

According to cross sectional studies 50-70% of patients with depression in primary care remain undetected, with somatisation being one of the most important single problems associated with a missed diagnosis.[5] Given that about two thirds of depressed patients present mainly with somatic symptoms,[6] detecting depression in connection with somatisation should be a core professional skill of doctors. During consultation the discussion should move away from somatic symptoms to emotional health by asking patients open questions on what they think is the cause of their physical symptoms. It is also worth inquiring about possible life events preceding the symptoms.

The detection of depression can be improved by training in mental health and screening.[5] Patients at high risk in both primary care and general hospital settings (for example, those with chronic medical illness, chronic pain syndromes, recent life events, fair or poor self rated health, and unexplained physical symptoms[7]) can be screened for depression by asking two questions on mood and interest (box 1).[8] Eventually, however, the diagnosis is a clinical one, which must be obtained through consultation to determine whether the criteria for depression are met (fig 1). Although drugs and general medical conditions such as hypothyroidism, hyperthyroidism, Huntington's disease, Cushing's disease, and Addison's disease do not represent a substantial public health problem as a causal

factor for depression, management, when appropriate, must be directed at the underlying condition rather than the depressive symptoms. More commonly several physical illnesses occur with depression; if so, treatment must be directed at the depression as well as the illness.[7] Depression also occurs commonly with anxiety disorders.[5] Depression requires treatment first when it is considered the primary diagnosis.

What should be taken into account while building a management plan?

Guidelines for depression emphasise the importance of an effective doctor-patient relationship while an appropriate and comprehensive management plan is being negotiated (box 2), and this relationship should continue throughout treatment. Factors that also need to be taken into account when designing the management plan and deciding on a treatment setting are patients' preferences, concomitant psychiatric and physical disorders, concurrent drugs, patients' experiences with previous treatments, the severity of depressive symptoms or subtypes of depression, risk of suicide, and availability of treatment options.[9][10][11]

As single component interventions, such as screening alone, have been shown to be ineffective in the management of depression in primary care, complex multifaceted educational and organisational interventions have been developed to improve outcomes.[4][5] A recent systematic review and metaregression found that the effective determinants of "collaborative care" (one particular multifaceted intervention), were systematic identification of patients, case managers with a professional background, and regular supervision of case managers by specialists.[12] Despite a lack of corresponding studies outside the United States[11][12] the collaborative care model seems promising for enhancing treatment outcomes and bridging the gap between primary and secondary care, given that it allows patients to be managed by case managers or primary care providers under specialist supervision without the need for treatment elsewhere.

Which treatment setting?

More than 80% of patients with depression are managed and treated in primary care.[11] The treatment of depressed patients in secondary care should be skewed towards those with more severe disease. Specialist treatment is indicated for patients displaying psychotic features or active suicidality. Moreover, specialists should be involved when patients are resistant to treatment or have recurrent depression. A stepped care model (fig 2), originally introduced by the National Institute for Health and Clinical Excellence (NICE), lists the needs associated with treating or managing depression at different service levels.[10][11]

How is depression managed in the acute phase?

Although most of the interventions for treating depression have been carried out in high income countries, an increasing amount of evidence comes from low income and middle income countries.[13] Whatever the treatment for depression the primary goal in the acute phase is remission

SUMMARY POINTS

- Somatisation is one of the most important single problems associated with a missed diagnosis of depression in primary care
- Depression should be managed comprehensively and the efficacy of treatment evaluated for the first time within one month
- When response to treatment is poor the diagnosis and compliance with treatment should be reassessed
- Psychosocial treatments are first line treatments for mild depression
- Structured psychological interventions, such as cognitive behaviour therapy and interpersonal therapy, and antidepressants are effective in moderate to severe depression
- Evidence suggests that combined antidepressant and cognitive behaviour therapy is more efficacious than antidepressants alone in moderate to severe depression and chronic depression

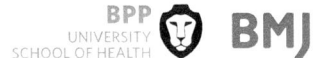

BOX 1 TWO SCREENING QUESTIONS FOR DEPRESSION

- During the past month have you often been bothered by feeling down, depressed, or hopeless?
- During the past month have you often been bothered by having little interest or pleasure in doing things?

If patients answer yes to either question then the specificity of screening can be further increased by asking them whether they want help with their problems

---

BOX 2 COMPONENTS OF A COMPREHENSIVE MANAGEMENT PLAN FOR DEPRESSION. ADAPTED FROM AMERICAN PSYCHIATRIC ASSOCIATION AND WORLD FEDERATION OF SOCIETIES OF BIOLOGICAL PSYCHIATRY GUIDELINES[9] [10]

- Determine the pharmacological or psychosocial treatment
- Determine the treatment setting
- Establish and maintain a therapeutic alliance
- Monitor and reassess the patient's psychiatric status in the course of treatment
- Monitor the patient's response to treatment
- Reassess the adequacy of diagnosis when appropriate
- Monitor possible side effects and physical condition
- Enhance treatment adherence
- Educate patients and their families about the nature of the illness (psychoeducation)

---

of symptoms,[9] [10] given that remission is associated with a better prognosis than the improvement of depressive symptoms without remission.[14]

Psychological treatments

In mild depression, based mostly on clinical experience, NICE recommends a further assessment within two weeks (watchful waiting) for those not agreeing to intervention and for those who healthcare professionals believe may recover spontaneously without intervention.[11] Otherwise the recommended first line treatments for mild depression on the basis of substantial research based evidence are guided self help as well as brief psychological interventions (6-8 sessions) including problem solving therapy, brief cognitive behaviour therapy, and counselling.[11] Evidence also shows that problem solving therapy, brief cognitive behaviour therapy, and counselling are effective in moderate depression.[11] On the basis of substantial evidence from a randomised controlled trial (274 participants), a NICE guideline recommends one of three types of computerised cognitive behaviour therapy as optional for the treatment of mild and moderate depression.[15] Antidepressants are not recommended for the initial treatment of mild depression because of minimal evidence to support their efficacy and a poor risk-benefit ratio.[10] [11]

Several structured psychological interventions (16-20 sessions) were found to be effective for moderate to severe depression. Firstly, research based evidence favouring individual cognitive behaviour therapy over a wait list control is good.[11] Secondly, in a small number of well designed randomised controlled trials interpersonal therapy was more effective than placebo or usual care by a general practitioner.[11] Group interpersonal therapy was also found to be efficacious in a randomised controlled trial in a low income country.[16] Finally, data from two small randomised controlled trials to treat depression suggest that marital therapy (treatment for couples with depressed spouses, when relationship problems are associated with depression) is more efficacious than no therapy,[17] but clear evidence is lacking for the efficacy of family therapy and short term psychodynamic psychotherapy.[9] [11] [18] Although patients generally prefer these psychological treatments, they are not always available.[19]

Pharmacological treatment

Robust evidence from numerous randomised controlled trials shows that tricyclic antidepressants, selective serotonin reuptake inhibitors (SSRIs), and selective serotonin and norepinephrine reuptake inhibitors are more efficacious than placebo for treating major depressive disorder.[10] Most of the investigations were, however, sponsored by the pharmaceutical industry.[11] [20] The evidence for serotonergic-noradrenergic mirtazapine is also well documented.[10] [11]

A Cochrane review and meta-analyses of 194 randomised controlled trials found that the tricyclic antidepressant amitriptyline (one of the reference compounds for pharmacological treatment of depression) can still be regarded at least as efficacious as other tricyclic antidepressants or SSRIs, although it is not as well tolerated as SSRIs.[21] Also, according to the few randomised controlled trials carried out in low income and middle income countries,[13] a multifaceted stepped care model including treatment with amitriptyline, imipramine, or fluoxetine for those with severe or persistent depression by structured pharmacotherapy programme,[22] and fluoxetine alone[23] have been shown to be efficacious in treating depression. Generally, strong evidence suggests that SSRIs are better tolerated than tricyclic antidepressants.[21] NICE recommends SSRIs as first choice drugs for depression.[11]

International classification of disease, 10th revision	Diagnostic and Statistical Manual of Mental Disorders, fourth edition
Depressive episode	**Major depressive episode**
Typical symptoms:	**A** Five (or more) of the following symptoms have been present during the same two week period and at least one of the symptoms is either depressed mood or loss of interest or pleasure. Each symptom should be present most of the day or nearly every day:
• Depressed mood	
• Loss of interest and enjoyment	
• Increased fatiguability	
	• Depressed mood
Common symptoms:	• Diminished interest or pleasure in almost all activities
• Reduced concentration and attention	• Significant weight loss or weight gain or decreased or increased appetite
• Reduced self esteem and self confidence	• Insomnia or hypersomnia
• Ideas of guilt and unworthiness	• Psychomotor agitation or retardation
• Bleak and pessimistic views of future	• Fatigue or loss of energy
• Ideas or acts of self harm or suicide	• Feeling of worthlessness or inappropriate guilt
• Disturbed sleep	• Diminished ability to think or concentrate or indecisiveness
• Diminished appetite	• Recurrent thoughts of death, suicidal ideation, suicide attempt, or suicide plan
F32.0 Mild depressive episode - at least two of the typical symptoms and at least two of the common symptoms, and none should present to an intense degree	**B** The symptoms do not meet criteria for a mixed episode
F32.1 Moderate depressive episode - at least two of the typical symptoms and at least three of the common symptoms	**C** The symptoms cause clinically significant distress or impairment in social, occupational, or other important areas of functioning
F32.2 Severe depressive episode - all the typical symptoms and at least four of the common symptoms, and some should be of severe intensity	**D** The symptoms are not due to the direct physiological effects of a substance (for example, a drug of misuse, a medication) or a general medical condition (for example, hypothyroidism)
F32.3 Severe depressive episode with psychotic symptoms - criteria given for F32.2 and in which delusions, hallucinations, or depressive stupors are present	**E** The symptoms are not better accounted for by bereavement
Minimum duration of an episode is about two weeks, and patient has never had a manic or hypomanic episode	**296.2x Major depressive disorder, single episode** • Presence of a single major depressive episode • The major depressive episode is not better accounted for by schizoaffective and is not superimposed on schizophrenia or schizophreform, delusional or psychotic disorder otherwise specified • A manic, a mixed, or a hypomanic episode has never occurred
Further depressive episodes should be classified under one of the subdivisions of recurrent depressive disorder (F33.1-3)	Presence of two or more major depressive episodes justifies a diagnosis of major depressive disorder, recurrent 296.3x

Fig 1 Classification criteria for depression

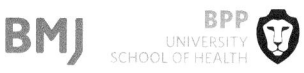

Severity	Responsibility	Focus	Interventions
	Inpatient care, crisis teams	Severe dysfunction, risk for life	Medication, combination treatments, electroconvulsive therapy
	Mental health specialist, including crisis teams	Treatment resistant, recurrent, atypical and psychotic depression, those with special risk	Medication, complex psychotherapeutic treatments, combination treatments
	Mental health specialist, general practitioner or primary care team	Moderate to severe depression	Medication or psychotherapeutic treatments, or both, psychosocial interventions
		Mild depression	Observation, psychoeducation, psychosocial interventions. Psychotherapeutic or biological treatments, or both (if appropriate)
	General practitioner or primary care doctor, practice nurse	Recognition	Assessment

Fig 2 Stepped care model for treatment and management of depression in primary care. Adapted from World Federation of Societies of Biological Psychiatry guideline, original idea from NICE guideline[10] [11]

A recent systematic review and meta-analysis of 93 published and unpublished randomised controlled trials showed that serotonergic-noradrenergic antidepressant drugs had a modest efficacy advantage over SSRIs, the number needed to treat to benefit being about 24.[24] Irreversible monoamine oxidase inhibitors, an older class of antidepressants, are not considered first line treatments because of their potentially fatal side effects.[10] We believe that moclobemide (a reversible monoamine oxidase inhibitor) is not suitable as first line treatment for depression owing to the potential risk of serotonergic syndrome and the unconditional need for a wash-out period while switching antidepressants.

All guidelines[9] [10] [11] emphasise the importance of clinical judgment when applying the evidence from clinical trials to individual patients. For example, participants in clinical trials are often free of common concomitant psychiatric or physical conditions, and thus the generalisability of the results to real world circumstances are questionable. When prescribing antidepressants, potential side effects and interactions with current drugs need to be considered along with a patients' preference and experience of previous treatments. Furthermore, antidepressants are associated with poor rates of remission—in one trial remission occurred in only 36.8% of participants treated with an SSRI.[14] Finally, the better treatment outcomes with multifaceted interventions rather than with treatments as usual[4] also highlight the importance of factors other than antidepressants in the management of depression.

Combination of pharmacological and psychological treatments

Strong evidence shows efficacy of combined antidepressant and cognitive behaviour therapy over antidepressant alone in moderate to severe depression and in chronic depression.[11] One relatively small randomised controlled trial found interpersonal therapy combined with antidepressants to be more efficacious than interpersonal therapy alone.[11]

How should treatment efficacy be evaluated?

Response to treatment must be carefully monitored irrespective of the chosen treatment modality, and structured measures of symptom severity and functional status can be used.[9] According to the World Federation of Societies of Biological Psychiatry guideline for primary care, the efficacy of antidepressant treatment should be evaluated 2-4 weeks after the primary care provider starts treatment, using patient self rating or observer rating scales (box 3).[10] This evaluation can also be done by other healthcare professionals in the primary care team.[4] [14] It should be remembered, however, that remission is a clinical judgment that cannot be replaced by rating scales.

What should be done if patients do not respond to treatment in the acute phase?

If the response to antidepressants is insufficient after 2-4 weeks then strategies to optimise treatment should be implemented.[10] Normal clinical practice at this point is to increase the antidepressant dose to the upper level of the standard dose.[10] [11] On the basis of a systematic review of eight randomised controlled trials on dose escalation, evidence is insufficient for dose escalation of SSRIs.[25]

If patients show no improvement after four weeks of pharmacological treatment[10] or at least moderate improvement after 4-8 weeks of psychological[9] treatment then the diagnosis and compliance to treatment should be reassessed. If the diagnosis is still depression, a new management plan must be negotiated, taking into account patients' preferences and availability of treatments: options to consider when psychological treatment has been part of the man agement plan are changing intensity or type of psychotherapy, changing to pharmacological treatment, and combining antidepressant with ongoing psychotherapy.[9] The general consensus on antidepressants is to switch to another one. A systematic review of eight randomised controlled trials and 23 open studies found that any switch within or between classes of antidepressants seems legitimate after the first use of an SSRI.[26]

How is depression treated in a continuation phase?

The goal of the continuation phase is to stabilise the remission and to prevent relapse.[10] Antidepressants should be continued for about six months after remission because strong evidence shows that this reduces the risk of relapse.[11] The antidepressant and dose successfully used in the acute phase should be given during the continuation phase.[10] If no relapse occurs and the patient does not need prophylactic treatment, then gradual discontinuation of the antidepressant over four weeks is recommended at the end of this phase,[9] [10] [11] with the patient being informed about possible discontinuation or withdrawal symptoms.

Studies of psychotherapies in continuation and maintenance phases are largely lacking.[9] A recent systematic review and meta-analysis of four clinical trials (three randomised controlled trials) found that cognitive behaviour therapy during the continuation phase significantly

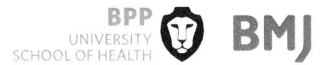

BOX 3 EVALUATING THE EFFICACY OF TREATMENT FOR DEPRESSION. ADAPTED FROM WORLD FEDERATION OF SOCIETIES OF BIOLOGICAL PSYCHIATRY GUIDELINE[10]

- Non-response—25% or less decrease in symptom severity compared with baseline
- Partial response—26-49% decrease in symptom severity compared with baseline
- Response—50% or greater decrease in severity of symptoms compared with baseline
- Remission—absence of symptoms defined by absolute scale (for example, score of ≤7 on Hamilton rating scale for depression)

Several patient self rating and observer rating scales are available—for example, Beck depression inventory, 16 item clinician rated quick inventory of depressive symptomatology, Hamilton rating scale for depression, Montgomery-Asberg depression rating scale

BOX 4 FACTORS ASSOCIATED WITH INCREASED RISK FOR DEPRESSION RECURRENCE. ADAPTED FROM WORLD FEDERATION OF SOCIETIES OF BIOLOGICAL PSYCHIATRY GUIDELINE[10]

- Three or more episodes of major depression
- High prior frequency of recurrence
- Previous episode in past year
- Residual symptoms during continuation phase treatment
- Severity of episodes (for example, suicidality and psychotic features)
- Long previous episodes
- Relapse after drug withdrawal

SOURCES AND SELECTION CRITERIA

We searched PubMed, the Cochrane database of systematic reviews, and citation lists of relevant publications using the subject headings and key words "depression", "major depression", "treatment", "management", "psychosocial", and "pharmacological." We also searched guidelines from the National Institute for Health and Clinical Excellence, the American Psychiatric Association, and the World Federation of Societies of Biological Psychiatry.

TIPS FOR NON-SPECIALISTS

- A definitive diagnosis of depression should be assessed within one or two weeks of the initial visit
- Rule out bipolar disorder by questioning whether mania or hypomania has occurred earlier in life
- In addition to suicidal ideas and intent ask patients directly about hallucinations and delusions
- Become familiar with the efficacy of some locally available first line and second line antidepressants and their short and long term side effects and interactions with other drugs
- A member of the primary care team should learn one of the observer rating scales for depression to evaluate the efficacy of treatment
- Patients should be seen weekly or biweekly during the acute phase and every month or bimonthly during the continuation phase

reduced the rate of relapse and recurrence compared with controls who received assessment only. The efficacy of the therapy, based on five small randomised controlled trials, was similar to that of other active treatments such as pharmacotherapy.[27]

ONGOING RESEARCH

- To identify the active elements of the multifaceted interventions in the management of depression
- In the Cochrane Collaboration, as part of the multiple meta-analyses of new generation antidepressants (MANGA) study, separate reviews are comparing the efficacy of commonly used new compounds with other antidepressants
- New antidepressants with novel mechanisms of action, such as melatonergic agomelatine, are being developed
- Ongoing research is investigating technological adaptations on psychotherapies, especially computerised cognitive behaviour psychotherapy
- A promising treatment for depression, transcranial magnetic stimulation, might have significant antidepressant effects, but larger multicentre studies are needed to assess this modality
- Therapeutic brain stimulation through delivery of pulsed electrical impulses to the left cervical vagus nerve, vagus nerve stimulation, is a novel approach for treatment resistant depression

ADDITIONAL EDUCATIONAL RESOURCES

- National Institute for Health and Clinical Excellence, Depression (http://guidance.nice.org.uk/CG23)
- Clinical guideline, based on the best available evidence, on the appropriate treatment within the National Health Service in England and Wales
- Royal College of Psychiatry (www.rcpsych.ac.uk)
- Structured leaflets on depression and related issues in different languages for patient education purposes
- Cochrane Database of Systematic Reviews (www3.interscience.wiley.com/cgi-bin/mrwhome/106568753/HOME)
- High quality, independent, systematic reviews on psychotherapies and pharmacotherapies

Information for patients

- National Institute for Health and Clinical Excellence. Depression: information for the public (amended) (http://guidance.nice.org.uk/CG23/publicinfo/pdf/English)
- Freely available information on the care people with depression can expect to receive from their general practitioner or other healthcare professionals
- Royal College of Psychiatry (www.rcpsych.ac.uk)
- Freely available information for the public on depression, in different languages

Which patients need maintenance or prophylactic treatment?

Given that depression has a strong tendency for recurrence (30-40% of patients with depression in primary care[28]), prophylactic therapy is indicated for patients at high risk of recurrence (box 4).[10] A consultant psychiatrist or specialist in secondary care should evaluate the need for maintenance or prophylactic treatment.[10 11]

We thank V Benno Meyer-Rochow for checking the English language of this paper.

Contributors: Both authors researched and drafted the sections with which they were most familiar. MT combined the separate sections. Both authors contributed to and approved all versions of the manuscript. MT is the guarantor.

Competing interests: MT has been reimbursed by GlaxoSmithKline, Eli Lilly, Novartis, and H Lundbeck for attending six conferences, was paid by Eli Lilly and Astra Zeneca for speaking on seven different occasions, and has served as coauthor or principal investigator in international multicentred placebo controlled clinical trials organised and financed by five different medical companies. TL has been reimbursed by H Lundbeck, Astra Zeneca, and Wyeth for attending

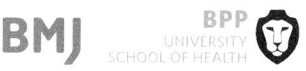

three conferences, has been paid for speaking on two occasions by Pfizer, and has received personal funds for research from H Lundbeck.

Provenance and peer review: Commissioned and externally peer reviewed.

1   Ustün TB, Ayuso-Mateos JL, Chatterji S, Mathers C, Murray CJ. Global burden of depressive disorders in the year 2000. *Br J Psychiatry* 2004;184:386-92.

2   Moussavi S, Chatterji S, Verdes E, Tandon A, Patel V, Ustun B. Depression, chronic diseases, and decrements in health: results from the world health surveys. *Lancet* 2007;370:851-8.

3   Katon WJ. Clinical and health services relationships between major depression, depressive symptoms, and general medical illness. *Biol Psychiatry* 2003;54:216-26.

4   Williams JW Jr, Gerrity M, Holsinger T, Dobscha S, Gaynes B, Dietrich A. Systematic review of multifaceted interventions to improve depression care. *Gen Hosp Psychiatry* 2007;29:91-116.

5   Tylee A, Walters P. Underrecognition of anxiety and mood disorders in primary care: why does the problem exist and what can be done? *J Clin Psychiatry* 2007;68(suppl 2):27-30.

6   Tylee A, Gandhi P. The importance of somatic symptoms in depression in primary care. *Prim Care Companion J Clin Psychiatry* 2005;7:167-76.

7   Williams JW Jr, Noël PH, Cordes JA, Ramirez G, Pignone M. Is this patient clinically depressed? *JAMA* 2002;287:1160-70.

8   Arroll B, Goodyear-Smith F, Kerse N, Fishman T, Gunn J. Effect of the addition of a "help" question to two screening questions on specificity for diagnosis of depression in general practice: diagnostic validity study. *BMJ* 2005;331:884-6.

9   American Psychiatric Association. Practice guideline for the treatment of patients with major depressive disorder (revision). *Am J Psychiatry* 2000;157(suppl 4):1-45.

10   Bauer M, Bschor T, Pfennig A, Whybrow PC, Angst J, Versiani M, et al. World Federation of Societies of Biological Psychiatry (WFSBP) guidelines for biological treatment of unipolar depressive disorders in primary care. *World J Biol Psychiatry* 2007;8:67-104.

11   National Institute for Clinical Excellence. *Depression: management of depression in primary and secondary care* . London: NICE, 2004. (National Clinical Practice Guideline No 23.)

12   Bower P, Gilbody S, Richards D, Fletcher J, Sutton A. Collaborative care for depression in primary care. Making sense of a complex intervention: systematic review and meta-regression. *Br J Psychiatry* 2006;189:484-93.

13   Patel V, Araya R, Chatterjee S, Chisholm D, Cohen A, De Silva M, et al. Treatment and prevention of mental disorders in low-income and middle-income countries. *Lancet* 2007;370:991-1005.

14   Rush AJ, Trivedi MH, Wisniewski SR, Nierenberg AA, Stewart JW, Warden D, et al. Acute and longer-term outcomes in depressed outpatients requiring one or several treatment steps: a STAR*D report. *Am J Psychiatry* 2006;163:1905-17.

15   National Institute for Health and Clinical Excellence. Technological Appraisal 97 Computerised cognitive behaviour therapy for depression and anxiety: Guidance. 22 Feb 2006. http://guidance.nice.org.uk/TA97/guidance/pdf/English.

16   Bolton P, Bass J, Neugebauer R, Verdeli H, Clougherty KF, Wickramaratne P, et al. Group interpersonal psychotherapy for depression in rural Uganda. *JAMA* 2003;289:3117-24.

17   Barbato A, D'Avanzo B. Marital therapy for depression. *Cochrane Database Syst Rev* 2006;(Issue 2):CD004188. doi: 10.1002/14651858.CD004188.pub2.

18   Henken HT, Huibers MJH, Churchill R, Restifo K, Roelofs J. Family therapy for depression. *Cochrane Database Syst Rev* 2007;(Issue 3):CD006728. doi: 10.1002/14651858.CD006728.

19   Wolf NJ, Hopko DR. Psychosocial and pharmacological interventions for depressed adults in primary care: a critical review. *Clin Psychol Rev* 2008;28:131-61.

20   Melander H, Ahlqvist-Rastad J, Meijer G, Beermann B. Evidence biased medicine—selective reporting from studies sponsored by pharmaceutical industry: review of studies in new drug applications. *BMJ* 2003;326:1171-3.

21   Guaiana G, Barbui C, Hotopf M. Amitriptyline for depression. *Cochrane Database Syst Rev* 2007;(Issue 3):CD004186. doi: 10.1002/14651858.CD004186.pub2.

22   Araya R, Rojas G, Fritsch R, Gaete J, Rojas M, Simon G, et al. Treating depression in primary care in low-income women in Santiago, Chile: a randomised controlled trial. *Lancet* 2003;361:995-1000.

23   Patel V, Chisholm D, Rabe-Hesketh S, Dias-Saxena F, Andrew G, Mann A. Efficacy and cost-effectiveness of drug and psychological treatments for common mental disorders in general health care in Goa, India: a randomised, controlled trial. *Lancet* 2003;361:33-9.

24   Papakostas GI, Thase ME, Fava M, Craig Nelson J, Shelton RC. Are antidepressant drugs that combine serotonergic and noradrenergic mechanisms of action more effective than the selective serotonin reuptake inhibitors in treating major depressive disorder? A meta-analysis of studies of newer agents. *Biol Psychiatry* 2007;62:1217-27.

25   Ruhé HG, Huyser J, Swinkels JA, Schene AH. Dose escalation for insufficient response to standard-dose selective serotonin reuptake inhibitors in major depressive disorder: systematic review. *Br J Psychiatry* 2006;189:309-16.

26   Ruhé HG, Huyser J, Swinkels JA, Schene AH. Switching antidepressants after a first selective serotonin reuptake inhibitor in major depressive disorder: a systematic review. *J Clin Psychiatry* 2006;67:1836-55.

27   Vittengl JR, Clark LA, Dunn TW, Jarret RB. Reducing relapse and recurrence in unipolar depression: comparative meta-analysis of cognitive-behavioural therapy's effects. *J Consult Clin Psychol* 2007;3:475-88.

28   Van Weel-Baumgarten EM, Schers HJ, van den Bosch WJ, van den Hoogen HJ, Zitman FG. Long-term follow-up of depression among patients in the community and in family practice settings. A systematic review. *J Fam Pract* 2000;49:1113-20.

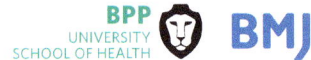

Long term treatment of depression with selective serotonin reuptake inhibitors and newer antidepressants

Steven Reid, consultant psychiatrist[1], Corrado Barbui, lecturer in psychiatry[2]

[1]Department of Liaison Psychiatry, St Mary's Hospital, London W2 1PF

[2]Department of Medicine and Public Health, Section of Psychiatry and Clinical Psychology, University of Verona, 37134 Verona, Italy

Correspondence to: S Reid steve. reid@nhs.net

Cite this as: BMJ 2010;340:c1468

DOI: 10.1136/bmj.c1468

http://www.bmj.com/content/340/bmj.c1468

The introduction of fluoxetine in 1987 marked the arrival of the selective serotonin reuptake inhibitors (SSRIs) for the treatment for depression. In the United States antidepressant prescriptions accounted for 2.6% of primary care visits in 1989, rising to 7.1% in 2000.[1] This pattern was reflected across Europe, where SSRIs are now the most commonly prescribed antidepressants. Newer antidepressants, such as the serotonin norepinephrine reuptake inhibitors, including venlafaxine and duloxetine, also contributed to the remarkable increase in antidepressant prescribing.[2]

Several reasons were put forward for this trend: improved tolerability; reduced lethality in overdose; the aggressive marketing of newly patented drugs; the wider range of available antidepressants; and ease of prescription. An analysis of the UK general practice research database showed that prescriptions almost doubled from 1993 to 2005.[3] However, the increase in antidepressant prescribing was not accounted for by new diagnoses but rather a rise in the number of prescriptions given for long term treatment: although the proportion of patients receiving short term treatment declined, the proportion of patients receiving continuing prescriptions for over five years increased. Another primary care study found that the mean duration of antidepressant prescriptions for depression was 4.8 years and 48% of the sample received treatment for more than two years.[4]

The early optimism accompanying SSRIs has faded amid controversy over their effectiveness and safety.[5] Recent meta-analyses have concluded that antidepressants have only a modest advantage over placebo, with the magnitude of benefit increasing with severity of depression.[6][7] Debate has persisted about the association between SSRIs and suicidal behaviour,[8] considerable disquiet has been expressed about the perceived medicalisation of social problems that really require social solutions. In this review we examine the evidence for the benefits and harms of long term use of SSRIs and newer antidepressants in adults with major depression.

Do SSRIs reduce the risk of relapse or recurrence of depression?

Depression is commonly a recurrent illness: over half of people with a diagnosis of major depression will go on to have a further episode, and the risk of future relapse rises, with 80% of those having a second episode going on to have a third.[9] Most clinical guidelines recommend that treatment with antidepressants should be continued for four to six months after recovery to reduce the risk of relapse (re-emergence of original symptoms) and recurrence (new episode of depression).[10][11] However, the benefits of long term or maintenance treatment are considered, particularly by clinicians, to be less certain.[12]

A systematic review included 31 randomised trials (4410 participants) investigating whether continuing treatment with antidepressants (of all classes, although most included either a tricyclic antidepressant or an SSRI) reduced the risk of relapse.[13] These trials were mainly discontinuation studies in which participants with depressive disorders who had responded to acute treatment were randomly assigned to continue drug treatment or receive a placebo.

Pooled results found that, compared with placebo, continuing antidepressant treatment after recovery markedly reduced the proportion of patients who relapsed over one to three years (pooled odds ratio for relapse 0.30; 95% confidence interval 0.22 to 0.38). A re-analysis of these data (shown in table 1), summarises the rates of relapse by length of follow-up.[14] While the absolute risk reduction progressively increased from six to 36 months of follow-up, the relative risk reduction was stable (from 60% at six months to 58% at 36 months), suggesting that continuing antidepressant treatment more than halved the average relapse rate regardless of the duration of treatment. The absolute risk reduction was similar at six and 12 months, although the larger sample size at 12 months provides a more precise estimate. On average four patients required antidepressant treatment to prevent one additional relapse. Further systematic reviews, restricted to data on SSRIs and newer antidepressants (bupropion, mirtazapine, nefazodone, and venlafaxine), produced similar findings: a risk reduction in the proportion of patients relapsing of about 50%.[15] These trials also indicate that the reduction in relapse rates with prophylactic antidepressants is greater for patients with single episodes (odds ratio for relapse 0.12; 0.06 to 0.26) than for those with recurrent episodes (0.37; 0.31 to 0.44).[16]

Discontinuation trials have been criticised as their results apply only to patients responding to treatment and not to those who experience spontaneous recovery.[17] In addition, discontinuation of treatment may result in withdrawal symptoms that mimic depression itself, leading to an overestimate of the true effect of the medication. A systematic review comprising continuation trials only—

SUMMARY POINTS

- The rise in the prescribing of antidepressants is largely accounted for by an increase in long term treatment
- Half of people with a diagnosis of major depression will go on to have a further episode, and risk of recurrence increases with each episode
- Evidence for the benefits of long term prescribing of antidepressants comes almost exclusively from secondary care settings
- Continuing antidepressant treatment roughly halves the absolute risk of relapse
- The increased risk of suicidal behaviour associated with selective serotonin reuptake inhibitors (SSRIs) is restricted to people aged under 25
- People with risk factors for relapse of depression should be advised to continue with SSRIs for at least 12 months and consider long term treatment

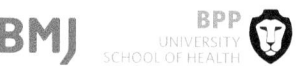

Table 1 Antidepressant drugs compared with placebo for preventing relapse in depression: summary measures by length of follow-up*

Follow-up (months)	Relapse rate in participants (%)		Relative risk reduction (%) (95% CI)	Absolute risk reduction (%) (95% CI)	Number needed to treat (95% CI)	No of studies (participants: antidepressant/ placebo)
	Antidepressant	Placebo				
6	14.7	36.8	60 (48 to 70)	22 (16 to 29)	4.5 (3.5 to 6.4)	9 (442/296)
12	17.1	37.0	54 (47 to 59)	20 (17 to 23)	5.0 (4.3 to 6.0)	12 (1604/1122)
18	16.2	47.9	66 (47 to 78)	32 (21 to 43)	3.1 (2.3 to 4.8)	3 (117/123)
24	28.4	60.8	53 (40 to 64)	32 (23 to 42)	3.1 (2.4 to 4.4)	6 (190/166)
36	29.8	71.5	58 (47 to 67)	42 (32 to 51)	2.4 (1.9 to 3.1)	5 (174/176)
Overall	19.1	43.0	55 (51 to 59)	24 (21 to 27)	4.2 (3.8 to 4.7)	35 (2525/1883)

95% CI= 95% confidence interval.

Absolute numbers were extracted from figure 1 of Furukawa et al.[14] Recalculations were performed using the spreadsheet available at www.ebpcenter.com/spreadsheets/index.html.

that is, trials in which participants with depression were randomly assigned to SSRIs or placebo, with longer term follow-up of those that responded—pooled results from six trials that comprised 1299 participants and found that SSRIs were significantly superior to placebo at six to eight months (odds ratio 1.66, 1.12 to 2.48), though a less dramatic effect than that observed in discontinuation trials.[18]

What are the potential harms of long term treatment with SSRIs?

Self harm and suicide

Systematic reviews of randomised trials suggest an increased risk of self harm in people prescribed SSRIs, particularly those aged under 25 years, but no clear relation with completed suicide.[8] The evidence from trials is limited, however, by short duration of follow-up, and as suicide is a rare outcome most trials lack sufficient power to measure an effect.

Observational studies with large populations offer an additional perspective and, importantly, include completed suicide as an outcome. A recent systematic review combined data from eight observational studies (over 200 000 patients) that reported data on completed or attempted suicide in depressed individuals who had taken SSRIs for depression and in individuals who had received no antidepressant treatment.[19] SSRIs increased the risk of completed or attempted suicide when prescribed for adolescents (odds ratio 1.92; 95% confidence interval 1.51 to 2.44) but reduced the risk when prescribed for adults (0.57; 0.47 to 0.70). In individuals aged 65 or above, exposure to SSRIs also had a protective effect (0.46; 0.27 to 0.79). These results are in line with the conclusions of the recent US Food and Drug Administration's re-analysis of clinical trial data, which showed that the risk of suicidal behaviour was raised in people aged under 25, not affected in those aged 25-64, and reduced in those aged 65 and older,[20] suggesting that prescribing SSRIs in adults with major depression may be considered a strategy for reducing suicide risk.

Discontinuation effects

Missed doses are common with any long term drug treatment, but with SSRIs and newer antidepressants abrupt interruption of treatment may lead to discontinuation symptoms.[21] These symptoms develop 24-72 hours after interruption and include dizziness, vertigo, nausea, fatigue, headache, anxiety, agitation, insomnia, irritability, akathisia, electric shock-like sensations, and, possibly, aggressive and impulsive behaviour. For most, discontinuation symptoms are mild and short lived, but they can sometimes be severe and prolonged. They may be mistaken for signs of physical

illness, or as they include psychological and behavioural symptoms they may be misinterpreted as early signs of relapse.

Data on SSRI discontinuation symptoms are mainly drawn from spontaneous reports of adverse drug reactions, but evidence from prospective studies shows that duration of treatment increases the risk of occurrence and that they are more likely after treatment with antidepressants that have a short half life, such as paroxetine and venlafaxine.[21] [22] Consequently, clinical guidelines recommend warning patients about the possibility of discontinuation symptoms and advising that antidepressants should not be stopped abruptly. Dose of treatment should be gradually reduced over at least four weeks.[21] [23]

Sexual dysfunction

Sexual dysfunction is a common though often neglected adverse effect of antidepressants. All three phases of the sexual response cycle may be affected: reduced interest and desire for sex; erectile dysfunction in men and diminished arousal in women; and difficulty in attaining orgasm in both sexes. A systematic review quantifying prevalence of sexual adverse effects emerging with use of antidepressants found rates of 4% to 80% after four to 12 weeks of treatment (table 2) compared with 14% associated with placebo.[24] Newer antidepressants were associated with the highest rates of sexual dysfunction,[24] a finding confirmed in a meta-analysis of 104 experimental and observational studies: citalopram (73%), paroxetine (71%), and venlafaxine (67%) had the highest incidence of sexual dysfunction, while mirtazapine (24%) and nefazodone (8%) had the lowest.[25] Evidence is lacking to support any strategy to manage sexual dysfunction caused by antidepressants. Spontaneous remission may occur, but for most patients sexual dysfunction persists during treatment.[26] Switching drugs is an option, but another drug may not be equally effective.

Pregnancy

The safety of antidepressants in pregnancy is an important consideration for women treated with SSRIs. A review of antenatal mental health care is beyond the scope of this article, but substantial literature is now available to support decision making.[27] SSRIs do not seem to increase the risk of birth defects after exposure during the first trimester; the exception is paroxetine, which is associated with a 1.5-fold increased risk for congenital heart defects. As a class, SSRIs taken after 20 weeks' gestation may be associated with an increased risk of persistent pulmonary hypertension in the neonate, and all antidepressants prescribed in the third trimester may cause discontinuation effects, notably

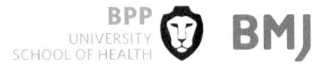

Table 2   Sexual dysfunction associated with four to 12 weeks of antidepressant use. Adapted from Serretti and Chiesa[24]

Drug	Prevalence (%)	Odds ratio (compared with placebo) (95% CI)
Citalopram	79	20.3 (14.6 to 29.9)
Duloxetine	42	4.3 (2.8 to 6.6)
Escitalopram	37	3.4 (2.3 to 5.1)
Fluoxetine	71	15.6 (13.0 to 18.8)
Imipramine	44	7.2 (2.6 to 20.1)
Mirtazapine	24	2.3 (0.8 to 6.8)
Moclobemide	4	0.2 (0 to 2.1)
Nefazodone	8	0.5 (0.1 to 1.6)
Paroxetine	71	16.9 (13.5 to 19.8)
Sertraline	80	27.4 (19.4 to 38.9)
Venlafaxine	80	24.8 (19.1 to 32.4)

95% CI= 95% confidence interval.

irritability, in the newborn, although these are usually mild and self limiting. Clinical guidelines recommend therefore that paroxetine should be stopped during pregnancy, and although SSRIs are not contraindicated, consideration should be given to use of tricyclic antidepressants, which have lower known risks in pregnancy.[28]

Bleeding disorders

Observational studies have shown that SSRIs and venlafaxine increase the risk of upper gastrointestinal haemorrhage and other bleeding disorders, probably by altering platelet function.[29] A case-control study using the UK Health Improvement Network's database (www.thin-uk.com/) estimated that 2000 patients a year would require treatment with SSRIs for one case of attributable upper gastrointestinal bleeding. This risk was modifiable, increasing considerably (number needed to harm 250) with concurrent use of low dose aspirin or non-steroidal anti-inflammatory drugs, but reduced by use of acid suppressing drugs.[30]

Hyponatraemia

Hyponatraemia is a potentially serious adverse effect, which has been associated with most antidepressants but reported most frequently with SSRIs.[31] Reported incidence rates suggest that three to five cases of hyponatraemia induced by SSRIs per 1000 patients a year may be expected, but substantially higher rates have been reported in older people, particularly women. Hyponatraemia manifests with muscle cramps, fatigue, and confusion, and it may result in seizures. When it is detected, antidepressants should be withdrawn immediately. Monitoring of serum sodium concentration is advisable in individuals aged 80 years or older, those with a history of hyponatraemia, or those receiving other drug treatments associated with hyponatraemia.[32]

Cardiovascular effects

In contrast to tricyclic antidepressants, SSRIs do not slow cardiac conduction, prolong the QT interval, or cause orthostatic hypotension[33] so are considered safe to use in cardiovascular disease. Observational evidence supports this, with no evidence of an increased risk of myocardial infarction or cardiovascular mortality with long term treatment.[34] Evidence from randomised trials has also shown no additional risk with SSRIs after myocardial infarction.[35]

An evidence based approach to long term treatment with SSRIs and newer antidepressants

In adults with depression who have benefited from treatment with an antidepressant good evidence exists that they are at high risk of relapse, particularly in the

---

SOURCES AND SELECTION CRITERIA

To identify relevant articles, we searched the Cochrane Library, Clinical Evidence, the National Institute for Health and Clinical Excellence's website, and Medline. We combined the search terms "major depressive disorder" and "antidepressant" with terms for adverse events ("adverse events", "harms", "drug reactions", "toxicity") and benefit ("efficacy", "effectiveness"). We gave priority to systematic reviews, meta-analyses, and evidence based clinical guidelines published within the past 10 years. When no report of those types was available, we considered individual randomised controlled trials or observational studies.

RISK FACTORS FOR RELAPSE OF MAJOR DEPRESSION

- Presence of residual symptoms
- Number of previous episodes
- Severity of most recent episode
- Duration of most recent episode
- Degree of treatment resistance in previous episode

---

first six months after recovery. Good evidence also exists that continuing antidepressant treatment reduces the absolute risk of relapse by about 50%. The trials on which guidelines are based come predominantly from secondary care settings with follow-up limited to three years. Longer term studies that include patients from primary care with less severe illness would inform clinical practice. Psychological treatments may augment the prophylactic effect of antidepressants, but much of the evidence for this has been incon clusive. Several studies have found that cognitive behavioural therapy combined with maintenance drug treatment significantly reduces rates of relapse compared with antidepressants alone, although whether this additional benefit is due to non-specific therapeutic effects is not clear.[36]

In summary, after a single depressive episode in the absence of specific risk factors for relapse (see the box on risk factors) people should be advised to continue treatment with antidepressants for 12 months after recovery. Treatment should be regularly re-evaluated, with the frequency determined by the severity of the episode. Individuals with risk factors for relapse, in particular those with several previous episodes or two episodes in the recent past, should be advised to continue with treatment for at least 12 months and consider long term maintenance treatment. With long term antidepressant treatment, regular reviews should take into consideration the social consequences of relapse for the individual, concurrent physical health problems, and the development of adverse effects, as well as patient preference.

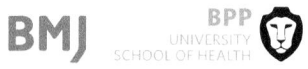
QUESTIONS FOR FUTURE RESEARCH

- Do selective serotonin reuptake inhibitors (SSRIs) continue to reduce the risk of relapse after three years?
- Do antidepressants differ in their effectiveness for preventing relapse?
- Are some subtypes of depression more responsive than others to treatment with selective serotonin reuptake inhibitors?
- How do psychological treatments compare with selective serotonin reuptake inhibitors in the prevention of relapse?

ADDITIONAL EDUCATIONAL RESOURCES

For healthcare professionals

- National Institute for Health and Clinical Excellence. Depression: the treatment and management of depression in adults (update). 2009. (Clinical guideline 90.) http://guidance.nice.org.uk/CG90
- National Institute for Health and Clinical Excellence. Depression in adults with a chronic physical health problem: treatment and management. 2009. (Clinical guideline 91.) http://guidance.nice.org.uk/CG91. This document gives a comprehensive summary of potential drug interactions
- British Association for Psychopharmacology (www.bap.org.uk)—Evidence based guidelines for treating depression
- Clinical Evidence (http://clinicalevidence.bmj.com/ceweb/index.jsp)—Up to date review of research evidence; registration required
- UK NHS Evidence—mental health (www.library.nhs.uk/mentalHealth/)—Evidence based reviews, updates and monthly newsletter
- Cochrane Collaboration (www.cochrane.org/)—International network for preparation and updating of reviews of interventions using the best available evidence

For patients

- Depression Alliance UK (www.depressionalliance.org/)—Help and information about depression
- Royal College of Psychiatrists (www.rcpsych.ac.uk/)—A range of information leaflets on depression in several languages

TIPS FOR NON-SPECIALISTS

- Treatment with selective serotonin reuptake inhibitors should be regularly reviewed
- Ask patients about adverse effects
- People with risk factors for relapse should continue treatment for at least 12 months
- When stopping a patient's treatment with selective serotonin reuptake inhibitors, gradually reduce the dose over four weeks

Contributors: Both authors reviewed the literature and drafted and amended the article. SR is the guarantor.

Provenance and peer review: Commissioned; externally peer reviewed.

Competing interests: Both authors have completed the Unified Competing Interest form at www.icmje.org/coi_disclosure.pdf (available on request from the corresponding author) (URL) and declare that all authors had (1) No financial support for the submitted work from anyone other than their employer; (2) No financial relationships with commercial entities that might have an interest in the submitted work; (3) No spouses, partners, or children with relationships with commercial entities that might have an interest in the submitted work; (4) SR is editor of the journal *Evidence-Based Mental Health*, and CB is a member of the editorial board of the Cochrane Collaboration Depression, Anxiety & Neurosis Group.

1. Pirraglia PA, Stafford RS, Singer DE. Trends in prescribing of selective serotonin reuptake inhibitors and other newer antidepressant agents in adult primary care. *Prim Care Companion J Clin Psychiatry* 2003;5:153-7.
2. Olfson M, Marcus SC. National patterns in antidepressant medication treatment. *Arch Gen Psychiatry* 2009;66:848-56.
3. Moore M, Yuen HM, Dunn N, Mullee MA, Maskell J, Kendrick T. Explaining the rise in antidepressant prescribing: a descriptive study using the general practice research database. *BMJ* 2009;339:b3999.
4. Petty DR, House A, Knapp P, Raynor T, Zermansky A. Prevalence, duration and indications for prescribing of antidepressants in primary care. *Age Ageing* 2006;35:523-6
5. Parker G. Antidepressants on trial: how valid is the evidence? *Br J Psychiatry* 2009;194:1-3.
6. Kirsch I, Deacon BJ,Huedo-Medina TB, Scoboria A, Moore TJ, Johnson BT. Initial severity and antidepressant benefits: a meta-analysis of data submitted to the Food and Drug Administration. *PLoS Med* 2008;5:e45.
7. Fournier JC, DeRubeis RJ, Hollon SD, Dimidjian S, Amsterdam JD, Shelton RC, et al. Antidepressant drug effects and depression severity: a patient-level meta-analysis. *JAMA* 2010;303:47-53.
8. Geddes J, Barbui C, Cipriani A. Risk of suicidal behaviour in adults taking antidepressants. *BMJ* 2009;339:b3066.
9. Kupfer DJ, Frank E, Wamhoff J. Mood disorders: update on prevention of recurrence. In: Mundt C, Goldstein MJ, eds. *Interpersonal factors in the origin and course of affective disorders* . Gaskell/Royal College of Psychiatrists, 1996:289-302.
10. National Institute for Health and Clinical Excellence. Depression: the treatment and management of depression in adults (update). 2009. (Clinical guideline 90.) http://guidance.nice.org.uk/CG90
11. Anderson IM, Ferrier IN, Baldwin RC, Cowen PC, Howard L, Lewis G, et al. Evidence-based guidelines for treating depressive disorders with antidepressants: a revision of the 2000 British Association for Psychopharmacology guidelines. *J Psychopharmacol* 2008;22:343-96.
12. Spence D. Black dog. *BMJ* 2009;339:b3995
13. Geddes JR, Carney SM, Davies C, Furukawa TA, Kupfer DJ, Frank E, et al. Relapse prevention with antidepressant drug treatment in depressive disorders: a systematic review. *Lancet* 2003;361:653-61.
14. Furukawa TA, Cipriani A, Barbui C, Geddes JR. Long-term treatment of depression with antidepressants: a systematic narrative review. *Can J Psychiatry* 2007;52:545-52.
15. Hansen R, Gaynes B, Thieda P, Gartlehner G, Veaugh-Geiss A, Krebs E, et al. Meta-analysis of major depressive disorder relapse and recurrence with second-generation antidepressants. *Psychiatr Serv* 2008;59:1121-30.
16. Kaymaz N, van OJ, Loonen AJ, Nolen WA. Evidence that patients with single versus recurrent depressive episodes are differentially sensitive to treatment discontinuation: a meta-analysis of placebo-controlled randomized trials. *J Clin Psychiatry* 2008;69:1423-36.
17. Deshauer D, Moher D, Fergusson D. Impact of study design on the results of continuation studies of antidepressants. *J Clin Psychopharmacol* 2008;28:467-8.
18. Deshauer D, Moher D, Fergusson D, Moher E, Sampson M, Grimshaw J. Selective serotonin reuptake inhibitors for unipolar depression: a systematic review of classic long-term randomized controlled trials. *CMAJ* 2008;178:1293-301.
19. Barbui C, Esposito E, Cipriani A. Selective serotonin reuptake inhibitors and risk of suicide: a systematic review of observational studies. *CMAJ* 2009;180:291-7.
20. Stone M, Laughren T, Jones L, Levenson M, Holland PC, Hughes A, et al. Risk of suicidality in clinical trials of antidepressants in adults: analysis of proprietary data submitted to US Food and Drug Administration. *BMJ* 2009;339:b2880.
21. Haddad P. Newer antidepressants and the discontinuation syndrome. *J Clin Psychiatry* 1997;58(suppl 7):17-21.
22. Coupland NJ, Bell CJ, Potokar JP. Serotonin reuptake inhibitor withdrawal. *J Clin Psychopharmacol* 1996;16:356-62.
23. Rosenbaum JF, Zajecka J. Clinical management of antidepressant discontinuation. *J Clin Psychiatry* 1997;58(suppl 7):37-40.
24. Serretti A, Chiesa A. Treatment-emergent sexual dysfunction related to antidepressants: a meta-analysis. *J Clin Psychopharmacol* 2009;29:259-66.
25. Gartlehner G, Thieda P, Hansen RA, Gaynes BN, Veaugh-Geiss A, Krebs EE, et al. Comparative risk for harms of second-generation antidepressants: a systematic review and meta-analysis. *Drug Saf* 2008;31:851-65.
26. Hu XH, Bull SA, Hunkeler EM, Ming E, Lee JY, Fireman B, et al. Incidence and duration of side effects and those rated as bothersome with selective serotonin reuptake inhibitor treatment for depression: patient report versus physician estimate. *J Clin Psychiatry* 2004;65:959-65.
27. Alwan S, Friedman JM. Safety of selective serotonin reuptake inhibitors in pregnancy. *CNS Drugs* 2009;23:493-509.
28. National Institute for Health and Clinical Excellence. Antenatal and postnatal mental health: clinical management and service guidance. 2007. (Clinical guideline 45.) http://guidance.nice.org.uk/CG45.
29. De Abajo FJ, Rodriguez LA, Montero D. Association between selective serotonin reuptake inhibitors and upper gastrointestinal bleeding: population based case-control study. *BMJ* 1999;319:1106-9.

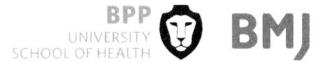

30 De Abajo FJ, Garcia-Rodriguez LA. Risk of upper gastrointestinal tract bleeding associated with selective serotonin reuptake inhibitors and venlafaxine therapy: interaction with nonsteroidal anti-inflammatory drugs and effect of acid-suppressing agents. *Arch Gen Psychiatry* 2008;65:795-803.

31 Wright SK, Schroeter S. Hyponatremia as a complication of selective serotonin reuptake inhibitors. *J Am Acad Nurse Pract* 2008;20(1):47-51.

32 Sharma H, Pompei P. Antidepressant-induced hyponatraemia in the aged. Avoidance and management strategies. *Drugs Aging* 1996;8:430-5.

33 Alvarez W, Jr, Pickworth KK. Safety of antidepressant drugs in the patient with cardiac disease: a review of the literature. *Pharmacotherapy* 2003;23(6):754-771.

34 Von Ruden AE, Adson DE, Kotlyar M. Effect of selective serotonin reuptake inhibitors on cardiovascular morbidity and mortality. *J Cardiovasc Pharmacol Ther* 2008;13(1):32-40.

35 Glassman AH, O'Connor CM, Califf RM, Swedberg K, Schwartz P, Bigger JT Jr, et al. Sertraline treatment of major depression in patients with acute MI or unstable angina. *JAMA* 2002;288:701-9.

36 Paykel ES. Cognitive therapy in relapse prevention in depression. *Int J Neuropsychopharmacol* 2007;10:131-6.

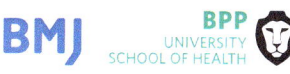

Generalized anxiety disorder: diagnosis and treatment

Elizabeth A Hoge, assistant in psychiatry[1][2][3], Ana Ivkovic, assistant in psychiatry[1], Gregory L Fricchione, associate chief of psychiatry[1][2]

[1]Department of Psychiatry, Massachusetts General Hospital, Boston, MA 02114, USA

[2]Benson-Henry Institute for Mind Body Medicine, Massachusetts General Hospital

[3]Center for Anxiety and Traumatic Stress Disorders, Massachusetts General Hospital

Correspondence to: G L Fricchione gfricchione@partners.org

Cite this as: BMJ 2012;345:e7500

DOI: 10.1136/bmj.e7500

http://www.bmj.com/content/345/bmj.e7500

Generalized anxiety disorder (GAD) is relatively common, with lifetime prevalence rates of 4-7%. It is a disorder of chronic uncontrollable worry, compounded by physiological symptoms such as disturbed sleep, muscle tension, and difficulty concentrating. The disorder is associated with seriously impaired social and occupational functioning, comorbidity with other disorders, and increased risk for suicide.[1] GAD can go undiagnosed because of a focus on physical symptoms and because of the stigma of mental illness. However, the disorder can be treated. This article reviews current knowledge about the diagnosis and treatment of GAD, including pharmacotherapy and psychosocial therapies.

What is generalized anxiety disorder?

GAD is characterized by excessive worry and symptoms of physiological arousal such as restlessness, insomnia, and muscle tension (box). To meet *Diagnostic and Statistical Manual of Mental Disorders*, fourth edition (DSM-IV) criteria for the disorder, the patient must have excessive and difficult to control anxiety about several different events or activities.[2] For example, anxiety confined to concern about personal safety would not qualify (but should elicit inquiries about symptoms of post-traumatic stress disorder or agoraphobia, for example). In addition to worry, patients must have at least three of the six physiological arousal symptoms listed in the box. These symptoms must not be caused by another psychiatric or medical disorder, or by the use of drugs, and they must cause serious distress or impairment for the clinical diagnosis to be made. The diagnostic criteria will probably be modified in the new DSM-V (for more information, see www.dsm5.org).

The ICD-10 (international classification of diseases, 10th revision) description of GAD contains slightly different description of symptoms. It focuses on physiological arousal such as trembling, sweating, palpitations, and dizziness and does not require symptoms to be present for six months. It is defined as: "Anxiety that is generalized and persistent but not restricted to, or even strongly predominating in, any particular environmental circumstances (it is "free-floating"). The dominant symptoms are variable but include complaints of persistent nervousness, trembling, muscular tensions, sweating, lightheadedness, palpitations, dizziness, and epigastric discomfort. Fears that the patient or a relative will shortly become ill or have an accident are often expressed." Because most clinical trials use DSM-IV criteria, we will focus on GAD as defined by the DSM-IV classification so that the reader can best evaluate the treatment trial data.

Who gets generalized anxiety disorder?

The lifetime prevalence was determined to be 5.7% in a sample from the United States, a similar rate to that found in other countries.[3] The highest prevalence (7.7%) occurred in the 45-59 year age range, and it was more common in women (7%) than in men (4%). Other predictors in a large epidemiological sample included being separated, widowed, divorced, unemployed, or being a homemaker.[4] In a study of children followed into adulthood, low socioeconomic status, childhood maltreatment, internalizing problems, and conduct problems in childhood were risk factors.[5] It is also associated with serious disability and impaired quality of life. In an international study of disability caused by mental illness, 38% of people with GAD had moderate to severe occupational role impairment, with an average of 6.3 days a month of missed work or loss of role functioning.[6]

How is generalized anxiety disorder diagnosed?

The disorder is not well recognized in primary care. In a large study of patients and their primary care physicians, physicians correctly recognized and diagnosed GAD only 34% of the time.[7] Part of the problem may be the misdiagnosis of anxiety as depression. In one primary care study, only 23% of the patients with pure anxiety were diagnosed with anxiety, compared with 65% of those with pure depression.[8] In other work, researchers examined patients who had been given a false positive diagnosis of depression: 27% of these patients had had an anxiety disorder instead.[9]

In addition, a focus on somatic symptoms may distract patients and doctors from the psychological symptoms; it is known that patients with GAD seek help from primary care more often than the general population. For example, a study of healthcare utilization patterns found that such patients visited primary care an average of 5.6 more times a year than age and sex matched controls without anxiety or depression.[10] Patients presenting with GAD also have higher rates of medical conditions. Associations have been found between GAD and increased rates of pain and gastrointestinal, cardiovascular, endocrine, and respiratory conditions.[11][12] Dysfunctional neural processing of emotional stimuli is thought to be involved in the pathophysiology of the disorder, but this area is poorly understood and research has been minimal.[13][14]

To improve detection and treatment, the International Consensus Group on Depression produced a consensus statement on GAD, which recommends two screening questions: "During the past four weeks, have you been bothered by feeling worried, tense, or anxious most of the time?" and "Are you frequently tense, irritable, and having trouble sleeping?"[15] However, it is not known how sensitive or specific these questions are.

SUMMARY POINTS

- Generalized anxiety disorder (GAD) is associated with substantial distress and disability
- GAD is often associated with other medical and psychiatric disorders
- Antidepressants, such as sertraline, are generally first line medical treatment options
- Psychotherapy and other psychosocial treatments can also be effective
- GAD increases the risk of major depression, so preventive approaches should be put in place

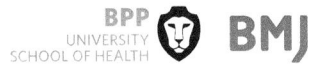

DSM-IV DIAGNOSTIC CRITERIA FOR GENERALIZED ANXIETY DISORDER

- Excessive anxiety and worry occurring more days than not for at least six months
- Worry that is difficult to control
- The anxiety or worry is associated with three or more of the following:
- Restlessness or feeling "keyed up" or on edge
- Being easily fatigued
- Difficulty concentrating or mind going blank
- Irritability
- Muscle tension
- Sleep disturbance
- The focus of the anxiety is not part of another disorder (such as fears of embarrassment in public in social anxiety disorder)

Does generalized anxiety disorder occur with other disorders?

Psychiatric comorbidity is common in GAD—29-62% of patients are estimated to have major depression.[4] [7] Other common comorbidities are social anxiety disorder (34%) and alcohol misuse (38%). Unfortunately, patients who also have comorbid psychiatric disorders are more impaired and have a less successful response to treatment than those with GAD alone.[16] The high comorbidity (and symptom overlap) with depression has contributed to the uncertainty about whether GAD is distinct from depression. However, symptoms unique to GAD—such as worry, differential response to benzodiazepines (not effective for depression), different patterns of REM sleep disturbance, and opposing patterns of response to emotional stimuli in the laboratory (relative insensitivity in depression and hyperactivity in GAD)—support it being a distinct disorder.[17] [18] When making a diagnosis in a patient with current depression, symptoms that overlap with depression—such as restlessness, difficulty concentrating, and sleep disturbance—cannot be used in the diagnosis of GAD. Ultimately, however, distinguishing between GAD and GAD with comorbidities should not overly concern the clinician because many treatment strategies are the same.

Although they may be distinct disorders, the presence of GAD predisposes to the subsequent development of major depression. One large prospective study of adolescents and adults found that GAD increased the odds of developing depression within four years 4.5-fold (odds ratio 4.5, 95% confidence interval 1.9 to 10.3).[19] Interestingly, drug treatment for GAD significantly lowers the risk of developing major depression.[20]

What is known about the causes?

Both genetic and environmental factors play a role in the development of GAD. In 2001, a meta-analysis of data from family and twin studies of several anxiety disorders found that GAD has a modest heritability (0.32, compared with 0.43 for panic disorder).[21] More recently, a case-control association study of 1059 Spanish primary care attendees found that a polymorphic variation at the serotonin 1-A receptor gene was associated with the common clinical presentation of comorbid major depression and GAD.[22] The above meta-analysis also found that environmental experiences are significantly associated with GAD, highlighting the importance of environmental stressors as a risk factor.

What are the treatment options?

Treatment options include psychological therapies and drugs. Psychological therapies include cognitive behavioral therapy (CBT), behavioral therapy, relaxation response training, and mindfulness meditation training. Of these, CBT is the most well studied and commonly used. Drugs include antidepressants, notably the serotonin reuptake inhibitors as first line agents, benzodiazepines, and the anticonvulsant pregabalin. National Institute for Health and Clinical Excellence (NICE) guidelines recommend treating patients with active substance dependence (different from non-harmful substance misuse) before starting treatment. Unfortunately, it is unclear whether psychotherapy or drugs should be tried first, with some studies showing a benefit of CBT over drugs,[23] and others showing a benefit of drugs, such as sertraline, over CBT.[24] The decision should be made after a discussion with the patient, during which the patient's values, attitudes, beliefs, preferences, and resources are reviewed. Furthermore, it is unclear whether the combination of drugs and psychotherapy is better than using one strategy alone.

What psychosocial treatments can be used?

Several types of psychotherapy have been used, with varying levels of empirical support. For anxiety disorders, CBT—a time limited symptom focused treatment—is the most well studied and highly utilized. Several well conducted meta-analyses have shown significant benefit of CBT compared with control groups,[25] [26] [27] and NICE guidelines recommend CBT as first line treatment.

This technique traditionally combines cognitive therapy—which focuses on monitoring thoughts and understanding self perpetuated cognitive distortions, habitual thought patterns, and subsequent behaviors—with behavioral therapy, which aims to expose the patient to feared experiences (originally, phobias). In GAD, targeted cognitions might, for example, be negative interpretations of neutral events that can be systematically evaluated and questioned. People with the disorder are more likely to see ambiguous or neutral stimuli as potentially threatening than those without an anxiety disorder,[28] [29] so automatic anxious thought patterns can be reduced by evaluating thoughts and impressions more objectively. Behavioral therapy is more difficult in GAD than with simple phobias, because worry based anxiety triggers for GAD are more difficult to target, more diffuse, and often shift. One approach has been to use exposure techniques to focus attention on the worries, which themselves may be serving as avoidance against more distressing emotions, such as anger or grief.[30] [31]

CBT is usually provided by a specially trained psychotherapist on an individual basis, with six to 12 sessions of one hour's duration as standard. Some studies suggest that CBT can be delivered over the internet, but how it compares to office based CBT is unclear. There is also preliminary evidence that internet based CBT administered by a non-clinician may be effective, although only one randomized controlled trial has been published to date and it was not tested against standard CBT.[32]

Several other psychotherapeutic approaches can be combined with CBT. For example, relaxation response training, in the form of progressive muscle relaxation or diaphragmatic breathing, has been added to CBT or used alone. Two small to medium sized randomized controlled studies comparing cognitive therapy alone with relaxation

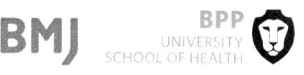

training alone found that they both significantly and equally reduce anxiety symptoms in GAD.[33 34] Meta-cognitive therapy uses similar techniques to those of cognitive therapy (working to correct automatic or distorted thinking) but also tackles the worry about worrying itself—for example, thoughts that the worrying will become uncontrollable or will cause negative consequences for the patient. The therapy focuses instead on changing beliefs about worry and guides patients away from a focus on attempts to control the worry.[35]

Two newer psychotherapies have recently been introduced for the treatment of GAD; both share a theoretical framework with CBT but include mindfulness training. Mindfulness was originally introduced in mental health treatment settings through meditation training strategies, such as mindfulness based stress reduction.[w1] Mindfulness teaches participants to increase awareness of present moment experiences, such as thoughts and emotions, without judgment or striving to make the experience last or disappear. One of these newer psychotherapies, which has support from a small but well conducted randomized controlled trial, is acceptance-based behavioral therapy. This therapy focuses on accepting problems rather than striving for immediate change, and uses mindfulness to help patients foster a compassionate and non-judgmental awareness of their experiences (which promotes clearer decision making) and a focus on present moment experiences rather than worries.[w2] Emotion regulation therapy also uses mindfulness training but focuses on addressing deficits in regulating emotions through additional techniques.[w3] The use of mindfulness meditation training for GAD is validated by a recent small randomized controlled trial, which found significant benefits compared with an active control class.[w4]

Traditional psychodynamic psychotherapy has been less well studied in GAD, possibly because of methodological challenges in studying a longer and less directed treatment in which the focus varies greatly among individuals. However, in one randomized controlled study from the United Kingdom, which measured the effect of analytically based psychotherapy for GAD, after just six months 42% of patients had "moderate" to "very considerable" improvements in symptoms.[w5] More recently, short term psychodynamic psychotherapy was compared with CBT in a group of 57 patients with GAD as part of a randomized controlled trial.[w6] Both treatments showed significant decreases in anxiety symptoms with no difference between the treatments in the primary outcome measure.

Although not a treatment for GAD by itself, education on sleep hygiene can be useful in primary care given the high frequency of sleep disturbance in this disorder. It is sometimes used with CBT to ensure the best possible sleep efficiency and quality. Advice includes going to bed and waking up at the same time each day, eliminating alcohol after 6 pm, and getting out of bed if unable to fall asleep, to avoid negative associations with the bed environment.[w7] In addition, although not widely studied in GAD, physical exercise decreased anxiety symptoms in at least one small randomised controlled trial.[w8] Lastly, self help books or manuals may be useful, according to a meta-analysis of six randomized controlled trials, two of which showed a benefit over a waiting list control.[w9-w11]

When should drugs be prescribed?

In 2011, NICE issued treatment guidelines outlining an algorithm for the treatment of GAD. It recommended drug treatment if symptoms cause marked functional impairment.

This was defined as self reported difficulty in functioning in the domains of work or school, social or leisure, and family life; higher scores on screening instruments such as the seven item "GAD-7"[w12]; or persistence of symptoms despite psychoeducation and low intensity psychological intervention (such as self help and psychoeducational groups). Currently, there is no clear time frame for exactly when drugs should be considered. One large open label study examining the duration of "untreated" GAD (no drug treatment) found that treatment (antidepressants) was more successful when started within one year, suggesting that drugs should be offered within one year of persistent symptoms.[w13] This treatment effect was not found with benzodiazepines.

Which drugs are effective?

Antidepressants have well documented efficacy in the treatment of GAD, regardless of the presence of comorbid depression.[w14] Treatment efficacy is measured by clinical response (defined in most studies as >50% reduction in HAM-A (Hamilton anxiety rating scale) score from baseline) or remission (defined as the proportion of patients with a final HAM-A score of ≤7). Selective serotonin reuptake inhibitors (SSRIs) and serotonin-norepinephrine (noradrenaline) reuptake inhibitors (SNRIs) are considered first line treatment options, largely because of their combined efficacy, tolerability, and safety profile. Response and remission rates vary across studies. A 2012 literature review of 50 studies attempted to clarify the expected clinical response and remission rates for GAD treated by drugs. The authors reported that the probability of a response with first line therapy is 67.7%, compared with 54.5% for second line therapy.[w15] Remission rates for first line therapy averaged 39.7%, but insufficient data were available in the reviewed studies on remission for second line therapy. "Second line therapy" in this study was diverse, including benzodiazepines, buspirone, and pregabalin, which limited the predictive value for this arm of the treatment. One review suggests that, although it is difficult to predict reliably which patients will respond to treatment, response to antidepressants is less likely if there is no evidence of an effect within four weeks.[w16] Others have suggested that a minimum trial period should be eight weeks or more, because 44% of patients with another anxiety disorder who did not respond to an SSRI at four weeks responded by 12 weeks.[w9 w11]

The SSRI, sertraline, is recommended by NICE as the initial treatment for GAD. This recommendation is based on its cost effectiveness (it is available as a generic). We are unaware of any head to head trial demonstrating an efficacy advantage for sertraline over other SSRIs or SNRIs for GAD. However, known clinical advantages of sertraline include its minimal drug-drug interactions (making it preferable to fluoxetine, paroxetine, and fluvoxamine), the lack of associated electrocardiographic changes (compared with citalopram), and its lower risk of symptoms on discontinuation compared with paroxetine and venlafaxine.

If no effect is seen after a four to eight week trial of an SSRI, consider switching to another SSRI or to the SNRI class of antidepressants. However, if a partial effect at is seen at four weeks, it is worth waiting until eight weeks because the effect of SSRIs can continue to increase during this period. The SNRIs, venlafaxine and duloxetine, can also be considered first line treatment options for GAD. Both are licensed in the UK for this indication. Their efficacy has been

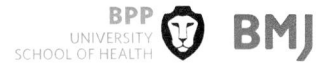

shown in several randomized placebo controlled studies of adult outpatients with GAD.[w17-w23] A large 24 week double blind placebo controlled study of venlafaxine for GAD in primary care patients with and without depression found a significant reduction in HAM-A score for depressed and non-depressed venlafaxine treated groups (a net decrease of 2.1 points) compared with placebo.[w22] Another large double blind placebo controlled study examined the efficacy and tolerability of duloxetine for the treatment of patients with GAD and found that duloxetine (at 60 mg/day and 120 mg/day) was efficacious, as measured by a significantly greater reduction in HAM-A score compared with placebo. Patients treated with duloxetine also had greater functional improvements as measured by scores on the Sheehan disability scale.[w17]

Pregabalin is an anticonvulsant and antineuralgic agent commonly prescribed for diabetic peripheral neuropathy and postherpetic neuralgia. Since 2000, several randomized placebo controlled studies have examined the efficacy of pregabalin for the treatment of GAD.[w24-w29] NICE guidance suggests that pregabalin be offered as an initial treatment option for patients with GAD who cannot tolerate SSRIs or SNRIs. Similar to benzodiazepines, pregabalin has a rapid onset of action, with anxiolysis occurring within one week of starting treatment. Sedation, dizzin ess, headache, and dry mouth are the most common side effects.[w30] Although pregabalin is generally not considered habit forming, there have been case reports of misuse and symptoms on withdrawal. Sudden discontinuation of pregabalin and other anticonvulsants has been associated with an acute confusional state, with reversible vasogenic edema of the splenium of the corpus callosum.[w31 w32] Gabapentin, another anticonvulsant drug often used for neuropathic pain, has also been used off label for the treatment of GAD, although evidence favors its use only for social anxiety.[w33]

Benzodiazepines have confirmed efficacy primarily for the short term treatment of GAD.[w34] Because of their habit forming potential and the availability of alternative non-habit forming drugs, NICE guidance recommends that they are offered for the treatment of GAD only as a short term measure in crises. Moreover, unwanted side effects (including sedation and psychomotor impairment) and the potential for withdrawal symptoms (necessitating a gradual discontinuation of treatment) limit their suitability. Short acting benzodiazepines such as alprazolam may lead to rebound anxiety, which can inadvertently promote long term use. Benzodiazepines (ideally longer acting ones like clonazepam) are mainly recommended as short term (≤1 month) treatment for acute anxiety. They can also be used as an initial adjunct to antidepressants given the delayed onset of action of these drugs and the ability of benzodiazepines to attenuate some of the initial side effects of SSRIs and SNRIs.[w35 w36]

Buspirone is a non-benzodiazepine anxiolytic that is effective in the treatment of GAD.[w37] A large well conducted placebo controlled trial of buspirone for the treatment of GAD with mild depressive symptoms showed a significant reduction in HAM-A scores compared with placebo.[w37] The efficacy of buspirone compared with antidepressants or pregabalin is unclear, given the current lack of head to head trials. Comparison studies of buspirone versus benzodiazepines have mixed results, although buspirone may be less effective in patients recently treated with benzodiazepines.[w38] The advantage of this drug over benzodiazepines is its lack of sedation, withdrawal symptoms, and physical or psychological dependence. Two to four weeks or longer are typically needed for a response.

Placebo has been used as the main comparator in most studies, and few head to head clinical studies exist. Thus, little is known about the comparable efficacy of the drugs used to treat GAD. A recent systematic review that pooled data from 27 randomized controlled trials of various drugs found a possible response and remission advantage for fluoxetine compared with all other treatments tested (benzodiazepines, buspirone, and quetiapine were not included).[w16] More head to head studies are needed. Augmentation pharmacotherapy for GAD is another area that requires further study.

Unlicensed treatments used in refractory GAD

If patients do not improve despite the use of treatments of adequate duration, consider unlicensed treatments as a possible next step. Unlicensed treatments should be initiated only by a specialist.

Recently there has been increased interest in the efficacy of second generation antipsychotics, both as monotherapy and as an augmentation strategy,[w39-w41] because only a minority of patients with GAD achieve remission despite current treatments. A recent systematic review and meta-analysis looked at augmentation with second generation antipsychotics and monotherapy in the treatment of GAD.[w42] The study reviewed five separate randomized placebo controlled augmentation studies (total of 912 patients), which failed to show a significant clinical advantage for second generation antipsychotics over placebo. Moreover, augmentation was associated with a higher dropout rate because of adverse effects. The same review found more promising results with studies of second generation antipsychotic monotherapy. Four randomized placebo controlled monotherapy studies (total of 1383 patients) showed significant efficacy of quetiapine monotherapy (up to 150 mg/day) over placebo. As with the augmentation studies, patients treated with quetiapine had an increased risk of all cause discontinuation and weight gain.[w42] Currently, antipsychotics should not be offered as an initial treatment option for GAD.[w43]

How long should drugs be continued?

If a particular drug is effective, the optimal treatment duration is generally one year,[w43] given the lower relapse rate for patients who continue on pharmacotherapy versus placebo.[w44] Treatment should also be continued for several months because a longer course of treatment increases the likelihood of remission.[w44 w45] This observation is supported by two double blind placebo controlled trials of extended release venlafaxine, which found higher response and remission rates when the initial eight week treatment course was extended to six months.[w46]

When should I refer?

GAD is more than just excessive worrying, and it is often a chronic disorder. In a group of older people with GAD who still remained symptomatic, the mean duration of the illness was 37 years.[w47] However, when successfully treated, the disorder can remit. A study that followed GAD patients, most of whom received treatment, over 22 years found that 63% had been symptom free for at least one year at the time of follow-up.[w48] This is similar to another study that found 58% recovery over 12 years. The course of GAD was longer in those with comorbid depression or substance use disorders.[w49]

Healthcare professionals should consider how long the worries have been present, whether they span

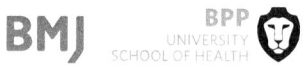

SOURCES AND SELECTION CRITERIA

We based this review on articles found by searching PubMed and the Cochrane Database of Systematic Reviews using the terms "generalized anxiety disorder" and "generalised anxiety disorder". Our search was limited to English language articles published between 2005 and 2012. Meta-analyses, reviews, and randomised controlled trials were prioritized.

TIPS FOR NON-SPECIALISTS

- Generalized anxiety disorder (GAD) is prevalent in primary care settings
- GAD is more than just a tendency to worry and should not be ignored
- There must be more than one topic of worry and the disorder must last for at least six months
- Onset after age 35 years, lack of history, and lack of stressors suggest a physical cause
- Consider GAD when patients present with unexplained somatic problems
- Recommend avoidance of nicotine and excess caffeine and alcohol
- Recommend exercise to help sleep and relieve tension
- Review the use of over the counter drugs regularly
- Individualize treatment on the basis of severity, arousal, somatization, comorbidities, and acceptability to the patient
- Discuss psychosocial and drug treatments with patients
- Antidepressants may take four weeks to take effect

ADDITIONAL EDUCATIONAL RESOURCES

Resources for healthcare professionals

- Anxiety and Depression Association of America (www.adaa.org/)—Provides research updates and free educational podcasts
- National Institute for Health and Clinical Excellence. Generalised anxiety disorder and panic disorder (with or without agoraphobia) in adults: management in primary, secondary and community care. 2007. http://publications.nice.org.uk/generalised-anxiety-disorder-and-panic-disorder-with-or-without-agoraphobia-in-adults-cg113

Resources for patients

- Anxiety and Depression Association of America (www.adaa.org/)—Educational resources about diagnosis and treatment, including real patient stories; registration not required
- Brain and Behavior Research Foundation (http://bbrfoundation.org/anxiety)—Resources and information about anxiety disorders and other comorbid disorders; includes recovery stories from patients with mental illness
- NHS Choices (www.nhs.uk/conditions/anxiety/pages/introduction.aspx)—UK website that describes the disorder along with its treatment and self help tips

several different topics of concern, and whether they are associated with the physical symptoms listed above. Physical examinations and laboratory testing can help rule out medical causes of anxiety or the physical symptoms associated with GAD. The possibility of thyroid dysfunction, hypoglycemia, hyperparathyroidism, arrhythmias, chronic obstructive pulmonary disease, seizure disorder, and more rarely pheochromocytoma should be investigated.

Investigate effects related to sympathomimetics, β adrenergic agonists, corticosteroids, thyroid hormone, and other drugs along with possible effects of substance use (such as caffeine, amphetamines, cocaine) and withdrawal (such as alcohol, sedative hypnotics). When no associated with other disorders, GAD can often be treated successfully in primary care with the first line drugs listed above or with referral to psychotherapy. Primary care providers can also successfully advise patients with sleep difficulties on sleep hygiene and teach some of the simple CBT skills.[w9] However, in the presence of comorbid depression, alcohol or substance misuse, or another anxiety disorder, referral to a psychiatrist may be indicated.

Contributors: EAH, AI, and GLF planned the organization, content, and structure of the paper. AI wrote the pharmacology section and EAH wrote the other sections. GLF organized the sections and provided crucial edits and additions. EAH is guarantor.

Competing interests: All authors have completed the ICMJE uniform disclosure form at www.icmje.org/coi_disclosure.pdf (available on request from the corresponding author) and declare: no support from any organisation for the submitted work; no financial relationships with any organisations that might have an interest in the submitted work in the previous three years; no other relationships or activities that could appear to have influenced the submitted work.

Provenance and peer review: Commissioned; externally peer reviewed.

1   Nepon J, Belik SL, Bolton J, Sareen J. The relationship between anxiety disorders and suicide attempts: findings from the national epidemiologic survey on alcohol and related conditions. *Depress Anxiety* 2010;27:791-8.

2   American Psychiatric Association Task Force on DSM-IV. Diagnostic and statistical manual of mental disorders: DSM-IV. APA, 1994.

3   Kessler RC, Berglund P, Demler O, Jin R, Merikangas KR, Walters EE. Lifetime prevalence and age-of-onset distributions of DSM-IV disorders in the national comorbidity survey replication. *Arch Gen Psychiatry* 2005;62:593-602.

4   Wittchen HU, Zhao S, Kessler RC, Eaton WW. DSM-III-R generalized anxiety disorder in the national comorbidity survey. *Arch Gen Psychiatry* 1994;51:355-64.

5   Moffitt TE, Caspi A, Harrington H, Milne BJ, Melchior M, Goldberg D, et al. Generalized anxiety disorder and depression: childhood risk factors in a birth cohort followed to age 32. *Psychol Med* 2007;37:441-52.

6   Ormel J, VonKorff M, Ustun TB, Pini S, Korten A, Oldehinkel T. Common mental disorders and disability across cultures. Results from the WHO Collaborative Study on Psychological Problems in General Health Care. *JAMA* 1994;272:1741-8.

7   Wittchen HU, Kessler RC, Beesdo K, Krause P, Hofler M, Hoyer J. Generalized anxiety and depression in primary care: prevalence, recognition, and management. *J Clin Psychiatry* 2002;63(suppl 8):24-34.

8   Ormel J, Koeter MW, van den Brink W, van de Willige G. Recognition, management, and course of anxiety and depression in general practice. *Arch Gen Psychiatry* 1991;48:700-6.

9   Nisenson LG, Pepper CM, Schwenk TL, Coyne JC. The nature and prevalence of anxiety disorders in primary care. *Gen Hosp Psychiatry* 1998;20:21-8.

10   Berger A, Dukes E, Wittchen HU, Morlock R, Edelsberg J, Oster G. Patterns of healthcare utilization in patients with generalized anxiety disorder in general practice in Germany. *Eur J Psychiatry* 2009;23:90-100.

11   Culpepper L. Generalized anxiety disorder and medical illness. *J Clin Psychiatry* 2009;70(suppl 2):20-4.

12   Kessler RC, Ormel J, Demler O, Stang PE. Comorbid mental disorders account for the role impairment of commonly occurring chronic physical disorders: results from the National Comorbidity Survey. *J Occup Environ Med* 2003;45:1257-66.

13   Strawn JR, Bitter SM, Weber WA, Chu WJ, Whitsel RM, Adler C, et al. Neurocircuitry of Generalized Anxiety Disorder in Adolescents: a pilot functional neuroimaging and functional connectivity study. *Depress Anxiety* 2012; published online 24 May.

14   Shin LM, Liberzon I. The neurocircuitry of fear, stress, and anxiety disorders. *Neuropsychopharmacology* 2010;35:169-91.

15   Ballenger JC, Davidson JR, Lecrubier Y, Nutt DJ, Borkovec TD, Rickels K, et al. Consensus statement on generalized anxiety disorder from the International Consensus Group on Depression and Anxiety. *J Clin Psychiatry* 2001;62(suppl 11):53-8.

16   Olfson M, Fireman B, Weissman MM, Leon AC, Sheehan DV, Kathol RG, et al. Mental disorders and disability among patients in a primary care group practice. *Am J Psychiatry* 1997;154:1734-40.

17   Hettema JM. The nosologic relationship between generalized anxiety disorder and major depression. *Depress Anxiety* 2008;25:300-16.

18   Mennin DS, Heimberg RG, Fresco DM, Ritter MR. Is generalized anxiety disorder an anxiety or mood disorder? Considering multiple factors as we ponder the fate of GAD. *Depress Anxiety* 2008;25:289-99.

19   Bittner A, Goodwin RD, Wittchen HU, Beesdo K, Hofler M, Lieb R. What characteristics of primary anxiety disorders predict subsequent major depressive disorder? *J Clin Psychiatry* 2004;65:618-26; quiz 730.

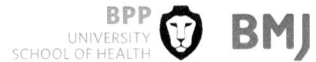

20 Goodwin RD, Gorman JM. Psychopharmacologic treatment of generalized anxiety disorder and the risk of major depression. *Am J Psychiatry* 2002;159:1935-7.

21 Hettema JM, Neale MC, Kendler KS. A review and meta-analysis of the genetic epidemiology of anxiety disorders. *Am J Psychiatry* 2001;158:1568-78.

22 Molina E, Cervilla J, Rivera M, Torres F, Bellon JA, Moreno B, et al. Polymorphic variation at the serotonin 1-A receptor gene is associated with comorbid depression and generalized anxiety. *Psychiatr Genet* 2011;21:195-201.

23 Power KG, Simpson RJ, Swanson V, Wallace LA, Feistner ATC, Sharp D. A controlled comparison of cognitive- behaviour therapy, diazepam, and placebo, alone and in combination, for the treatment of generalised anxiety disorder. *J Anxiety Disord* 1990;4:267-92.

24 Schuurmans J, Comijs H, Emmelkamp PM, Gundy CM, Weijnen I, van den Hout M, et al. A randomized, controlled trial of the effectiveness of cognitive-behavioral therapy and sertraline versus a waitlist control group for anxiety disorders in older adults. *Am J Geriatr Psychiatry* 2006;14:255-63.

25 Mitte K. Meta-analysis of cognitive-behavioral treatments for generalized anxiety disorder: a comparison with pharmacotherapy. *Psychol Bull* 2005;131:785-95.

26 Hofmann SG, Smits JA. Cognitive-behavioral therapy for adult anxiety disorders: a meta-analysis of randomized placebo-controlled trials. *J Clin Psychiatry* 2008;69:621-32.

27 Hunot V, Churchill R, Silva de Lima M, Teixeira V. Psychological therapies for generalised anxiety disorder. *Cochrane Database Syst Rev* 2007;1:CD001848.

28 Aikins DE, Craske MG. Cognitive theories of generalized anxiety disorder. *Psychiatr Clin North Am* 2001;24:57-74; vi.

29 Mathews A, Richards A, Eysenck M. Interpretation of homophones related to threat in anxiety states. *J Abnorm Psychol* 1989;98:31-4.

30 Borkovec TD, Whisman MA. Psychosocial treatment for generalized anxiety disorder. In: Mavissakalian MR, Prien RF, eds. Long-term treatments of anxiety disorders. American Psychiatric Press, 1996:171-99.

31 Borkovec TD, Newman MG, Castonguay LG. Cognitive-behavioral therapy for generalized anxiety disorder with integrations from interpersonal and experiential therapies. *CNS Spectr* 2003;8:382-9.

32 Robinson E, Titov N, Andrews G, McIntyre K, Schwencke G, Solley K. Internet treatment for generalized anxiety disorder: a randomized controlled trial comparing clinician vs. technician assistance. *PLoS One* 2010;5:e10942.

33 Ost LG, Breitholtz E. Applied relaxation vs. cognitive therapy in the treatment of generalized anxiety disorder. *Behav Res Ther* 2000;38:777-90.

34 Arntz A. Cognitive therapy versus applied relaxation as treatment of generalized anxiety disorder. *Behav Res Ther* 2003;41:633-46.

35 Hoyer J, Gloster AT. Psychotherapy for generalized anxiety disorder: don't worry, it works! *Psychiatr Clin North Am* 2009;32:629-40.

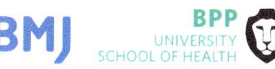

Post-traumatic stress disorder

Jonathan I Bisson, professor of psychiatry, Sarah Cosgrove, public representative, Catrin Lewis, research psychologist, Neil P Robert, consultant clinical psychologist

Division of Psychological Medicine and Clinical Neurosciences, School of Medicine, Cardiff University, Cardiff, UK

Correspondence to: J I Bisson
BissonJI@cardiff.ac.uk

Cite this as: *BMJ* 2015;351:h6161

DOI: 10.1136/bmj.h6161

http://www.bmj.com/content/351/bmj.h6161

What is post-traumatic stress disorder (PTSD)?

PTSD is a mental disorder that may develop after exposure to exceptionally threatening or horrifying events. Many people show remarkable resilience and capacity to recover following exposure to trauma.[1] PTSD can occur after a single traumatic event or from prolonged exposure to trauma, such as sexual abuse in childhood. Predicting who will go on to develop PTSD is a challenge.[2]

Patients with PTSD are at increased risk of experiencing poor physical health, including somatoform, cardiorespiratory, musculoskeletal, gastrointestinal, and immunological disorders.[3][4] It is also associated with substantial psychiatric comorbidity,[5] increased risk of suicide,[6] and considerable economic burden.[7][8]

PTSD is a widely accepted diagnosis[9] but some believe that the term medicalises understandable responses to catastrophic events and further disempowers those who are already disempowered.[10]

How common is PTSD?

About 3% of the adult population has PTSD at any one time.[11] Lifetime prevalence is between 1.9%[12] and 8.8%,[7] but this rate doubles in populations affected by conflict[13] and reaches more than 50% in survivors of rape.[5]

How does PTSD present?

Symptoms include persistent intrusive recollections, avoidance of stimuli related to the trauma, negative alterations in cognitions and mood, and hyperarousal (table).[14][15] A diagnosis can be made in someone whose ability to function normally has been noticeably impaired for one month according to DSM-5 criteria. Delayed presentation (sometimes years later) is common,[7] including where the effects are severe.[16]

How is PTSD diagnosed?

Box 1 describes the nature of the traumatic event(s) required by DSM-5 (diagnostic and statistical manual of mental disorders, fifth edition)[14] for diagnosis and the proposed criteria by ICD-11 (international classification of diseases, 11th revision).[17] Some events such as bullying, divorce, death of a pet, and learning about a diagnosis of cancer in a close family member are not deemed extreme enough to precipitate PTSD. However, they can result in almost identical symptoms and raise questions about the validity of the definitions for traumatic events.[18]

DSM-5 lists the 20 symptoms required for PTSD to be diagnosed,[14] separated into four groups (table). All symptoms must be associated with the traumatic event. In the proposed criteria by ICD-11,[17] PTSD will be diagnosed according to six criteria (table). To reflect the heterogeneity of PTSD, ICD-11 will introduce a new complex PTSD diagnosis (table). This requires satisfaction of the criteria for PTSD plus symptoms of mood dysregulation, negative self concept, and persistent difficulty in sustaining relationships and feeling close to others. Service users may meet the diagnostic criteria in one system but not in the other owing to the differences.[19]

Can PTSD be prevented?

Psychological interventions

Psychological interventions have been evaluated after traumas concerning a single incident, such as a road traffic crash and physical or sexual assaults. Meta-analyses show that brief, trauma focused, cognitive behavioural interventions can reduce the severity of symptoms when the intervention is targeted at those with early symptoms.[20][21] However, non-targeted interventions (including psychoeducation, psychological debriefing, individual and group counselling, cognitive behavioural therapy (CBT) based programmes, and collaborative care based approaches) are largely ineffective.[22][23][24][25]

Drug interventions

No robust evidence supports the use of drug interventions.[26]

Prevention after large scale traumatic events

Evidence to support routine intervention after traumatic events involving many people (for example, terrorist attacks and natural disasters) is lacking. However, some evidence suggests that high levels of social support are perceived as protective.[27] Consensus guidelines recommend supportive, practical, and pragmatic input but avoidance of formal clinical interventions unless indicated.[28][29][30]

Can PTSD be treated?

Psychological therapy

Clinical guidelines recommend trauma focused psychological therapies based on evidence from systematic reviews and meta-analyses.[31][32][33] Individual trauma focused CBT and eye movement desensitisation and reprocessing (EMDR) (box 2) have been found to be equally effective.[34]

Group trauma focused CBT is also effective, but fewer studies have focused on this method.[35] Non-trauma focused CBT—including components such as grounding techniques to manage flashbacks (for example, focusing on the here and now by describing items in a room), relaxation training (for example, controlled breathing and progressive muscle relaxation), positive thinking and self talk (for example,

WHAT YOU NEED TO KNOW

- Individual reactions to traumatic events vary greatly and most people do not develop a mental disorder after exposure to trauma
- PTSD should be considered in any patient exposed to a major traumatic event
- Up to 3% of adults has PTSD at any one time. Lifetime prevalence rates are between 1.9% and 8.8%
- Psychological treatments, particularly trauma focused psychological therapies, can be effective
- Although the effect sizes are not as high as for psychological therapies, drug treatments can be effective
- Patients with complex PTSD should receive specialist multidisciplinary care

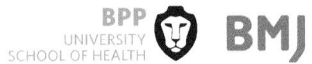

Symptoms required for diagnosis of PTSD

DSM-5 criteria[14]	Proposed ICD-11 criteria[17]
Intrusion symptoms	
Recurrent, involuntary and intrusive distressing memoriesRecurrent distressing dreams (content and/or affect related) Dissociative reaction (acting or feeling as if event is recurring)Intense or prolonged psychological distress to cuesNoticeable physiological reactions to cues	Vivid intrusive memories, flashbacks, or nightmares, typically accompanied by strong and overwhelming emotions such as fear or horror, and strong physical sensations
Avoidance	
Avoidance or efforts to avoid distressing thoughts or feelings about or closely associated with the traumaAvoidance or efforts to avoid external reminders (people, places, conversations, activities, objects, situations)	Avoidance of thoughts and memories of the event or eventsAvoidance of activities, situations, or people reminiscent of the event or events
Negative alterations in cognitions and mood	
Inability to remember an important aspect (typically due to dissociative amnesia)Persistent and exaggerated negative beliefs or expectations about oneself, others, or the world (for example, "I am bad," "No one can be trusted," "The world is completely dangerous")Persistent, distorted cognitions about the cause or consequences that lead to self blame or the blame of othersPersistent negative emotional state (for example, fear, horror, anger, guilt, shame)Noticeably diminished interest or participation in important activitiesFeelings of detachment or estrangement from othersPersistent inability to experience positive emotions (for example, happiness, satisfaction, love)	Not applicable
Alterations in arousal and reactivity	
Irritable behaviour and angry outbursts (with little or no provocation)Reckless or self destructive behaviourHypervigilanceExaggerated startle responseProblems with concentrationSleep disturbance	Persistent perceptions of heightened current threat—for example, as indicated by hypervigilance or an enhanced startle reaction to stimuli such as unexpected noises
Additional criteria for complex PTSD	
Not applicable	Severe and pervasive problems in affect regulationPersistent beliefs about oneself as diminished, defeated, or worthless, accompanied by deep and pervasive feelings of shame, guilt, or failure related to the stressorPersistent difficulties in sustaining relationships and in feeling close to others

---

BOX 1 TRAUMATIC EVENT(S) REQUIRED FOR DIAGNOSIS OF PTSD

DSM-5 criteria[14]

- Exposure to actual or threatened death, serious injury, or sexual violation, in one or more of the following ways:
- Directly experiencing the traumatic event(s)
- Witnessing traumatic event(s) in others
- Learning that the traumatic event(s) occurred to a close family member or close friend; cases of actual or threatened death must have been violent or unintentional
- Experiencing repeated or extreme exposure to aversive details of the traumatic event(s) (for example, first responders collecting human remains; police officers repeatedly exposed to details of child abuse); this does not apply to exposure through electronic media, television, movies, or pictures, unless this exposure is work related

Proposed ICD-11 criterion[17]

- Exposure to an extremely threatening or horrific event or series of events

---

BOX 2 TRAUMA FOCUSED EXPOSURE THERAPY, CBT AND EMDR

Exposure therapy

- Therapists help patients to confront their traumatic memories through written or verbal narrative, detailed recounting of the traumatic experience, and repeated exposure to trauma related situations that were being avoided or evoked fear but are now safe (for example, driving a car where the road traffic incident occurred or walking in the busy park where an assault occurred)

Cognitive therapy

- Focuses on identifying and modifying misinterpretations that led patients to overestimate the current threat (for example, patients who think assault is almost inevitable if they leave the house)
- Focuses on modifying beliefs and how patients interpret their behaviour during the trauma, including problems with guilt and shame

EMDR

- Standardised, trauma focused procedure. Involves the use of bilateral physical stimulation (eye movements, taps, or tones), hypothesised to stimulate the patient's information processing to help integrate the targeted event as an adaptive contextualised memory

---

repeating positive phrases such as "I can deal with this")—has been found to be superior to waiting list control groups and has shown similar efficacy to trauma focused CBT and EMDR immediately after treatment, but this is not maintained at follow-up.[34] Non-trauma focused CBT offers a valid alternative to trauma focused therapy if the latter is poorly tolerated, contraindicated, or unavailable. It is unclear whether specific therapies are more or less effective for particular subgroups or trauma types.[36 37]

Research on interventions for more complex presentations of PTSD is limited.[38] Evidence suggests that phased approaches may be beneficial for more complex presentations of PTSD.[39] Phase based approaches target problems such as affect dysregulation, dissociation, and somatic symptoms to promote adaptive coping, a sense of safety, and stabilisation before undertaking any trauma focused intervention.

Self help programmes

Guided self help interventions for depression and anxiety disorders are being used as an alternative to face to face therapy as these interventions offer enhanced access to cost effective treatment.[40] Some evidence suggests that internet based guided self help therapies effectively alleviate the symptoms of traumatic stress, but randomised controlled trials (RCTs) have historically been limited to subsyndromal populations.[41 42] More recent evidence supports the efficacy of guided self help for people meeting diagnostic criteria for PTSD,[43 44 45] but no head to head trials have compared guided self help with trauma focused psychological therapy administered by a therapist.

Drug treatment

The National Institute for Health and Care Excellence and World Health Organization recommend drug treatment second to trauma focused therapy.[33 46] The effect sizes for drug treatments compared with placebo are inferior to those reported for psychological treatments with a trauma focus over waiting list or treatment as usual controls.[33 47] Effect sizes with drug treatment are similar to those observed from use of antidepressants for depression compared with placebo.[48] A recent systematic review and meta-analysis found statistically significant evidence (when at least two RCTs were available) of reduction in severity of PTSD symptoms for four drugs (fluoxetine, paroxetine, sertraline, and venlafaxine) versus placebo.[47] In single RCTs, amitriptyline, GR205171 (a neurokinin-1 antagonist),

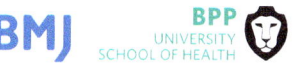

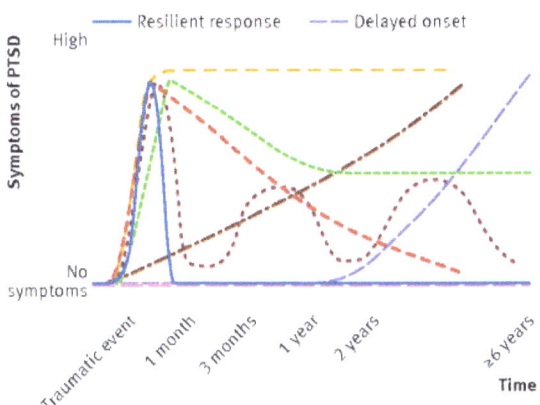

Examples of the many different trajectories of PTSD symptoms after exposure to trauma

mirtazapine, and phenelzine have shown superiority over placebo in reducing the symptoms of PTSD.

In an RCT the α 1 adrenoceptor antagonist prazosin was found to reduce nightmares in veterans with PTSD,[49] and a further RCT in veterans showed reduction in overall symptom severity.[50] This suggests a possible role for α 1 adrenoceptor blockers in PTSD, although further research is needed. Olanzapine, in contrast with another antipsychotic, risperidone, has been shown to accentuate the effects of antidepressants when resistance to treatment is encountered.[51] [52]

Combination therapy

Evidence to support the use of pharmacotherapy combined with psychological therapy over either treatment method separately is insufficient.[53]

How should PTSD and comorbidity be managed?

PTSD is associated with depression, anxiety disorders, and drug and alcohol use disorders. Little evidence exists for the effectiveness of psychological interventions for PTSD with comorbid substance use disorders. Some evidence suggests that trauma focused CBT can be effective with concomitant interventions to stabilise drug or alcohol use, but treatment effects are not as large as for PTSD in the absence of drug or alcohol misuse.[54]

What is the prognosis in PTSD?

Few longitudinal follow-up studies have been done of PTSD, but for many patients PTSD is severe and enduring.[5] There is, however, good evidence that patients may benefit from treatment even when the symptoms have been present for many years.[34]

Are there emerging options to prevent and treat PTSD?

Several experimental studies provide hope that better or alternative ways to prevent and treat PTSD are on the way. Simple visuospatial tasks such as playing a computer game shortly after a traumatic experience reduce re-experiencing.[55] For established PTSD, interest in using drugs to augment psychological therapy is increasing. The results of a recent RCT of the psychedelic 3,4-methylenedioxymethylamphetamine with psychotherapy for treatment resistant PTSD have been promising.[56] [57] These approaches remain in their infancy, and further well designed clinical studies are required to determine if they will live up to their early promise.

Contributors: JB, CL, and NR planned, conducted reviews, and drafted the article. SC drafted the patient's perspective box and commented on and amended the initial draft. All authors reviewed and agreed the final draft. JB is the guarantor.

HOW WERE PATIENTS INVOLVED IN THIS CLINICAL REVIEW?

Sarah Cosgrove is a former patient with PTSD and a representative of the public in Cardiff University's Traumatic Stress Research Group. Sarah is a coauthor of the paper and provides an account of her experiences in the patient's perspective box.

A PATIENT'S PERSPECTIVE

I was diagnosed with PTSD in November 2013 in the aftermath of a violent assault. From the time of the attack to the case coming to court, I had support from police and victim services enabling me to face my assailant in court with courage and conviction.

But in the weeks after the judicial process had concluded, I started to unravel. Naturally a glass half full sort of person, I slid into a state of great anxiety, frightened to be alone, scared to be in a group, reluctant to go out, and terrified of staying at home. I knew something was very wrong. I had gone from being confident and outgoing, to not being able to sleep, being tearful, and experiencing episodes of unparalleled low mood. My GP immediately diagnosed PTSD. Being able to put a label on what I was going through was so helpful—it meant that there was something wrong.

Fortunately, I was offered the chance to participate in a trial of a guided self help programme for sufferers of PTSD. This enabled me to both confront my experience and desensitise it, and within a few months I felt stronger than I had ever been. The programme has given me a coping strategy to employ whenever I get negative thoughts or flashbacks. It may have saved my life; at the very least it got me back to the person I used to be.

TIPS FOR NON-SPECIALISTS

- A traumatic event can precipitate conditions other than PTSD, such as depression, phobic anxiety, and substance use disorders
- PTSD is associated with comorbidity
- Sensitive questioning is required to elicit symptoms of PTSD as patients may avoid volunteering their traumatic experience(s)
- Patients with PTSD may present in primary care with physical symptoms that are difficult to explain
- Trauma focused psychological therapy is the treatment of choice for PTSD, although drugs and other forms of psychological treatment can help
- Patient choice and availability of psychological therapy will influence the treatment given

---

WHEN TO SUSPECT PTSD

- When patients present with mental or physical symptoms that cannot be fully explained after a traumatic event
- When patients present with characteristic symptoms of PTSD—re-experiencing, avoidance, and hyperarousal
- When patients disclose a history of involvement in a traumatic event
- When patients present with mental or physical symptoms that are difficult to explain in the absence of a disclosed traumatic event

Competing interests: We have read and understood the BMJ policy on declaration of interests and declare the following: JB, CL, and NR have undertaken systematic reviews, meta-analyses, randomised controlled trials, and other research in the specialty of traumatic stress, some of which is referred to in the manuscript. JB, CL, and NR are members of a research team that developed a web based guided self help programme to treat PTSD. The programme is likely to be marketed in the future. Royalties will be payable to Cardiff University, with a proportion of these being shared with the research team in line with Cardiff University's rules.

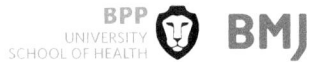

ADDITIONAL EDUCATIONAL RESOURCES

Information for healthcare professionals

- Websites providing information on the assessment and treatment of PTSD:
- International Society for Traumatic Stress Studies (www.istss.org)
- US Department of Veterans Affairs, National Centre for PTSD (www.ptsd.va.gov)

Information for patients

- Websites providing information on symptoms of PTSD and treatment options:
- NHS Choices PTSD (www.nhs.uk/Conditions/Post-traumatic-stress-disorder/Pages/Introduction.aspx)
- Royal College of Psychiatrists (www.rcpsych.ac.uk/expertadvice/problemsdisorders/posttraumaticstressdisorder.aspx)
- International Society for Traumatic Stress Studies (www.istss.org)
- National Centre for Mental Health (http://ncmh.info/conditions/post-traumatic-stress-disorder-ptsd/)
- US Department of Veterans Affairs, National Centre for PTSD (www.ptsd.va.gov/public/pages/fslist-self-help-cope.asp)—provides information on the symptoms of PTSD, self help, and treatment options

SOURCES AND SELECTION CRITERIA

We identified Cochrane and other relevant systematic reviews and meta-analyses, and supplemented these with additional searches and our knowledge of the subject. Wherever possible, we used evidence from recent meta-analyses of randomised trials.

Provenance and peer review: Commissioned; externally peer reviewed.

1 Bonanno GA. Loss, trauma, and human resilience: have we underestimated the human capacity to thrive after extremely aversive events? Am Psychol2004;59:20-8.

2 Karstoft K, Galatzer-Levy IR, Statnikov A, Li Z, Shalev AY. Bridging a translational gap: using machine learning to improve the prediction of PTSD. BMC Psychiatry2015;15:30.

3 Schnurr PP, Green BL, Kaltman, S. Trauma exposure and physical health. In: Friedman MJ, Keane TM, Resick PA, eds. Handbook of PTSD: science and practice. Guilford Press, 2007.

4 Gupta MA. Review of somatic symptoms in post-traumatic stress disorder. Int Rev Psychiatry2013;25:86-99.

5 Kessler RC, Sonnega A, Bromet E, Hughes M, Nelson CB. Posttraumatic stress disorder in the national comorbidity survey. Arch Gen Psychiatry1995;52:1048-60.

6 Sareen J, Cox BJ, Stein MB, Afifi TO, Fleet C, Asmundson GJG. Physical and mental comorbidity, disability, and suicidal behavior associated with posttraumatic stress disorder in a large community sample. Psychosom Med2007;69:242-8.

7 Ferry F, Bolton D, Bunting B, O'Neill S, Murphy S, Devine B. Economic impact of post traumatic stress in Northern Ireland. Northern Ireland Centre for Trauma and Transformation and University of Ulster Psychology Research Institute, 2010.

8 Tanielian TL, Jaycox LH, eds. Invisible wounds of war: psychological and cognitive injuries, their consequences. RAND, 2009.

9 Bisson J. Post-traumatic stress disorder. BMJ2007;334:789-93.

10 Muldoon OT, Lowe RD. Social identity, groups, and post traumatic stress disorder. Polit Psychol2012;33:259-73.

11 McManus S, Meltzer H, Brugha T, Bebbington P, Jenkins R, eds. Adult psychiatric morbidity in England, 2007: results of a household survey. NHS Information Centre for Health and Social Care, 2008.

12 Alonso J, Angermeyer MC, Lépine JP. The European Study of the Epidemiology of Mental Disorders (ESEMeD) project: an epidemiological basis for informing mental health policies in Europe. Acta Psychiatr Scand2004;109(s420):5-7.

13 Steel Z, Chey T, Silove D, Marnane C, Bryant RA, van Ommeren M. Association of torture and other potentially traumatic events with mental health outcomes among populations exposed to mass conflict and displacement: a systematic review and meta-analysis. JAMA2009;302:537-49.

14 American Psychiatric Association. Diagnostic and statistical manual of mental disorders, 5th edn. American Psychiatric Publishing, 2013.

15 World Health Organization. The ICD-10 classification of mental and behavioural disorders: clinical descriptions and diagnostic guidelines. WHO, 1992.

16 Brewin CR, Fuchkan N, Huntley Z, et al. Outreach and screening following the 2005 London bombings: usage and outcomes. Psychol Med2010:40;2049-57.

17 Maercker A, Brewin CR, Bryant RA, et al. Proposals for mental disorders specifically associated with stress in the International Classification of Diseases-11. Lancet2013;381:1683-5.

18 White J, Pearce J, Morrison S, Dunstan F, Bisson JI, Fone DL. Risk of post traumatic stress disorder following traumatic events in a community sample. Epidemiol Psychiatr Sci2015;24:249-57.

19 Bisson JI. What happened to harmonisation of the PTSD diagnosis? The divergence of ICD11 and DSM5. Epidemiol Psychiatr Sci2013;22:205-7.

20 Kleim S, Kroger C. Prevention of chronic PTSD with early cognitive behavioral therapy. A meta-analysis using mixed-effects modeling. Behav Res Ther2013;51:753-61.

21 Roberts NP, Kitchiner NJ, Kenardy J, Bisson JI. Early psychological interventions to treat acute traumatic stress symptoms. Cochrane Database Syst Rev2010;3:CD007944.

22 Bastos MH, Furuta M, Small R, McKenzie-McHarg K, Bick D. Debriefing interventions for the prevention of psychological trauma in women following childbirth. Cochrane Database Syst Rev2015;4:CD007194.

23 Gartlehner G, Forneris CA, Brownley KA, et al. Interventions for the prevention of Posttraumatic Stress Disorder (PTSD) in adults After exposure to psychological trauma. Comparative Effectiveness Review No 109. AHRQ Publication No 13-EHC062-EF. Agency for Healthcare Research and Quality, Apr 2013. www.effectivehealthcare.ahrq.gov/reports/final.cfm.

24 Roberts NP, Kitchiner NJ, Kenardy J, Bisson JI. Multiple session early psychological interventions for the prevention of post-traumatic stress disorder. Cochrane Database Syst Rev2009;3:CD006869.

25 Rose S, Bisson J, Churchill R, Wessely S. Psychological debriefing for preventing post traumatic stress disorder (PTSD). Cochrane Database Syst Rev2002;2:CD000560.

26 Sijbrandij M, Kleiboer A, Bisson JI, Barbui C, Cuijpers P. Pharmacological prevention of Posttraumatic Stress Disorder and Acute Stress Disorder: a systematic review and meta-analysis. Lancet Psychiatry2015;2:413-21.

27 Brewin CR, Andrews B, Valentine JD. Meta-analysis of risk factors for posttraumatic stress disorder in trauma-exposed adults. J Consult Clin Psychol2000;68:748-66.

28 Inter-Agency Standing Committee. IASC guidelines on mental health and psychosocial support in emergency settings. IASC, 2007.

29 Bisson JI, Tavakoly B, Witteveen AB, et al. TENTS guidelines: development of post-disaster psychosocial care guidelines through a Delphi process. Br J Psychiatry2010:196:69-74.

30 Williams R, Bisson J, Kemp V. Principles for responding to people's psychosocial and mental health needs after disasters. OP94. Royal College of Psychiatrists, 2014.

31 American Psychiatric Association. Practice guidelines for the treatment of patients with acute stress disorder and posttraumatic stress disorder. APA, 2004.

32 Australian Centre for Posttraumatic Mental Health. Australian guidelines for the treatment of adults with acute stress disorder and posttraumatic stress disorder. ACPMH, 2007.

33 National Collaborating Centre for Mental Health. Post-traumatic stress disorder (PTSD): the management of PTSD in adults and children in primary and secondary care—national cost impact report. National Institute for Health and Clinical Excellence, 2005.

34 Bisson J, Roberts N, Andrew M, Cooper R, Lewis C. Psychological therapies for chronic post-traumatic stress disorder (PTSD) in adults (Review). Cochrane Database Syst Rev2013;12:CD003388.

35 Barrera TLM. A meta-analytic review of exposure in group cognitive behavioral therapy for posttraumatic stress disorder. Clin Psychol Rev2013;33:24-32.

36 Health Technology Assessment database. Comparative effectiveness of psychological treatments and pharmacological treatments for adults with posttraumatic stress disorder. 2011. www.effectivehealthcare.ahrq.gov/index.cfm/search-for-guides-reviews-and-reports/?pageaction=displaytopic&.

37 Jonas D, Cusack K, Forneris C, et al. Psychological and pharmacological treatments for adults with posttraumatic stress disorder (PTSD). AHRQ Comparative Effectiveness Review 2013, Report No: 13-EHC011-EF.

38 Courtois CA, Ford JD. Treating complex traumatic stress disorders: an evidenced-based guide. Guilford Press, 2009.

39 Cloitre M, Courtois CA, Charuvastra A, Carapezza R, Stolbach BC, Green BL. Treatment of complex PTSD: Results of the ISTSS expert clinician survey on best practices. J Trauma Stress2011;24:615-27.

40 Lewis G, Araya R, Elgie R, Harrison G, Proudfoot J. Self help interventions for mental health problems. In: Briefing DoHE, ed, 2003.

41 Kar N. Cognitive behavioral therapy for the treatment of post-traumatic stress disorder: A review. Neuropsychiatr Dis Treat2011;7:167-81.

42 Van Emmerik AAP. Writing therapy for posttraumatic stress: a meta-analysis. Psychother Psychosom2013;82:82-8.

43 Ivarsson D, Blom M, Hesser H, et al. Guided internet-delivered cognitive behavior therapy for post-traumatic stress disorder: A randomized controlled trial. Internet Interv2014;1:33-40.

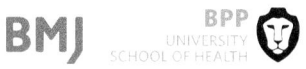

44 Litz BT, Engel CC, Bryant RA, et al. A randomized, controlled proof-of-concept trial of an Internet-based, therapist-assisted self-management treatment for posttraumatic stress disorder. Am J Psychiatry2007;164:1676-83.

45 Spence J, Titov N, Dear BF, et al. Randomized controlled trial of Internet delivered cognitive behavioral therapy for posttraumatic stress disorder. Depress Anxiety2011;28:541-50.

46 World Health Organization. WHO guidelines on conditions specifically related to stress. Geneva: WHO, 2013.

47 Hoskins M, Pearce J, Bethell A, et al. Pharmacotherapy for post-traumatic stress disorder: systematic review and meta-analysis. Br J Psychiatry2015;206:93-100.

48 Leucht S, Hierl S, Kissling W, Dold M, Davis JM. Putting the efficacy of psychiatric and general medicine medication into perspective: review of meta-analyses. Br J Psychiatry2012;200:97-106.

49 Raskind MA, Peskind ER, Hoff DJ, et al. A parallel group placebo controlled study of prazosin for trauma nightmares and sleep disturbance in combat veterans with post-traumatic stress disorder. Biol Psychiatry2007;61:928-34.

50 Raskind MA, Peterson K, Williams T, et al. A trial of prazosin for combat trauma PTSD with nightmares in active-duty soldiers returned from Iraq and Afghanistan. Am J Psychiatry2013;170:1003-10.

51 Stein MB, Kline NA, Matloff JC. Adjunctive olanzapine for SSRI-resistant combat-related PTSD: a double-blind, placebo-controlled study. Am J Psychiatry2002;159:1777-9.

52 Krystal JH, Rosenheck RA, Cramer JA, et al. Adjunctive risperidone treatment for antidepressant-resistant symptoms of chronic military service-related PTSD: a randomized trial. JAMA2011;306:493-502.

53 Hetrick SE, Purcell R, Garner B, Parslow R. Combined pharmacotherapy and psychological therapies for post traumatic stress disorder (PTSD). Cochrane Database Syst Rev2010;7:CD007316.

54 Roberts NP, Roberts PA, Jones N, Bisson JI. Psychological interventions for post-traumatic stress disorder and comorbid substance use disorder: a systematic review and meta-analysis. Clin Psychol Rev2015;38:25-38.

55 James EL, Bonsall MB, Hoppitt L, et al. Computer game play reduces intrusive memories of experimental trauma via reconsolidation-update mechanisms. Psychol Sci2015;26:1201-15.

56 Mithoefer MC, Wagner TM, Mithoefer AT, Jerome L, Doblin R. The safety and efficacy of ±3,4-methylenedioxymethamphetamine-assisted psychotherapy in subjects with chronic, treatment-resistant posttraumatic stress disorder: the first randomized controlled pilot study. J Psychopharmacol2011;25:439-52.

57 Mithoefer MC, Wagner MT, Mithoefer AT, et al. Durability of improvement in post-traumatic stress disorder symptoms and absence of harmful effects or drug dependency after 3,4-methylenedioxymethamphetamine-assisted psychotherapy: a prospective long-term follow- up study. J Psychopharmacol2013;27:28-39.

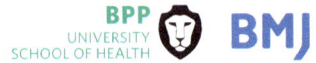

Management of seasonal affective disorder

Drug and Therapeutics Bulletin

Drug and Therapeutics Bulletin
Editorial Office, London WC1H 9JR

Correspondence to: dtb@bmjgroup.com

Cite this as: BMJ 2010;340:c2135

DOI: 10.1136/bmj.c2135

http://www.bmj.com/content/340/bmj.c2135

Low mood associated with a certain season (usually winter) is very common. For example, in the UK, up to 6% of adults have "recurrent major depressive episodes with seasonal pattern", commonly known as seasonal affective disorder (SAD).[1][2][3] People with SAD consult in primary care more often than age- and gender-matched control groups; patients also receive more prescriptions and are referred more often to secondary care.[4] Around 6-35% of patients require hospitalisation for SAD at some point.[5] Here we discuss the management of adults with SAD, and in particular light therapy.

About SAD

SAD involves symptoms typical for depression (eg, lowered mood, energy loss, fatigue) and also atypical symptoms (eg, hypersomnia, increased appetite and eating, carbohydrate craving, weight gain).[1][2][6] Some specialists have questioned the value of considering "SAD" as a separate diagnostic category from non-seasonal depression;[7] and of note it is classified as a subset of recurrent major depressive or bipolar disorder rather than as a separate category by both the Diagnostic and Statistical Manual of Mental Disorders (DSM-IV; see box 1) and the World Health Organization's International Statistical Classification of Diseases and Related Health Problems (ICD-10).[1][8]

What causes SAD?

Evidence suggests that SAD has a genetic element, with genes affecting serotonin metabolism (which has a seasonal pattern) being implicated in seasonal mood variations.[9][10] Melatonin, a hormone secreted by the pineal gland during darkness, has also been implicated in the aetiology of SAD. It is important in the regulation of daily or 'circadian' rhythms (eg, the sleep-wake cycle) and seasonal or 'circannual' rhythms (eg, regulating reproduction in many mammals).[11] The time at which the plasma melatonin concentration rises occurs later in patients with than without SAD.[12] Nocturnal melatonin secretion can be suppressed by light (eg, a light intensity of around 3000 lux suppresses melatonin secretion by around 70%; see box 2 for examples of light intensities measured in lux).[13][14]

Who gets SAD?

The mean age of onset of SAD is around 27 years; it can occur in childhood, when rates among girls and boys are similar.[5][16] Women are up to four times more likely than men to be affected during the reproductive years.[9][17] In older adults, prevalence rates decline and the genders are equally likely to be affected.

Clinical course

Episodes of SAD last around 4 months.[5][18] Around 60% of patients diagnosed with SAD continue to have a seasonal disturbance of mood and/or behaviour in the long term, while around 20% have complete remission within several years of first diagnosis.[9] Some patients have manic or hypomanic episodes in spring and summer.[19] SAD can markedly impair quality of life in winter, but this may return to normal in summer.[20][21]

Diagnosis

Various rating scales have been used to measure symptoms in SAD (eg, the 21-item and 17-item versions of the Hamilton Depression Rating Scale [HAM-D21 and HAM-D17, respectively] and the six-item depression subscale [HAM-D6]).[18] The gold standard of diagnosis is a structured interview to determine whether patients fulfil DSM-IV criteria (see box 3).[9]

Conventional antidepressants

Acute treatment of SAD

The suggestion that serotonin metabolism is disordered in SAD underlies the use of selective serotonin reuptake inhibitors (SSRIs) for acute treatment of patients with the condition; however, there have been few good-quality clinical trials of such intervention.[26]

One five-week randomised placebo-controlled trial, involving 68 adults with SAD, found a higher response rate with fluoxetine 20 mg daily (59% v 34% with placebo, P<0.05).[27] A second, eight-week, placebo-controlled trial, involving 187 adults with SAD and a mean baseline HAM-D29 of around 36, found a greater change in mean HAM-D29 with sertraline 50-200 mg daily (-17.90 v -13.39 with placebo, difference 4.51, 95% CI 0.76 to 8.28).[23]

Fluoxetine and sertraline are licensed for major depressive episodes, although SAD is not specifically mentioned in the summaries of product characteristics (SPCs) for these drugs.[28][29]

Prevention of SAD episodes

Given that SAD may recur, long-term and maintenance treatment may be needed.[30]

Pooled data from three randomised trials, involving a total of 1042 patients who started treatment before onset of SAD symptoms in autumn, suggested that compared with people on placebo, there was a lower recurrence rate among those on bupropion 150-300 mg daily (a noradrenaline and dopamine reuptake inhibitor not licensed in the UK for this indication, and not commonly used for SAD in UK practice; 16% v 28%; relative risk [RR] 0.56).[5][31] However, no P values were stated for this difference.

Light therapy

Why use light therapy?

No clear mechanism of action has been established for light therapy in SAD. One theory is that morning bright light counters disordered circadian rhythms in patients with SAD.[32][33] Other theories suggest that light may also have direct effects on some neurotransmitters (eg, serotonin).[10]

What does light therapy involve?

Light therapy involves daily scheduled exposure to fluorescent light boxes, dawn simulators (devices that slowly increase the room illumination over a period of around 90 minutes during sleep), or incandescent light visors (shaped like baseball caps with light sources shining from the brim down into the wearer's eyes). The "dose"

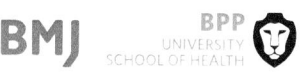

BOX 1 DSM-IV CRITERIA FOR "WITH SEASONAL PATTERN" WITHIN RECURRENT MAJOR DEPRESSIVE DISORDER OR MAJOR DEPRESSIVE EPISODES IN BIPOLAR DISORDER[1]

- Regular temporal relationship between the onset of major depressive episodes and a particular time of the year (eg, fall [autumn] or winter)
- Full remissions (or a change from depression to mania or hypomania) at a characteristic time of year (eg, spring)
- In the last two years, two major depressive episodes that demonstrate the seasonal relationship and no non-seasonal episodes
- Seasonal episodes substantially outnumber non-seasonal episodes that may have occurred over the individual's lifetime

BOX 2 EXAMPLES OF LIGHT INTENSITIES MEASURED IN LUX[14 15]

Moonlight: 0.2 lux
Winter's day: 20000 lux
Bright sunny summer's day: 100000 lux

BOX 3 STRUCTURED INTERVIEW GUIDE HAMILTON DEPRESSION RATING SEASONAL AFFECTIVE DISORDER (SIGH-SAD): AN INTERVIEW COVERING HAM-D21 PLUS ATYPICAL DEPRESSION SUPPLEMENT OF 8 ITEMS GIVING HAM-D29[22 23 24]

- Current SAD episode criteria: total SIGH-SAD 20 or more, including HAM-D21 10 or more and Atypical Depression Supplement 5 or more
- Response: a reduction of at least 50% from baseline
- Remission: score falls to below 8[25]

of light is determined by the intensity and duration of exposure.[34]

Assessing light therapy

Methodological difficulties

Several factors make designing trials of light therapy difficult. For example, the appropriate "minimum dose" of treatment is unclear, and it is hard to find a credible control condition since patients are not "blind" to therapy, and treatment expectations may contribute to a positive outcome.[34 35] The acceptable maximum dose for a low-light control is not known.

In addition, it is difficult to combine the results of light therapy trials in a meta-analysis due to differences between studies in terms of the doses of light used; the methods of delivery (eg, light box, dawn simulation or visor); comparator treatments; and populations.[36]

Clinical efficacy of light therapy

A systematic review of randomised controlled trials of bright light therapy (at least 3000 lux-hours daily) for SAD found eight studies involving a total of 360 patients with a maximum of 300 lux for controls, and lasting 7-42 days.[37] The effect sizes for a significant reduction in depression symptom severity with bright light were consistently positive across the studies. However, there was significant heterogeneity among the studies, indicating that they should probably not be combined statistically.

The same review also identified five randomised controlled trials (involving a total of 133 patients) assessing dawn simulation (increasing light exposure from 0 lux to around 200-300 lux, over 1.5-2.5 hours) with controls receiving less than 5 lux and/or less than 15 minutes of treatment; the

effect size for a significant reduction in symptom severity was reported as moderate to large.[37]

In a meta-analysis of five randomised controlled trials of light visors, no difference between light intensities of 3500-7600 lux, 400-650 lux, and under 100 lux was found; however, the authors stated that the combined statistical power of the studies was insufficient to demonstrate a significant effect.[35]

A recent update of the National Institute for Health and Clinical Excellence (NICE) guideline on the management of depression in adults has reviewed the data on light therapy for depression with a seasonal pattern.[36] This review included 20 randomised controlled trials, comparing light therapy (ranging from 176 lux to 15000 lux daily) with waiting list control management, "attentional" control (eg, sham light box), or active treatment controls (eg, cognitive behavioural therapy [CBT], fluoxetine). Compared with waiting-list control, bright light reduced depressive symptoms more (eg, weighted mean difference [WMD] in SIGH-SAD score -10.4, 95% CI -15.99 to -4.81); however, bright light did not differ significantly from attentional control or active treatments. The review concluded that it was unclear whether the superior effectiveness of the light therapy compared with waiting list management was more than a placebo effect. Another possibility is that light therapy was as effective as fluoxetine or CBT. The NICE review also concluded that dawn simulation did not reduce symptoms more than attentional control.[36]

No published randomised controlled trials have assessed the combination of light therapy and antidepressants in SAD.[33]

Unwanted effects of light therapy

Unwanted effects of light therapy include eye strain or visual disturbances (in 19-27% of patients), headache (13-21%), agitation (6-13%), nausea (7%), sweating (7%) and sedation (6-7%).[9] These effects are generally mild and subside with time or with reduction of the dose.[9] Hypomania can also occur.[9 24]

Practicalities of light therapy

Regulations

Light therapy devices intended as treatment for disease, which do not achieve their principal intended action on the human body by pharmacological, immunological or metabolic means, come within the scope of the Medical Device Directive and should carry a CE mark.[38]

Cost

Light boxes and other appliances are available for sale or hire in the UK both online and in high street stores (at around £200), but are not currently available on prescription in the NHS.[39] People defined as "chronically sick or disabled" do not have to pay VAT when they buy equipment (relating to the specific disability) supplied for their personal or domestic use.[40 41] Where required for treating SAD, light boxes are classified as zero-rated for VAT.[40 41]

Stopping and restarting light therapy

There are few data on stopping and restarting light therapy. Specialists suggest that patients on light therapy generally continue treatment until the time of their usual spontaneous remission; it can be stopped abruptly.[24] In rare cases where

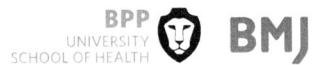

a patient experiences a relapse, treatment can be resumed for several weeks.

If light therapy is felt to be effective, it can be resumed in subsequent years before, or with the appearance of, the first symptoms (eg, difficulty waking, daytime fatigue, carbohydrate craving) prior to the onset of depression. However, this may be unnecessary, as patients do not always become depressed every winter.

Other treatments

Cognitive behavioural therapy

Two randomised controlled trials of CBT in patients with SAD have been published.[42] [43]

The first was a pilot study involving 23 patients who received group CBT tailored to SAD (1.5 hour sessions twice weekly, with four to six participants per group), light therapy (10 000 lux for 45 minutes in the morning and 45 minutes in the evening), or both, for six weeks.[42] SIGH-SAD scores improved from pre- to post-treatment with no significant difference between groups (only graphical information presented). At the 1 year follow-up, no patients treated with CBT (with or without light therapy) the previous winter met SIGH-SAD criteria for relapse, compared with 62.5% of patients who had received light therapy only (P=0.005).

The second study, involving 61 patients with a mean pre-treatment SIGH-SAD score of around 28.6, compared four strategies for SAD: CBT (1.5 hour sessions twice weekly, with four to eight participants per group, for six weeks); light therapy (10 000 lux for 45 minutes in the morning and 45 minutes in the evening for one week, then flexible dosing for five weeks); both of these treatments for six weeks; and waiting list control management (minimal contact monitoring for six weeks; then treatment with light therapy).[43] All three active-treatment groups had a significant fall in SIGH-SAD scores (post-treatment scores: CBT only 12.9; light only 12.7; CBT plus light 8.5) and scores in all these groups were lower than that in the waiting list control group (23.1; P<0.05 for each active treatment).

Self-help and complementary treatments

An NHS Direct patient leaflet on SAD recommends lifestyle changes to reduce symptoms, including exercise, a healthy diet and trying to get as much natural sunlight as possible.[39]

A systematic review of complementary and self-help treatments for depression identified one randomised controlled trial that assessed vitamin D therapy as treatment for SAD (involving only 15 patients but suggesting the treatment was more effective than light therapy); one that assessed vitamin B12 as treatment for SAD (involving 27 patients, which found no benefit); and one that assessed ginkgo biloba for prevention of SAD relapse (involving 27 patients, which also found no benefit).[44]

One randomised trial, involving 27 patients with SAD, compared bright light (2500 lux between 2pm and 4pm daily), physical exercise (training on a stationary bicycle between 1pm and 2pm daily), and "no treatment" for one week.[45] The two active treatments reduced depressive symptoms (HAM-D21 fell by 64.5% with light and 68.5% with exercise, each P<0.001 v baseline) while "no treatment" did not (change in score 4.9%, not significant).

Negative ion generators

The environmental concentration of negative air ions varies greatly (for example, it is higher in humid, vegetated environments and at the seashore, and lower in urban environments and heated or air conditioned interiors).[24] It is thought that sustained exposure to negative air ionisation may elevate mood, although no definitive mechanism of action for this effect has been established.[25]

One double-blind randomised controlled trial involved only 25 patients with SAD, who received negative ions from an electronic device for 30 minutes shortly after rising (between 5.30am and 8.30am), for 20 days, at one of two doses.[46] More of those who received the higher density of ions achieved remission (58% with 2.7×10^6 ions/cm^3 v 15% with 104 ions/cm^3, P=0.025).

What do guidelines say?

American Psychiatric Association guidelines published in 2000 suggest that the entire range of treatments for major depressive disorder may also be used to treat patients with SAD, either in combination with, or as an alternative to, light therapy.[47] As first-line treatment, the guidelines recommend light therapy as a time-limited trial, primarily in out-patients with clear seasonal patterns of symptoms. For patients with more severe depression, the guidelines recommend light therapy as a potential adjunct to psychopharmacologic intervention.

British Association for Psychopharmacology guidelines published in 2008 state that antidepressants are a first-line treatment for moderate and severe major depression in adults irrespective of depression type, and that CBT may be used in addition.[26] For SAD, the guidelines state that light therapy is a first-line acute treatment but that effective prophylaxis against relapse is then needed, including consideration of an antidepressant. The limited evidence available suggests that bupropion or CBT helps to prevent recurrence the following winter.

Canadian Network for Mood and Anxiety Treatments (CANMAT) guidelines published in October 2009 recommend "second-generation" antidepressants (eg, SSRIs) or CBT first line for major depressive disorder, and medication plus CBT as second-line treatment.[48] [49] For SAD, they recommend light therapy first-line.[33]

The final draft of the NICE guideline on depression in adults, updated for publication in October 2009, suggests that people with depression with a seasonal pattern should be treated according to the strategy offered in the guideline for major depressive disorder in general.[36] Recommendations include an antidepressant (normally an SSRI) or CBT for mild to moderate depression, or both for moderate or severe depression; and that CBT should be offered for relapse prevention. The draft guideline also states that although there are a large number of studies that address the efficacy of light therapy in people with seasonal depression, they are difficult to interpret due to methodological differences. It goes on to propose that patients with winter depression who wish to try light therapy in preference to antidepressant or psychological treatment should be advised that the evidence for the efficacy of such therapy is uncertain.

The various guidelines appear to have reached different conclusions about light therapy because they included different studies and analysed primary data or published meta-analyses.[50]

Conclusion

Seasonal affective disorder (SAD) describes a subtype of major depression which has a seasonal pattern (usually winter depression and remission or hypomania during spring and summer). It includes atypical symptoms such as hypersomnia, carbohydrate craving and weight

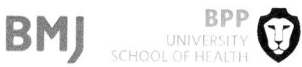

- This article was originally published in *Drug and Therapeutics Bulletin* (*DTB* 2009;47:128-32).
- *DTB* is a highly regarded source of unbiased, evidence based information and practical advice for healthcare professionals. It is independent of the pharmaceutical industry, government, and regulatory authorities, and is free of advertising.
- *DTB* is available online at http://dtb.bmj.com.

gain. A common approach is to treat the condition as for non-seasonal depression, for example, using SSRI antidepressants and/or cognitive behavioural therapy (CBT).

Light therapy has been suggested for treating people with SAD. Trials of such therapy are complex as they need a plausible control arm, and methodological differences between published trials have made the results hard to interpret. In addition, reviews and guidelines of light therapy have included different trials and reached contradictory conclusions. Nevertheless, bright light therapy in the early morning, using a light box or dawn simulation, appears to be a reasonable first-line approach to relieve depressive symptoms, instead of, or as well as, drug therapy and/or CBT when the patient has mild or moderate symptoms; people with more severe symptoms should be treated with antidepressant drugs, with or without light therapy and/or CBT.

For prevention of subsequent episodes, there is limited evidence for a benefit of CBT or bupropion (an unlicensed indication in the UK).

1 American Psychiatric Association. *Diagnostic and Statistical Manual of Mental Disorders* . 4th ed, text revision. American Psychiatric Association, 2000.
2 Michalak EE Wilkinson C, Dowrick C, Wilkinson G. Seasonal affective disorder: prevalence, detection and current treatment in North Wales. *Br J Psychiatry* 2001;179:31-4.
3 Thompson C, Thompson S, Smith R. Prevalence of seasonal affective disorder in primary care; a comparison of the seasonal health questionnaire and the seasonal pattern assessment questionnaire. *J Affect Disord* 2004;78:219-26.
4 Eagles JM, Howie FL, Cameron IM, Wileman SM, Andrew JE, Robertson C, et al. Use of health care services in seasonal affective disorder. *Br J Psychiatry* 2002;180:449-54.
5 Modell JG,.Rosenthal NE, Harriett AE, Krishen A, Asgharian A, Foster VJ, et al. Seasonal affective disorder and its prevention by anticipatory treatment with bupropion XL. *Biol Psychiatry* 2005;58:658-67.
6 Rosenthal NE, Sack DA, Gillin JC, Lewy AJ, Goodwin FK, Davenport Y, et al. Seasonal affective disorder: a description of the syndrome and preliminary findings with light therapy. *Arch Gen Psychiatry* 1984;41:72-80.
7 Hansen V, Skre I, Lund E. What is this thing called "SAD"? A critique of the concept of seasonal affective disorder. *Epidemiol Psichiatr Soc* 2008;17:120-7.
8 World Health Organization. International statistical classification of diseases and related health problems 10th revision, version for 2007 (ICD-10). 2007. http://apps.who.int/classifications/apps/icd/icd10online.
9 Lam RW, Levitt AJ, eds. Canadian consensus guidelines for the treatment of seasonal affective disorder. 1999. http://ubcsad.bc-alter.net/CCG%20SAD%201999.pdf.
10 Sohn CH, Lam RW. Update on the biology of seasonal affective disorder. *CNS Spectr* 2005;10:635-46.
11 European Medicines Agency. Assessment report for Circadin. 2007. www.emea.europa.eu/humandocs/PDFs/EPAR/circadin/H-695-en6.pdf.
12 Lewy AJ, Bauer VK, Cutler NL, Sack RL, Ahmed S, Thomas KH, et al. Morning vs evening light treatment of patients with winter depression. *Arch Gen Psychiatry* 1998;55:890-6.
13 Macchi MM, Bruce JN. Human pineal physiology and functional significance of melatonin. *Front Neuroendocrinol* 2004;25:177-95.
14 McIntyre IM, Norman TR, Burrows GD, Armstrong SM. Human melatonin suppression by light is intensity dependent. *J Pineal Res* 1989;6:149-56.
15 Avery DH, Eder DN, Bolte MA, Hellekson CJ, Dunner DL, Vitiello MV, et al. Dawn simulation and bright light in the treatment of SAD: a controlled study. *Biol Psychiatry* 2001;50:205-16.
16 Swedo SE, Pleeter JD, Richter DM, Hoffman CL, Allen AJ, Hamburger SD, et al. Rates of seasonal affective disorder in children and adolescents. *Am J Psychiatry* 1995;152:1016-9.
17 Magnusson A, Stefansson JG. Prevalence of seasonal affective disorder in Iceland. *Arch Gen Psychiatry* 1993;50:941-6.
18 Martiny K, Lunde M, Simonsen C, Clemmensen L, Poulsen DL, Solstad K, et al. Relapse prevention by citalopram in SAD patients responding to 1 week of light therapy. A placebo-controlled study. *Acta Psychiatr Scand* 2004;109:230-4.
19 Magnusson A, Partonen T. The diagnosis, symptomatology, and epidemiology of seasonal affective disorder. *CNS Spectr* 2005;10:625-34.
20 Michalak EE, Tam EM, Manjunath CV, Solomons K, Levitt AJ, Levitan R, et al. Generic and health-related quality of life in patients with seasonal and nonseasonal depression. *Psychiatry Res* 2004;128:245-51.
21 Michalak EE, Murray G, Levitt AJ, Levitan RD, Enns MW, Morehouse R, et al. Quality of life as an outcome indicator in patients with seasonal affective disorder: results from the Can-SAD study. *Psychol Med* 2007;37:727-36.
22 Williams JBW. A structured interview guide for the Hamilton Depression Rating Scale. *Arch Gen Psychiatry* 1988;45:742-7.
23 Moscovitch A, Blashko CA, Eagles JM, Darcourt G, Thompson C, Kasper S, et al. A placebo-controlled study of sertraline in the treatment of outpatients with seasonal affective disorder. *Psychopharmacology* 2004;171:390-7.
24 Terman M, Terman JS. Light therapy for seasonal and nonseasonal depression: efficacy, protocol, safety, and side effects. *CNS Spectr* 2005;10:647-63.
25 Terman M, Terman JS, Ross DC. A controlled trial of timed bright light and negative air ionization for treatment of winter depression. *Arch Gen Psychiatry* 1998;55:875-82.
26 Anderson IM, Ferrier IN, Baldwin RC, Cowen PJ, Howard L, Lewis G, et al. Evidence-based guidelines for treating depressive disorders with antidepressants: a revision of the 2000 British Association for Psychopharmacology guidelines. *J Psychopharmacol* 2008;22:343-96.
27 Lam RW, Gorman CP, Michalon M, Steiner M, Levitt AJ, Corral MR, et al. Multicenter, placebo-controlled study of fluoxetine in seasonal affective disorder. *Am J Psychiatry* 1995;152:1765-70.
28 Eli Lilly and Company Limited. Prozac 20 mg hard capsules, and 20 mg per 5 ml oral liquid. Summary of product characteristics, UK. Eli Lilly and Company Limited, 2009.
29 Wockhardt UK Ltd. Sertraline 50 mg and 100 mg film-coated tablets. Summary of product characteristics, UK. Wockhardt UK Ltd, 2009.
30 Westrin A, Lam RW. Long-term and preventative treatment for seasonal affective disorder. *CNS Drugs* 2007;21:901-9.
31 Terman JS, Terman M, Lo ES, Cooper TB. Circadian time of morning light administration and therapeutic response in winter depression. *Arch Gen Psychiatry* 2001;58:69-75.
32 GlaxoSmithKline UK. Zyban 150 mg prolonged release film-coated tablets. Summary of product characteristics. GlaxoSmithKline UK, 2009.
33 Ravindran AV, Lam RW, Filteau MJ, Lespérance F, Kennedy SH, Parikh SV, et al. Canadian Network for Mood and Anxiety Treatments (CANMAT) clinical guidelines for the management of major depressive disorder in adults. V. Complementary and alternative medicine treatments. *J Affect Disord* 2009;117:S54-64.
34 Eastman CI. Is bright light therapy a placebo? In: Partonen T, Magnusson A, eds. Seasonal affective disorder, practice and research. Oxford University Press, 2001.
35 Thompson C. Evidence-based treatment. In: Partonen T, Magnusson A, eds. Seasonal affective disorder: practice and research. Oxford University Press, 2001.
36 National Institute for Health and Clinical Excellence. Depression in adults (update). 2009. www.nice.org.uk/nicemedia/pdf/DepressionUpdateFullGuideline.pdf.
37 Golden RN, Gaynes BN, Ekstrom RD, Hamer RM, Jacobsen FM, Suppes T, et al. The efficacy of light therapy in the treatment of mood disorders: a review and meta-analysis of the evidence. *Am J Psychiatry* 2005;162:656-62.
38 EurLex. 31993L0042. Council directive 93/42/EEC of 14 June 1993 concerning medical devices. 1993. http://eur-lex.europa.eu/LexUriServ/LexUriServ.do?uri=CELEX:31993L0042:EN:HTML.
39 NHS Direct. Seasonal affective disorder. http://cks.library.nhs.uk/patient_information_leaflet/seasonal_affective_disorder.
40 Directgov. 2009. VAT relief on products and services for disabled people. www.direct.gov.uk/en/DisabledPeople/FinancialSupport/Taxreliefandreductions/DG_10028495.
41 National Light Hire. VAT exemption. 2009. www.sad-lighthire.co.uk/exemption.html.
42 Rohan KJ, Roecklein KA, Tierney Lindsey K, Johnson LG, Lippy RD, Lacy TJ, et al. A randomized controlled trial of cognitive-behavioral therapy, light therapy, and their combination for seasonal affective disorder. *J Consult Clin Psychol* 2007;75:489-500.
43 Rohan KJ, Lindsey KT, Roecklein KA, Lacy TJ. Cognitive-behavioral therapy, light therapy, and their combination in treating seasonal affective disorder. *J Affect Disord* 2004;80:273-83.
44 Jorm AF, Christensen H, Griffiths KM, Rodgers B. Effectiveness of complementary and self-help treatments for depression. *MJA* 2002;176:S84-96.
45 Pinchasov BB, Shurgaja AM, Grischin OV, Putilov AA. Mood and energy regulation in seasonal and non-seasonal depression before and after

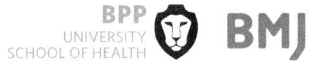

midday treatment with physical exercise or bright light. *Psychiatry Res* 2000;94:29-42.

46 Terman M, Terman JS. Treatment of seasonal affective disorder with a high-output negative ionizer. *J Altern Complement Med* 1995;1: 87-92.

47 American Psychiatry Association. Practice guideline for the treatment of patients with major depressive disorder (revision). *Am J Psychiatry* 2000;157(4 suppl):1-45.

48 Parikh SV, Segal ZV, Grigoriadis S, Ravindran AV, Kennedy SH, Lam RW, et al. Canadian Network for Mood and Anxiety Treatments (CANMAT) clinical guidelines for the management of major depressive disorder in adults. II. Psychotherapy alone or in combination with antidepressant medication. *J Affect Disord* 2009;117:S15-25.

49 Lam RW, Kennedy SH, Grigoriadis S, McIntyre RS, Milev R, Ramasubbu R, et al. Canadian Network for Mood and Anxiety Treatments (CANMAT) clinical guidelines for the management of major depressive disorder in adults. III. Pharmacotherapy. *J Affect Disord* 2009;117:S26-43.

50 Anderson IM, Haddad PM. CANMAT guidelines for depression: clear and user-friendly. *J Affect Disord* 2009;117:S3-4

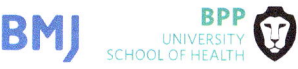

Obsessive-compulsive disorder

David Veale, consultant psychiatrist[1], reader in cognitive behaviour therapy[2],
Alison Roberts, clinical psychologist[1]

[1]Centre for Anxiety Disorders and Trauma, South London and Maudsley NHS Foundation Trust, London SE5 8AZ, UK

[2]Anxiety Disorders Residential Unit, South London and Maudsley NHS Foundation Trust and Institute of Psychiatry, King's College London

Correspondence to: D Veale david.veale@kcl.ac.uk

Cite this as: BMJ 2014;348:g2183

DOI: 10.1136/bmj.g2183

http://www.bmj.com/content/348/bmj.g2183

Obsessive-compulsive disorder (OCD) is characterised by the presence of obsessions or compulsions, or commonly of both. OCD is the fourth most common mental disorder after depression, alcohol/substance misuse, and social phobia, with a lifetime prevalence in community surveys of 1.6%.[1] The severity of OCD differs markedly from one person to another. People are often able to hide their OCD, even from their own family, although it can cause problems in relationships and interfere with the ability to study or work. Health consequences can also occur: fear of contamination can, for example, prevent the accessing of appropriate health services or lead to dermatitis from excessive washing. When the disorder starts in childhood or adolescence, young people may avoid socialising with peers or become unable to live independently. The World Health Organization ranks OCD as one of the 10 most handicapping conditions by lost income and decreased quality of life.[2] This clinical review summarises the evidence on how to recognise, assess, and manage people with OCD.

Who gets OCD?

OCD occurs all over the world, although cultural factors may shape the content. (For example, religious obsessions are more common in some communities.) The sex ratio in epidemiological surveys across the world is equal,[1] but more women have compulsive washing, and more men have sexual obsessions, magical numbers, or obsessional slowness.

The mean age of onset is late adolescence for men and the early 20s for women. However, OCD can also present in older people, either after a long history of the condition hitherto undiagnosed or with symptoms that are more recent in onset. OCD occurs with a point prevalence of about 1% of the population.[3] [4] Children and adolescents can also have OCD, with a prevalence of about 0.25% in 5-15 year olds.[5] They have a similar presentation to adults.[6] The differences reflect developmental stages (for example, more sexual and religious obsessions in adolescents than in children and more fears of death of a parent for young people than for adults).[6] Rarely, children may develop a sudden onset of obsessive-compulsive symptoms with an episodic course and the presence of motor tics, hyperactivity, or choreiform movements. This is associated with various infectious agents and other environmental factors in several case series of children with OCD.[7]

What are obsessions and compulsions?

An obsession is defined as an unwanted intrusive thought, doubt, image, or urge that repeatedly enters the mind. Obsessions are distressing and ego-dystonic (that is, they are repugnant or inconsistent with the person's values). The person usually regards the intrusions as unreasonable or excessive and tries to resist them. A minority of obsessions are regarded as overvalued ideas and, rarely, delusions.[8] Obsessions do not concern day to day worries, which occur in generalised anxiety disorder; perceived defects in appearance, which occur in body dysmorphic disorder; or fear of having a serious disease, which occurs in health anxiety.

Compulsions are repetitive behaviours or mental acts that a person feels driven to perform in response to an obsession. They are largely involuntary and are seldom resisted. A compulsion can take the form of either an overt action observable by others (such as checking that a door is locked) or a covert mental act that cannot be observed (such as repeating a certain phrase in the mind). Covert or mental compulsions are generally more difficult to resist or monitor than overt ones, as they are "portable" and easier to perform. The table lists common obsessions and compulsions. A compulsion in OCD is not in itself pleasurable, which differentiates it from impulsive acts such as shopping, gambling, or paraphilias that are associated with immediate gratification.

The term "ritual" is synonymous with compulsion but usually refers to motor acts. "Rumination" in OCD refers to mental acts repeated endlessly in response to intrusive ideas and doubts. The term "pure O" is sometimes used by patients to describe ruminations without observable compulsions. To warrant a diagnosis of OCD, obsessions and compulsions must be time consuming (for example, more than one hour a day) or cause significant distress or functional impairment (see box).[9] [10] Hoarding is a compulsion in OCD, but "hoarding disorder" is now planned to be a separate diagnosis in ICD-11 (international classification of diseases, 11th revision). It refers to the excessive acquisition and marked difficulty in discarding of items, regardless of their actual value, leading to significant distress or handicap.

Although tics may be mistaken for compulsions, they can be differentiated by the focal uncomfortable somatic sensations that precede and are relieved by the tic. Motor tics vary from simple abrupt movements to more complex and apparently purposive behaviours (such as clapping or touching an object). Phonic or vocal tics range from simple throat clearing sounds to more complex vocalisations in speech. The behaviour is considered a compulsion rather than a tic if it is performed a certain number of times or in a certain order or at a particular time of day, is done in response to an obsession, and is intended to reduce

SUMMARY POINTS

- The World Health Organization ranks obsessive-compulsive disorder (OCD) as one of the 10 most handicapping conditions by lost income and decreased quality of life
- OCD occurs across all ages but most commonly presents in young people
- Shame often prevents people with OCD seeking help and causes delays in effective treatment
- Non-specialists should ask screening questions if OCD is suspected
- OCD is a treatable condition—children and adults should initially be offered cognitive behavioural therapy
- For moderate to severe OCD in children and adults, selective serotonin reuptake inhibitors may also be offered

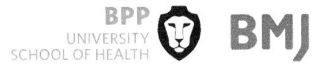

Common obsessions and compulsions

Obsessions	Related compulsions
Fears of contamination from dirt, germs, bodily fluids or faeces, chemicals, or dangerous material (for example, asbestos)	Washing and cleaning compulsions and avoidance of triggers
Fears of causing harm to self or others	Checking (for example, doors being locked) and reassurance compulsions
Excessive concern with symmetry or being "just so"	Ordering and repeating compulsions
Forbidden thoughts or images (for example, being a paedophile, blasphemy, or violence such as stabbing one's baby)	Checking one's memory and avoidance of triggers

anxiety or prevent harm. However, the boundaries between a complex tic and a tic-like compulsion can be blurred.[11]

How can we identify and diagnose obsessive-compulsive symptoms?

Simple screening questions for OCD take only a few minutes and may indicate a need for onward referral. Guidance from the National Institute for Health and Care Excellence (NICE)[12] suggests that the following questions can be used clinically to help to diagnose OCD when the symptoms are significantly distressing or interfering in a person's life:

- Do you wash or clean a lot?
- Do you check things a lot?
- Is there any thought that keeps bothering you that you would like to get rid of but cannot?
- Do your daily activities take a long time to finish?
- Are you concerned about putting things in a special order or are you very upset by mess?
- Do these problems trouble you?

If a person responds affirmatively to one of the above questions, a more formal diagnostic interview would be conducted. The diagnosis of OCD uses the ICD-10 criteria (see box). This will not fundamentally change in ICD-11.

Some people's OCD symptoms are easily observed or reported. They may wash repeatedly to prevent contamination, check plugs to prevent fire, or avoid harm in more idiosyncratic ways, using symmetry, order, or actions repeated to a lucky number. Some patients do not realise that they have OCD or feel too ashamed and stigmatised to seek help. They may present to a general practitioner with dermatological symptoms (from excessive washing), genital or anal symptoms (from excessive checking and washing), general stress (for example, from losing a job as a result of repeated lateness), or doubts about contracting HIV.

Other themes concern intrusions about sexuality, blasphemy, morality, or mistakes. OCD is more difficult to recognise when the compulsions are covert or stigmatising. Observers may notice simply that the person seems preoccupied or anxious or takes a long time to respond to questions. They would not be able to see the person trying mentally to replace unacceptable sexual thoughts with "safe" or "correct" thoughts, praying, or trying to reassure him or herself that a particular action is safe. Thus OCD is often hidden, as patients believe that their own intrusive thoughts or images are too shameful. They may refuse to reveal the content of their intrusive thoughts to a health professional, owing to the fear of being misunderstood or being reported to social services. Generalists may not need to know the exact content of intrusive thoughts, and reassuring a person with OCD that having unacceptable or senseless thoughts is extremely normal may be sufficient before onward referral.

Health visitors or social workers may, however, raise concerns about whether sexual or violent thoughts might mean that a person with OCD is dangerous. Each case needs to be assessed individually, but no recorded cases exist of people with OCD acting on their thoughts. In these situations, it is more important that health professionals assess the unintended risk (for example, a parent neglecting to change a nappy owing to fears of being a paedophile).[13]

A person with OCD is likely to terminate a compulsion when he or she feels "comfortable" or "just right." In the long term, this is a criterion that may be impossible to achieve or take a very long time to obtain. What is important in recognising and understanding OCD is not the behaviour but the intended aim of the behaviour. Thus the intended aim of a compulsion in OCD is to verify whether a threat exists (for example, a checking ritual) or to get rid of a threat by "undoing" it (for example, by compulsive washing or replacing a thought).

Avoidance is an integral part of OCD. Common examples are taking care not to touch toilet seats, door handles, or taps used by others; hiding all sharp objects or knives; and making sure never to be left alone with a child or suppressing intrusive unwanted images of having sex with a child if there are fears of being a paedophile. As well as anxiety, associated emotions in OCD include disgust (especially in contamination OCD), shame (especially with forbidden thoughts), and a distressing sense of "incompleteness" until things feel "just right."

Generalists should also assess the degree of family involvement in the OCD, attitudes to treatment, and any restrictions that have been placed on family members—being banned from using certain rooms, for example, or having to change clothes and shower when they enter the house. More often, patients are engaged in endless seeking of reassurance about whether an activity is safe. Relatives may accommodate the person's OCD or be overprotective, aggressive, dismissive, or avoidant. People with OCD may also react with aggression when a family member does not adhere to their compulsions. Family members are likely to use different ways of coping, resulting in further discord. Finally, the family may seek help for the patient, who may be unwilling to take this step him or herself.

What causes OCD?

A genetic predisposition to OCD is likely on the basis of twin and genome-wide linkage studies.[14] Developmental factors may include emotional, physical, and sexual abuse or neglect, social isolation, teasing, or bullying.[15] [16] Psychological factors that maintain OCD include an over-inflated sense of responsibility and magical thinking, an intolerance of uncertainty, and a belief in the controllability of intrusive thoughts.[17] Stressors include pregnancy and the postnatal period.[18] Examples of postnatal obsessions are worries about harming or abusing the baby or not being careful enough (for example, with bottle sterilisation). Common avoidance behaviour and compulsions include hiding knives, repeatedly seeking reassurance, or checking that the baby is still breathing while asleep. Compulsions and avoidance then "work" by reducing anxiety and perceived harm in the short term (and are therefore reinforcing), but this become a vicious circle with unintended consequences in the long term.

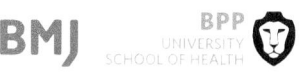

Very rarely, obsessive-compulsive symptoms can present in adults as a consequence of certain neurological conditions such as a brain tumour, Sydenham's chorea, Huntington's chorea, or frontotemporal dementia or as a complication of brain injury to the frontal lobe or basal skull. A rare presentation of OCD has also been described in children (paediatric autoimmune neuropsychiatric disorders associated with streptococcal infection, or PANDAS). It is characterised by a rapid onset and fluctuating symptoms of OCD or a broader set of neuropsychiatric symptoms, and it may be mediated by autoimmune antibodies in the basal ganglia after a streptococcal infection. However, no laboratory tests are available to help to make the diagnosis.[19] [20]

What other conditions are associated with OCD?

The most common comorbid diagnoses in surveys of people with OCD are depression (in about a third), social phobia (in a third), alcohol misuse (in a quarter), specific phobias (in a quarter), generalised anxiety disorder (in about 10%), and other related obsessive-compulsive disorders such as body dysmorphic disorder (in about 10%).[21] OCD is more common than would be expected in people with schizophrenia (in about 10%),[22] bipolar disorder (in about 10%),[23] anorexia and bulimia nervosa (in about 20%),[24] and Tourette's disorder (in about 20%).[23] Lastly, OCD symptoms are common in autistic spectrum disorder, but such patients are more likely to have repeating, hoarding, touching, tapping, and self damaging behaviours compared with those without autistic spectrum disorder.[25] However, symptoms of OCD in autistic spectrum disorder can also be confused with symptoms of excessive rigidity and a need to maintain "sameness," which is not fear driven as in OCD.

What treatments are available and how successful are they?

Research shows that people can spend 10 years or more struggling with OCD before they get the appropriate help.[26] The role of shame and stigma is common to many mental health problems but can be particularly problematic for people with OCD who have ego-dystonic sexual or violent thoughts. People with OCD also describe getting very skilled at hiding their compulsions in an attempt to carry on functioning as normal.

Psychological treatment

NICE's guidance on efficacy and tolerability is based on 17 controlled studies and concludes that cognitive behavioural therapy that includes "exposure and response prevention" is an effective treatment for OCD.[12] [27] A key message to people with OCD is that it is not their fault that they have developed OCD and that this is a recognised condition that can be treated. Therapy fundamentally consists of patients repeatedly testing out their fears and expectations and learning to tolerate anxiety, while not performing any compulsive or safety seeking behaviour. This can be done gradually as planned exposure or as part of a behavioural experiment to test whether the results best fit the theory that they have a problem with worrying that a bad event will happen (rather than a problem with causing a bad event to happen). Good quality cognitive behavioural therapy will provide this in the context of a supportive and empathic relationship and a shared understanding of the problem (for example, having a good understanding about how the things people do to keep themselves feeling safe are actually counterproductive and make things worse).[17]

Follow-up studies of cognitive behavioural therapy show that about 30% of people refuse treatment, leave early, or do not respond.[28] Other studies have shown that up to 50% of people have residual symptoms after treatment.[29] A recent systematic review attempted to identify predictors of drop-out and poor response, but only hoarding was a poor predictor.[30] A common belief exists that people who have had the problem for a long time need very long term treatment, but a recent meta-analysis found that the duration of treatment was unrelated to outcome.[30] No evidence of efficacy or effectiveness exists for psychoanalysis in the treatment of OCD, and insufficient evidence is available to support the use of other psychological therapies, hypnosis, or homeopathy.[12]

Drug treatment

Good evidence exists for the benefit of selective serotonin reuptake inhibitors (SSRIs) and clomipramine in the short term and in the longer term for prevention of relapse. SSRIs are acknowledged as the first line drug treatment of choice because of better tolerability than clomipramine. A dose-response relation exists with SSRIs, so that higher doses are better for OCD than is the standard dose of an SSRI needed for depression. A trial of an SSRI at the highest tolerated dose lasts for at least 12 weeks. However, discontinuation of an SSRI or clomipramine, in the absence of cognitive behavioural therapy, usually leads to a high rate of relapse.

Drug treatments beyond SSRIs are unlicensed and should be preceded by specialist assessment. For those patients for whom SSRIs and cognitive behavioural therapy have been ineffective, the evidence for adjunctive antipsychotic drugs in the short term is weak and an increased risk of adverse events is seen in the long term. Thus a recent controlled trial of patients resistant to one SSRI found that cognitive behavioural therapy was more effective than either risperidone or a placebo.[31] Meta-analyses show no significant benefit for augmentation with quietapine or olanzapine, a small effect size for risperidone, and a modest effect size for aripiprazole.[32] Antipsychotics are thus recommended only in patients who are refractory to cognitive behavioural therapy and SSRIs. When an antipsychotic is prescribed, it should be given at a low dose for a four week trial to determine whether it is effective. Novel compounds with some evidence for refractory cases include lamotrogine, topiramate, and acetylcysteine.[33]

Other treatment

Ablative lesion neurosurgery is used very rarely for extremely refractory patients, although no controlled trials have been done. Deep brain stimulation is being investigated as an alternative to ablative neurosurgery for very severe refractory cases. A systematic review of transcranial magnetic stimulation found it to be ineffective in OCD.[12] No evidence exists of a benefit of antibiotics in children with PANDAS, as the antibodies are the cause of the problem not the bacteria themselves. Plasma exchange or immunoglobulin might be used in the most severe children only.[34]

Where and how do I refer?

The NICE guidelines on OCD suggest that the first point of referral is to a service where people may be offered either low intensity interventions such as guided self help or computerised cognitive behavioural therapy with a psychological wellbeing practitioner.[35] [36] However, most

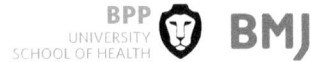

QUESTIONS FOR FUTURE RESEARCH

- Is low intensity or computerised cognitive behavioural therapy effective for mild to moderate obsessive-compulsive disorder (OCD)?

- Is intensive cognitive behavioural therapy (same duration delivered over one week) as effective as standard cognitive behavioural therapy (delivered once a week)?

- What are the most effective treatments for severe OCD refractory to treatment?

- What is the best way help a family cope with OCD?

- How can we predict who will respond to cognitive behavioural therapy or drug treatment?

- How can the risk of relapse be reduced (given the chronic and fluctuating course in some people with OCD)?

ADDITIONAL EDUCATIONAL RESOURCES

Resources for health professionals

- Veale D, Freeston M, Krebs G, Heyman I, Salkovskis P. Risk assessment and management in obsessive-compulsive disorder. *Adv Psychiatr Treat* 2009;15;332-43 (http://apt.rcpsych.org/content/15/5/332.full)—Describes risk assessment in OCD

- NICE guidelines on treating obsessive-compulsive disorder (OCD) and body dysmorphic disorder (2005) (http://publications.nice.org.uk/obsessive-compulsive-disorder-cg31)—Remains the best resource for treating OCD using stepped care

- NICE evidence update on OCD (2013) (http://arms.evidence.nhs.uk/resources/hub/1028833/attachment)—Latest update on treating OCD

Websites for people with OCD and their carers

- Maternal OCD (www.maternalocd.org)—Information on OCD presenting in the perinatal period

- OCD Action (www.ocdaction.org.uk)—National charity in the UK

- Obsessive Compulsive Foundation (www.ocfoundation.org)—US national charity

- OCD UK (www.ocduk.org)—National charity in the UK

- OCD Youth (www.ocdyouth.info)—Information on OCD for young people and their carers

Books for people with OCD and their carers

- Challacombe F, Oldfield V, Salkovskis P. Break free from OCD. Vermilion, 2011

- Derisley J, Heyman I, Robinson S, Turner C. Breaking free from OCD: a CBT guide for young people and their families. Jessica Kinglsey, 2008

- Veale D, Willson R. Overcoming OCD: a self-help guide using cognitive behavioural techniques. Robinson, 2009

---

patients would be offered 12 to 20 sessions of individual cognitive behavioural therapy.

People who have failed a course of cognitive behavioural therapy or SSRI (or a combination of the two), or who have more complex OCD or present with significant risks, should be referred to secondary care under the principle of stepped care. A stepped care model seeks to treat patients at the lowest appropriate service tier in the first instance, only "stepping up" to a specialist service when clinically required. This does not mean that everyone has to slavishly start at the lowest level of intervention, as sometimes immediate referral to a secondary care is clinically appropriate. If secondary care is ineffective, they should be referred to specialist outpatient services where particular emphasis should be put on prolonged, active exposure and experiments with the therapist, including home based treatment, which local, non-specialist services often do not have the capacity to deliver. Alternatively, the patient may benefit from more intensive cognitive behavioural therapy in a specialist residential or inpatient setting.[37] OCD can have a chronic and fluctuating course, so if someone has been previously seen for treatment they should be re-referred as a priority.[12]

DV acknowledges salary support from the National Institute for Health Research (NIHR) Biomedical Research Centre for Mental Health at South London and Maudsley NHS Foundation Trust and the Institute of Psychiatry, King's College London.

Contributors: Both DV and AR contributed to writing the manuscript. DV is the guarantor.

Competing interests: We have read and understood the BMJ Group policy on declaration of interests and declare the following interests: DV is an author of one of the recommended books.

Provenance and peer review: Commissioned; externally peer reviewed.

SOURCES AND SELECTION CRITERIA

We referred to published systematic reviews, including the treatment guideline from the National Institute for Health and Care Excellence (2005) and the obsessive compulsive disorder evidence update (2013). We identified reviews by searches for "compulsive behavior", "obsessive-compulsive disorder", "obsessive behavior", "compulsions", "obsessions", "obsessive compulsive neurosis", "scrupulosity", "symmetry", "recur$ adj obsession$", "recurr$ adj thought$", "symmetr$ or count$ or arrang$ or order$ or wash$ or repeat$ or hoard$ or clean$ or check$ (adj compulsi$)"

---

1 Kessler RC, Berglund P, Demler O, Jin R, Merikangas KR, Walters EE. Lifetime prevalence and age-of-onset distributions of DSM-IV disorders in the National Comorbidity Survey Replication. *Arch Gen Psychiatry* 2005;62:593-602.

2 Bobes J, Gonzalez MP, Bascaran MT, Arango C, Saiz PA, Bousono M. Quality of life and disability in patients with obsessive-compulsive disorder. *Eur Psychiatry* 2001;16:239-45.

3 Kessler RC, Chiu WT, Demler O, Merikangas KR, Walters EE. Prevalence, severity, and comorbidity of 12-month DSM-IV disorders in the National Comorbidity Survey Replication. *Arch Gen Psychiatry* 2005;62:617-27.

4 Wittchen HU, Jacobi F. Size and burden of mental disorders in Europe—a critical review and appraisal of 27 studies. *Eur Neuropsychopharmacol* 2005;15:357-76.

5 Heyman I, Fombonne E, Simmons H, Ford T, Meltzer H, Goodman R. Prevalence of obsessive-compulsive disorder in the British nationwide survey of child mental health. *Br J Psychiatry* 2001;179:324-9.

6 Kalra SK, Swedo SE. Children with obsessive-compulsive disorder: are they just "little adults"? *J Clin Invest* 2009;119:737-46.

7 Singer HS, Gilbert DL, Wolf DS, Mink JW, Kurlan R. Moving from PANDAS to CANS. *J Pediatr* 2012;160:725-31.

8 Veale D. Over-valued ideas: a conceptual analysis. *Behav Res Ther* 2002;40:383-400.

9 American Psychiatric Association. DSM 5. APA, 2013.

10 World Health Organization. International statistical classification of diseases and related health problems. 10th revision. WHO, 1992.

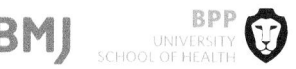

11 Palumbo D, Kurlan R. Complex obsessive compulsive and impulsive symptoms in Tourette's syndrome. *Neuropsychiatr Dis Treat* 2007;3:687-93.

12 National Institute for Health and Clinical Excellence. Obsessive-compulsive disorder: core interventions in the treatment of obsessive-compulsive disorder and body dysmorphic disorder. NICE, 2005.

13 Veale D, Freeston M, Krebs G, Heyman I, Salkovskis P. Risk assessment and management in obsessive-compulsive disorder. *Adv Psychiatr Treat* 2009;15:332-43.

14 Pauls DL. The genetics of obsessive-compulsive disorder: a review. *Dialogues Clin Neurosci* 2010;12:149-63.

15 Grisham JR, Fullana MA, Mataix-Cols D, Moffitt TE, Caspi A, Poulton R. Risk factors prospectively associated with adult obsessive-compulsive symptom dimensions and obsessive-compulsive disorder. *Psychol Med* 2011;41:2495-506.

16 Pace SM, Thwaites R, Freeston MH. Exploring the role of external criticism in obsessive compulsive disorder: a narrative review. *Clin Psychol Rev* 2011;31:361-70.

17 Obsessive Compulsive Cognitions Working Group. Cognitive assessment of obsessive-compulsive disorder. *Behav Res Ther* 1997;35:667-81.

18 Russell EJ, Fawcett JM, Mazmanian D. Risk of obsessive-compulsive disorder in pregnant and postpartum women: a meta-analysis. *J Clin Psychiatry* 2013;74:377-85.

19 Swedo SE, Leonard HL, Rapoport JL. The pediatric autoimmune neuropsychiatric disorders associated with streptococcal infection (PANDAS) subgroup: separating fact from fiction. *Pediatrics* 2004;113:907-11.

20 Susan E. From research subgroup to clinical syndrome: modifying the PANDAS criteria to describe PANS (pediatric acute-onset neuropsychiatric syndrome). *Pediatr Therapeut* 2012;2:113.

21 Murphy DL, Timpano KR, Wheaton MG, Greenberg BD, Miguel EC. Obsessive-compulsive disorder and its related disorders: a reappraisal of obsessive-compulsive spectrum concepts. *Dialogues Clin Neurosci* 2010;12:131-48.

22 Achim AM, Maziade M, Raymond E, Olivier D, Merette C, Roy MA. How prevalent are anxiety disorders in schizophrenia? A meta-analysis and critical review on a significant association. *Schizophr Bull* 2011;37:811-21.

23 Pallanti S, Grassi G, Sarrecchia ED, Cantisani A, Pellegrini M. Obsessive-compulsive disorder comorbidity: clinical assessment and therapeutic implications. *Front Psychiatry* 2011;2:70.

24 Kaye WH, Bulik CM, Thornton L, Barbarich N, Masters K. Comorbidity of anxiety disorders with anorexia and bulimia nervosa. *Am J Psychiatry* 2004;161:2215-21.

25 Russell AJ, Mataix-Cols D, Anson M, Murphy DG. Obsessions and compulsions in Asperger syndrome and high-functioning autism. *Br J Psychiatry* 2005;186:525-8.

26 Hollander E, Stein D, Kwon J, Rowland C, Wong C, Broatch J, et al. Psychosocial function and economic costs of obsessive-compulsive disorder. *CNS Spectrum* 1997;2:15-25.

27 Roth AFP. What works for whom? A critical review of psychotherapy research. Guilford Press, 1996.

28 Foa EB, Emmelkamp PMG. Failures in behaviour therapy. Wiley, 1983.

29 Abramowitz JS. The psychological treatment of obsessive-compulsive disorder. *Can J Psychiatry* 2006;51:407-16.

30 Olatunji BO, Davis ML, Powers MB, Smits JA. Cognitive-behavioral therapy for obsessive-compulsive disorder: a meta-analysis of treatment outcome and moderators. *J Psychiatr Res* 2013;47:33-41.

31 Simpson HB, Foa EB, Liebowitz MR, Huppert JD, Cahill S, Maher MJ, et al. Cognitive-behavioral therapy vs risperidone for augmenting serotonin reuptake inhibitors in obsessive-compulsive disorder: a randomized clinical trial. *JAMA Psychiatry* 2013;70:1190-9.

32 Komossa K, Depping AM, Meyer M, Kissling W, Leucht S. Second-generation antipsychotics for obsessive compulsive disorder. *Cochrane Database Syst Rev* 2010;(12):CD008141.

33 National Institute for Health and Care Excellence. Obsessive-compulsive disorder: evidence update 2013. NICE, 2013.

34 Perlmutter SJ, Leitman SF, Garvey MA, Hamburger S, Feldman E, Leonard HL, et al. Therapeutic plasma exchange and intravenous immunoglobulin for obsessive-compulsive disorder and tic disorders in childhood. *Lancet* 1999;354:1153-8.

35 Lovell K, Bee P. Optimising treatment resources for OCD: a review of the evidence base for technology-enhanced delivery. *J Ment Health* 2011;20:525-42.

36 Herbst N, Voderholzer U, Stelzer N, Knaevelsrud C, Hertenstein E, Schlegl S, et al. The potential of telemental health applications for obsessive-compulsive disorder. *Clin Psychol Rev* 2012;32:454-66.

37 Oldfield VB, Salkovskis PM, Taylor T. Time-intensive cognitive behaviour therapy for obsessive-compulsive disorder: a case series and matched comparison group. *Br J Clin Psychol* 2011;50:7-18.

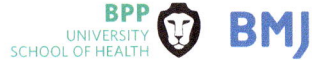

Bipolar disorder

Ian M Anderson, professor of psychiatry[1], Peter M Haddad, consultant psychiatrist and honorary reader in psychiatry[1 2], Jan Scott, professor of psychological medicine[3 4]

[1]Neuroscience and Psychiatry Unit, University of Manchester, Manchester M13 9PT, UK

[2]Greater Manchester West Mental Health NHS Foundation Trust, Manchester, UK

[3]Academic Psychiatry, Wolfson Unit Campus for Vitality and Ageing, Newcastle University, UK

[4]Fondation Fondamental and Universite-Paris-Est-Creteil, Paris, France

Correspondence to: I M Anderson
ian.anderson@manchester.ac.uk

Cite this as: *BMJ* 2012;345:e8508

DOI: 10.1136/bmj.e8508

http://www.bmj.com/content/345/bmj.e8508

Bipolar (affective) disorder, originally called manic depressive illness, is one of the most challenging psychiatric disorders to manage. Although it has been associated with creativity, it has a negative impact on the lives of most patients and more than 6% die through suicide in the two decades after diagnosis.[1] Organisational change means that specialist services mostly treat acute episodes, leaving primary care with long term management. This review summarises current best practice in the diagnosis and management of bipolar disorder, signposting areas of uncertainty.

What is bipolar disorder?

Bipolar disorders are characterised by recurrent episodes of elevated mood and depression, which are accompanied by changes in activity or energy and associated with characteristic cognitive, physical, and behavioural symptoms (fig 1). The term mania is used when elevated mood is severe and sustained or associated with psychotic symptoms, leading to marked disturbance of behaviour and function. Hypomania refers to less severe elevations in mood, which may be fairly brief, with a lower level of disturbance that usually does not bring the person to medical attention; however, hypomania may progress to mania. Bipolar disorders are divided into bipolar I disorder with episodes of mania and bipolar II disorder in which only episodes of hypomania occur (fig 1). Although traditionally viewed as opposite poles, manic and depressive symptoms often co-occur, giving rise to "mixed" states.[2]

In community samples, as many people experience milder episodic highs (subthreshold) as those who meet the criteria for bipolar disorder,[3] and together they form the bipolar spectrum. Cyclothymia refers to a subset of milder disorders with repeated short cycles of hypomania and mildly lowered mood occurring regularly over two or more years. There is controversy about whether these milder disorders, which can overlap with personality characteristics, should be included under the diagnosis of bipolar disorder,[4] and where to set the threshold between unipolar and bipolar disorder for those with episodes of depression and mild symptoms of hypomania.[5]

Who gets bipolar disorder?

A recent worldwide survey in 11 countries found a median age of onset of about 25 years,[3] with an overall lifetime prevalence of 0.6% for bipolar I disorder (male predominance, although an equal sex ratio has been found in other studies) and 0.4% for bipolar II disorder (female predominance). Milder subthreshold disorders had a worldwide lifetime prevalence of 1.4%. The highest values were found in the United States (1.0%, 1.1%, and 2.4% respectively).[3] Prepubertal mania is rare; typically, minor mood disturbance in adolescence progresses to episodes of depression and then to mania in adult life.[6]

What causes bipolar disorder?

Bipolar I disorder has a heritability of 0.75 explained largely by common variant alleles, which partly overlap with those for schizophrenia.[7] Its phenotypic expression is a result of interacting genetic and environmental factors. Physical or sexual abuse in childhood is nearly twice as common as in healthy people and is associated with an earlier onset and more severe illness course.[8] Life events and chronic stressors are important in precipitating and perpetuating mood episodes.[9]

What makes bipolar disorder so challenging?

Comorbid psychiatric disorders, most often anxiety disorders, are common (box 1).[3] Over a third of cases, especially those with early onset disorder, also have an alcohol or drug disorder, either as a precipitant or secondary complication.

Poor insight into being ill and rejection of help are more common in acute mania than in other phases of illness. This can necessitate compulsory treatment and make collaborative management difficult, even after recovery from acute episodes.[10] Disinhibited and violent behaviour in mania may lead to risk or harm to others and involvement of the criminal justice system. By contrast, hypomania often escapes medical attention and, even if recognised, there can be a reluctance to seek treatment or prevent recurrence. The patient may view hypomania as positive and associated with increased energy and productivity. Episodes of hypomania or mania nearly always have negative social, financial, and occupational consequences, which can be long lasting and, particularly with mania, devastating.

When help is sought for depression, which is more common than elevated mood,[11] previous episodes of hypomania are often not detected. Diagnosis may be delayed for many years after the first mood symptoms, which can lead to ineffective, or even harmful, treatment.[12] The "conversion rate" from depression to bipolar disorder is estimated at 1% a year,[13] and high rates of unrecognised bipolar disorder have been found in depressed patients who respond poorly to antidepressants.[14]

The disorder's variable course, ranging from isolated brief or infrequent episodes with full inter-episode recovery to severe persistent or chaotic illness, poses major challenges

---

SUMMARY POINTS

- Bipolar disorder is characterised by recurrent episodes of elevated mood and depression, together with changes in activity levels
- Elevated mood is severe and sustained (mania) in bipolar I disorder and less severe (hypomania) in bipolar II disorder
- Depression is usually more common and longer lasting than elevated mood, and—together with inter-episode milder symptoms—contributes most to overall morbidity
- Other psychiatric disorders, such as anxiety disorder and alcohol and drug misuse, are common
- Risk of death from suicide and from natural causes, most often cardiovascular disease, is increased
- Treatment is with drugs and supplemental psychotherapies; for both acute episodes and maintenance, treatment is guided by whether mania or depression predominates

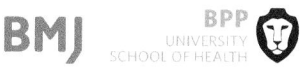

for management. Rapid cycling (four or more mood episodes each year) is a marker of severity and poor treatment response. Mild to moderate cognitive deficits such as impaired verbal learning, memory, and executive function can be present even when patients are euthymic and may lead to impaired functioning.[15]

Deliberate self harm—particularly associated with depressive and mixed episodes, psychosis, and substance misuse—occurs in 30-40% of patients.[16] The completed suicide rate in a recent large prospective study was 7.8% in men and 4.8% in women over a median 18 year follow-up after first psychiatric contact, higher than for depression or schizophrenia.[1] In addition, the standardised mortality ratio for natural causes of death is about 2.[17] Cardiovascular illness is the most common cause and is linked to lifestyle, obesity, and other components of the metabolic syndrome.

BOX 1 DIFFERENTIAL DIAGNOSIS OF BIPOLAR DISORDER

- Unipolar depression: Have a high index of suspicion of bipolar disorder in early onset severe depression or if there is a strong family history. Look for a history of elevated mood and remember that irritable agitation can be a presenting feature of bipolar disorder
- Reaction to stress*: Check for associated symptoms suggestive of bipolar disorder when prominent fluctuating mood arises from stressful life events
- Substance misuse*: Check whether mood changes came before or after an increase in drug or alcohol use because elevated mood can lead to loss of control of drug or alcohol intake
- Personality disorders, traits, or cyclothymia*: Should be suspected if there is a long history of relatively mild, brief, and often rapidly varying mood fluctuation starting in adolescence, without definite episodes of mania or hypomania or long periods of stable mood
- Attention deficit hyperactivity disorder (ADHD)*: ADHD and bipolar disorder have similar symptoms; because ADHD is more common, bipolar disorder should not be diagnosed before adulthood unless there are clear episodes of euphoric mood
- Schizophrenia or schizoaffective disorder: Prominent psychotic symptoms, especially if bizarre or not congruent with elevated or depressed mood, should raise the possibility of schizophrenia or schizoaffective disorder, particularly if the psychotic symptoms pre-date, or dominate, the mood symptoms
- Medical and organic brain conditions*: Suspect an underlying organic cause in atypical or fluctuating presentations or when manic-like or depressive symptoms occur in the context of illnesses or drugs known to cause behavioural change. These include neurological conditions, cerebrovascular disease, dementia and confusional states, endocrine disorders, and after administration of steroids.

* Comorbidity with bipolar disorder must also be considered.

How is bipolar disorder diagnosed?

The key to diagnosis is the presence or history of hypomania or mania. Of note, a predominantly irritable mood may mask an underlying manic picture, and psychotic symptoms can be mistaken for schizophrenia. Take a careful history and perform a mental state examination (fig 1 and box 2), and supplement this with collateral information. Be aware that elevated mood may be denied or not reported. Hypomania may not be obvious without previous knowledge of the person and may come to medical attention only after repeated episodes, adverse consequences, or pressure from others. The overlap with other disorders (box 1) can lead to a missed diagnosis if comorbidity with bipolar disorder is not considered.

To avoid overdiagnosis, in children and adolescents the diagnosis of bipolar disorder requires the presence of mania with unequivocal euphoria (not just irritability) and an episodic course.[16 18 19]

Self rating questionnaires, such as the mood disorder questionnaire (fig 2) or the hypomania checklist,[20 21] can help identify previous hypomanic or manic episodes with reasonable sensitivity but low specificity in general populations.

How do I distinguish between bipolar and unipolar depression?

Depression occurring in bipolar disorder cannot be reliably distinguished from unipolar depression on the basis of symptoms alone. In the absence of a history of elevated mood, a comprehensive review of studies comparing depression in the two disorders has proposed an approach based on symptom profile, family history, and illness course (box 3).[22]

How is bipolar disorder managed?

Acute treatment of episodes of illness aims to resolve symptoms and reduce immediate risk to self or others. Long term treatment aims to prevent future episodes of illness and help regain a premorbid level of functioning, improve physical health, and reduce longer term suicide

---

Effective treatments for bipolar disorder[18 19 23-32]

Indication	Treatment*	
	Drugs†	Adjunctive psychotherapy
Mania and mixed states	Good evidence: antipsychotics as a class, valproate, lithium, combined antipsychotics + lithium or valproate	Low stimulus environment (clinical experience)
	Suggestive evidence: carbamazepine	
	Short term benzodiazepines are clinically used for treating agitation and insomnia	
Depression	Good evidence: quetiapine	Good evidence: cognitive behavioural therapy, family focused therapy
	Suggestive evidence: olanzapine + fluoxetine‡, olanzapine, lamotrigine, lithium, valproate	
	Evidence for efficacy of antidepressants is poor	Suggestive evidence: interpersonal and social rhythm therapy
Maintenance and prevention of relapse§	Good evidence: monotherapy with lithium (mania and depression), antipsychotics as a class (mania), quetiapine (depression and mania), olanzapine (mania more than depression), lamotrigine (depression more than mania); combination therapy with antipsychotics + lithium or valproate (better than lithium or valproate alone for mania), lithium + valproate (better than valproate for overall relapse), quetiapine + lithium or valproate (better than lithium or valproate alone for mania and depression)	Good evidence: group psychoeducation (mania more than depression), family focused therapy
	Suggestive evidence: valproate (depression more than mania)	Suggestive evidence: cognitive behavioural therapy (especially less frequent relapsers), interpersonal and social rhythm therapy, cognitive remediation (cognitive impairment)
	Carbamazepine lacks an evidence base	

*Good evidence: meta-analysis and better quality randomised controlled trials against placebo unless otherwise stated; suggestive evidence: inconsistent or weak effects from meta-analysis or poorer quality randomised controlled trials against placebo.

†Inclusion of a drug in this table does not mean that the drug is licensed for the relevant indication; check approval status in your country.

‡Available as a single tablet in the United States.

§Most studies have been done in "enriched samples" where patients have responded to initial treatment with the drug(s) being investigated.

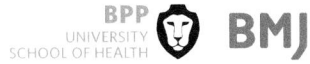

risk. Patients cycling between mania or hypomania and depression are especially difficult to treat, and stabilising mood is as important as treating the acute episode.

Diagnostic criteria for bipolar disorder (based on DSM-IV)

Bipolar I disorder*: Presence, or history of, at least one manic (or mixed) episode

Bipolar II disorder*: Presence, or history of, at least one major depressive episode and at least one hypomanic episode (with no history of a manic or mixed episode)

The symptoms are not attributable to physical illness or physiological effects of a drug or other substance and are not better accounted for by another psychiatric disorder

Manic symptoms	Depressive symptoms
Elevated, expansive, or irritable mood	Depressed mood
Increased activity that is goal directed or psychomotor agitation	Markedly reduced interest in nearly all activities
Reduced need for sleep	Increased or decreased appetite or weight
Excessive involvement in pleasurable activities with likely adverse consequences	Insomnia or hypersomnia
Inflated self esteem or grandiosity	Psychomotor retardation or agitation
Increased or pressured speech	Fatigue or loss of energy
Flight of ideas or racing thoughts	Feelings of excessive worthlessness or guilt
Distractibility	Impaired concentration or indecisiveness
	Recurrent thoughts or actions of death or suicide

Manic episode: At least four manic symptoms including altered mood that persists for at least a week and causes marked functional impairment, hospital admission, or there are psychotic symptoms

Hypomanic episode: As for manic episode but less severe; symptoms persist for at least four days and functioning is noticeably altered but not enough to lead to hospital admission or to greatly impair function. There are no psychotic symptoms

Major depressive episode: Five or more persistent depressive symptoms (which must include depressed mood or diminished interest), which last for at least two weeks and occur on most days, and that cause serious distress or functional impairment

Mixed episode: Persistent mood symptoms for at least a week that meet criteria (apart from duration) for both a manic and major depressive episode, which occur at different times or rapidly alternate

Psychotic symptoms: These may occur during manic episodes in bipolar I disorder (but by definition not during hypomanic episodes) and during depressive episodes in either bipolar I or bipolar II disorder

*The World Health Organization classification ICD-10 does not distinguish between bipolar I and bipolar II disorder and requires another mood episode in addition to a single manic episode

Fig 1 Diagnostic criteria for bipolar disorder. DSM-IV=*Diagnostic and Statistical Manual of Mental Disorders*, fourth edition; ICD-10=international classification of diseases, 10th revision

Mood disorder questionnaire to screen for previous episodes of elevated mood[20]

1 Has there ever been a period of time when you were not your usual self and...

...you felt so good or so hyper that other people thought you were not your normal self or you were so hyper that you got into trouble?	Yes/No
...you were so irritable that you shouted at people or started fights or arguments?	Yes/No
...you felt much more self confident that usual?	Yes/No
...you got much less sleep than usual and found that you didn't really miss it?	Yes/No
...you were much more talkative or spoke faster than usual?	Yes/No
...thoughts raced round your head or you couldn't slow your mind down?	Yes/No
...you were so easily distracted by things around you that you had trouble concentrating or keeping on track?	Yes/No
...you had much more energy than usual?	Yes/No
...you were much more active or did many more things than usual?	Yes/No
...you were much more social or outgoing than usual; for example, you telephoned friends in the middle of the night?	Yes/No
...you were much more interested in sex than usual?	Yes/No
...you did things that were unusual for you or that other people might have thought were excessive, foolish, or risky?	Yes/No
...spending money got you or your family into trouble?	Yes/No

2 If you checked YES to more than one of the above, have several of these ever happened during the same period of time? *Please circle one response only.*

Yes   No

3 How much of a problem did any of these cause you - like being unable to work; having family, money, or legal troubles; getting into arguments or fights? Please circle one response only.

No problem   Minor problem   Moderate problem   Serious problem

Scoring: Likely bipolar disorder if at least 7 symptoms from section 1 are answered YES together with YES in section 2 and moderate or serious problem in section 3

Fig 2 Mood disorder questionnaire

Drugs form the mainstay of treatment for bipolar I and II disorders but their role in milder disorders is less well established (table). Specific psychotherapies are important adjuncts in reducing relapse, treating depression, and improving function (table). Other crucial elements include ensuring a strong therapeutic alliance with treating clinicians, maintaining continuity of care, and tackling comorbid disorders and risk factors for relapse, including alcohol and substance misuse and disrupted circadian rhythms.

Given the lack of evidence on how to treat comorbid psychiatric disorders (such as anxiety), usual practice is to stabilise mood and then carefully treat the specific disorder.

What drugs are effective?

Most evidence concerns the treatment of mania and bipolar depression, with less evidence on hypomania and milder mood fluctuations. Many drugs are more effective for one

---

BOX 2 CLINICAL ASSESSMENT OF BIPOLAR DISORDER

Observe the patient for changes in psychomotor activity and behaviour:

- In hypomania or mania there may be obvious elation, with flamboyant gestures and dress as well as increased activity and speed of movements, with the patient having difficulty staying still. Speech may be rapid and difficult to interrupt, moving rapidly from one topic to another, with a grandiose flavour to the content. Irritability may be close to the surface or even prominent
- In depression distress may be obvious; eyes may be downcast and tears present, movements may be slow, or agitation may be present and speech similarly affected. The content of speech typically has negative themes about self, relationships with others, and the world

Take a full history of depressive and manic symptoms in current and previous episodes (including inter-episode symptoms)

Screening questions for hypomania and mania

- Do you currently (or have you in the past) experienced mood that is (was) higher than normal, or do you feel (have felt) much more irritable than usual, and that others have noticed?
- At the same time do (did) you have an increase in your energy levels so that you are (were) much more active or don't (didn't) need as much sleep?

If the answer to both of these is yes ask about other symptoms of mania (fig 1)

Screening questions for depression

- In the past month have you often been bothered by feeling down, depressed, or hopeless?
- During the past month have you often been bothered by having little interest or pleasure in doing things?

If the answer to either of these is yes ask about other symptoms of depression (fig 1)

Ask about a family history of psychiatric disorder, especially bipolar disorder

Assess

- Triggers to episodes and current psychosocial stressors
- Effects on social, personal, and occupational functioning
- Comorbidities including substance misuse, anxiety, and physical illness
- Risk of suicide or harm to others
- Obtain a corroborative history where possible
- Consider using a self rating scale to assess previous episodes of elevated mood

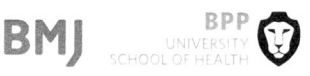

pole of the illness (table), so patients on "mood stabilisers" (usually referring to lithium or an anticonvulsant) may not be treated equally for both poles.

The details of effective drugs and the strength of the evidence in the table are based on recent evidence based guidelines and meta-analyses of randomised controlled trials (licensing varies by country).[18 19 23 24 25 26 27 28 29]

What is the role of psychotherapy?

Persistent or recurrent symptoms, functional impairment, comorbidity, and the contribution of environmental factors have stimulated interest in adjunctive psychotherapies. The current evidence based treatments, the stage of illness at which they are used, and the strength of evidence shown in the table are based on evidence based reviews and guidelines.[18 19 30 31 32] Definitive evidence about which treatment to choose is lacking. The treatments each have specific approaches but all deal with education about the illness, adherence to treatment, lifestyle regularity, and relapse prevention strategies.[33] Cognitive behavioural therapy helps identify and tackle harmful thought patterns and behaviours; family focused therapy aims to improve family communication patterns and strengthen problem solving and coping strategies; interpersonal and social rhythm therapy deals with problems with relationships and daily routines; psychoeducation provides information about bipolar disorder and enhances self management and early identification of relapse. We also now have evidence that cognitive remediation (behavioural training to improve cognitive performance) benefits people with bipolar disorder as well as those with schizophrenia.[32] The current challenge is how to match treatment to an individual patient's needs.

When should I refer and how should care be shared?

Box 4 shows indications for referral to specialist care; mood episodes always need specialist referral or involvement. Although some may need long term psychiatric care, many stable and well patients can be managed in primary care. Debate continues about models of psychiatric service delivery and its boundary with primary care. Whichever model is adopted, good communication and the provision of early and rapid psychiatric advice and referral are essential.[19]

How are episodes of elevated mood managed?

Mania often requires inpatient care to manage risk and allow treatment. This can require compulsory admission, and highly disturbed behaviour may need to be acutely treated with antipsychotics or benzodiazepines, or both (rapid tranquillisation). Excess stimulation must be avoided and a calm environment provided. Milder degrees of mania may be treated with intensive community support from specialist services. Mixed episodes are treated as manic episodes. Hypomania is often untreated and self limiting, but more intensive support and treatment adjustment may be needed to prevent escalation to mania in bipolar I disorder. The emphasis in bipolar II disorder is usually the management of recurrent depressive episodes.

The first step is to identify and treat any medical causes and deal with precipitants such as cessation of maintenance drugs, illicit drug use, and stressful life events. Prescribed antidepressants should be withdrawn because they may be exacerbating the elevated mood.[18 19 34] The efficacy and tolerability of any treatments for past episodes should be reviewed and current long term treatment optimised or restarted if it had been stopped.[18 19]

Antipsychotics are first line treatment for mania, particularly if severe.[18 19] A multiple treatments meta-analysis of 68 randomised controlled trials (RCTs) including both direct and indirect comparisons in the acute treatment of mania found that antipsychotics, lithium, valproate, and carbamazepine were more effective than placebo.[23] The most effective drugs were haloperidol (standardised mean difference v placebo −0.56, 95% confidence interval −0.69 to −0.43), risperidone (−0.50, −0.63 to −0.38), and olanzapine (−0.43, −0.54 to −0.32); all were more effective than valproate, with haloperidol also being more effective than lithium. The second generation antipsychotics risperidone, olanzapine, and quetiapine had the fewest overall dropouts.

If monotherapy with an antipsychotic, valproate, or lithium is insufficiently effective they can be combined. A meta-analysis of eight RCTs found combination therapy with an antipsychotic and lithium or valproate more effective than valproate or lithium alone,[24] and one RCT found that a valproate-antipsychotic combination was more effective than an antipsychotic alone.[35] Benzodiazepines may be needed short term for the management of agitation and insomnia, but they lack intrinsic antimanic properties.

BOX 3 DISTINGUISHING BETWEEN BIPOLAR I DEPRESSION AND UNIPOLAR DEPRESSION*

Clinical suspicion increases with the number of features present for both types of depression

Greater likelihood of bipolar I depression

- Atypical depressive features (hypersomnia, increased appetite, feeling of "leaden paralysis"—feeling that the body or limbs are extremely heavy and difficult to move)
- Mood lability
- Psychotic features or pathological guilt
- Psychomotor retardation
- Early onset of depression (<25 years)
- Multiple episodes of depression
- Family history of bipolar disorder

Greater likelihood of unipolar depression

- Reduced sleep or initial insomnia
- Loss of appetite or weight (or both)
- Normal or increased activity levels
- Somatic (bodily) problems
- Later onset of depression (>25 years)
- Longer duration of depressive episode (>6 months)
- No family history of bipolar disorder

Based on a comprehensive review of studies comparing the clinical features of depression in the two disorders[22]

BOX 4 REFERRAL TO SPECIALIST CARE

During acute episodes of illness refer all patients with known or suspected bipolar disorder to specialist care (or if currently under a specialist team ensure access to care) to:

- Treat the acute episode
- Assess and manage risk
- Confirm the diagnosis (if necessary)
- Establish or review the longer term management plan

Patients with an established diagnosis of bipolar disorder should remain under specialist care if they:

- Have difficulty engaging with services or adhering to treatment
- Have frequent relapses, poorly controlled illness, or persistent symptoms
- Have severe psychiatric comorbidity, including anxiety disorders or alcohol or drug misuse
- Require management of suicide risk or risk to others

Stable patients with bipolar disorder not currently under specialist care should be referred if they:

- Are considering getting pregnant or if they are pregnant
- Have side effects or complications from treatment that may require a change in drugs
- Are considering altering or stopping treatment
- Require access to specific psychotherapies

How is depression managed in people with bipolar disorder? As for mania, identify and remove any precipitants and establish the treatment history. Choice of drugs (table) is informed by the drug history and the need to avoid a switch to elevated mood. For patients on long term treatments with mild depression, guidelines recommend optimising their dose and monitoring mood initially.[18] [19] There are a limited number of evidence based treatments for bipolar depression (table).

A meta-analysis of 19 RCTs in bipolar depression found the best evidence of efficacy against placebo for quetiapine (five trials). Olanzapine and combined olanzapine and fluoxetine were each effective in single trials and lamotrigine was effective but with a small effect size (five trials).[25] A recent meta-analysis of 15 RCTs found no significant benefit for antidepressants over placebo in the treatment of bipolar depression.[26] Guidelines recommend that antidepressants should always be combined with an antimanic drug to reduce the risk of destabilising mood. Selective serotonin reuptake inhibitors are the drugs of choice,[18] [19] because they are least likely to cause a switch to mania.[34] Unless the history shows benefit from continuing antidepressant drugs, guidelines recommend considering withdrawal after the resolution of depressive symptoms.[18] [19]

Consider effective psychological treatments (table) alongside drugs, especially if depression is prolonged or recurrent or mild symptoms persist.

How should maintenance or prophylactic treatment be approached?
It is crucial that patients are engaged and enabled to make informed choices. This requires an understanding of the disorder and treatment that is tailored to individual circumstances. Patients should be enabled to identify triggers for relapse, understand the role of drugs for prevention and treatment of exacerbation, and identify functional and symptomatic goals. Stigma remains a major problem for many.

It is often difficult for patients to accept the need for long term treatment. A large study that assessed adherence by prescription collection found that only 54% of patients were fully adherent to maintenance drugs and 21% were non-adherent.[36] Overall benefit is unclear after an initial episode when the course of illness is uncertain and side effects of drugs (including weight gain) need to be balanced against the detrimental effect of further episodes.[18] The National Institute for Health and Clinical Excellence (NICE) recommends considering long term treatment in bipolar I disorder after two acute episodes, or a single manic episode with severe consequences, and in bipolar II disorder if there are frequent relapses, functional impairment, or suicide risk.[19]

Choice of drug(s) for maintenance or prophylaxis (table) is informed by the predominant pattern of relapse. A meta-analysis of 20 RCTs of maintenance treatment,[27] and a subsequent large RCT with lithium and quetiapine,[37] found that lithium and antipsychotic monotherapy and combined antipsychotics and lithium or valproate were effective against manic relapse. Quetiapine as monotherapy or combined with lithium and valproate was effective against depressive relapse.

In a pooled analysis of two placebo controlled RCTs, lamotrigine was effective against depressive—and to a lesser degree manic—relapse.[28] A recent open label RCT found that valproate monotherapy was less effective than lithium

or combined lithium-valproate in preventing emergent mood episodes.[29] Meta-analytical evidence also shows that lithium reduces suicide when used in maintenance treatment of mood disorders.[38] Such treatment has a low therapeutic index, however, and requires regular monitoring of serum lithium concentration every three months and renal and thyroid function six monthly.[19] [39] Rapid withdrawal can trigger relapse, so lithium should be stopped over several months.[40] For many patients polypharmacy is unavoidable but associated with problems with tolerability and adherence; it therefore needs to be planned rather than drugs just accumulating over time. If long term treatment is stopped, it must be done gradually over months and under specialist supervision. Close follow-up is needed to detect early signs of relapse.

Offer all patients who need long term treatment psychoeducation (see above). Other psychological treatments are indicated for inter-episodic and comorbid symptoms such as anxiety; repeated relapse; or persisting social, functional, or cognitive impairment (table).

What are the implications of bipolar disorder for women of childbearing age?
Women of childbearing age with bipolar disorder should be referred for specialist preconception advice if they are considering pregnancy and managed jointly between psychiatric and obstetric services if they are pregnant. A large retrospective study found that 23% of women with bipolar disorder relapsed during pregnancy. This figure was even higher (52%) in the postpartum period, with most relapses being depressive.[41] Risk is increased if mood stabilisers are stopped during pregnancy—two prospective studies reported that 85-100% of women relapsed compared with 30-37% if mood stabilisers were continued.[41] Lithium and anticonvulsants are associated with an increased risk of teratogenicity. The risk is greatest with valproate, which also causes later neurodevelopmental delay in children exposed prenatally.[19] Current guidance is that valproate is contraindicated in women of childbearing age and, if used, effective contraception is needed.[19] Valproate is contraindicated in pregnancy, and other anticonvulsants are contraindicated in the first trimester; lithium should be used only under obstetric supervision and, if possible, avoided during the first trimester. Antipsychotics are the antimanic treatment of choice during pregnancy, and cognitive therapy is preferred over antidepressants for depression.[19] After delivery, consider reinstating or starting drugs to prevent relapse. Breastfeeding is contraindicated for women on lithium, lamotrigine, and clozapine.[19]

What are the options when treatments don't seem to help?
For poor response to treatment review the diagnosis and attempt to identify and deal with any co-occurring disorders, drug or alcohol misuse, and non-adherence with treatment, which is reported in nearly half of patients with bipolar disorder.[36]

Next, increase the dose of current drugs within licensed limits and tolerability, then switch or add an alternative evidence based drug. Consider adjunctive psychotherapy and tackle environmental factors where possible. A meta-analysis of six cohort studies found that electroconvulsive therapy was as effective for bipolar depression as for unipolar depression,[42] making it an option for severe bipolar depression and when other treatments have failed; it is also an option for treatment resistant mania.[19] Clozapine can be

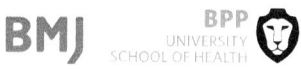
QUESTIONS FOR FUTURE RESEARCH

- How can we best conceptualise the different types of bipolar disorder, their relation to bipolar spectrum disorder, and the distinction from unipolar depression?
- What is the best method of early identification and treatment of children and adolescents at high risk of bipolar disorder?
- What is the best way to treat bipolar II and bipolar spectrum disorders?
- What is the best way to treat comorbid conditions, such as anxiety disorders?
- What treatments are effective for bipolar depression?
- What is the best way to treat poorly responsive bipolar disorder, including patients with rapid cycling and unstable illness?
- How can we choose which adjunctive psychotherapy meets an individual patient's needs?
- What are the most effective long term drug treatments for bipolar disorder?
- What is the most effective way to deliver services to patients with bipolar disorder?

TIPS FOR NON-SPECIALISTS

- Always check for a past (and family) history of elevated mood and increased energy or activity levels in patients presenting with depression
- Never treat patients with bipolar disorder with antidepressant drugs alone; an effective antimanic agent must also be prescribed
- In patients who respond poorly to treatment use non-judgmental questioning to assess the contribution of treatment non-adherence or drug and alcohol misuse
- In patients prescribed lithium, check serum lithium concentrations every three months and renal and thyroid function six monthly. Ensure that patients know the signs of lithium toxicity and the drugs that should be avoided (such as non-steroidal anti-inflammatory drugs) because they can interact with lithium
- Do not prescribe valproate to pregnant women and prescribe this drug to those of child bearing potential only if no effective alternative is available. A full discussion of the risks and effective use of contraception are required
- Refer women who want to get pregnant for specialist preconception counselling because of the risks to both mother and fetus
- Decide the duration of, and changes to, treatment in consultation with a specialist. Never stop long term drugs without specialist advice and support. Closely monitor for relapse if treatment is altered or stopped
- Be aware of the high risk of suicide and the potential for rapid escalation of mania; ensure that early and rapid specialist help is available if needed
- Include people with a diagnosis of bipolar disorder on a severe mental illness case register and monitor and treat physical health problems (such as obesity and other components of the metabolic syndrome)

ADDITIONAL EDUCATIONAL RESOURCES

Resources for healthcare professionals

- National Institute for Health and Clinical Excellence (www.nice.org.uk/cg38)—Clinical guideline 38 on the management of bipolar disorder. This guideline is about to be updated but sets UK standards
- British Association for Psychopharmacology (www.bap.org.uk/pdfs/Bipolar_guidelines.pdf)—Up to date UK evidence based guidelines for treating bipolar disorder
- British Association for Psychopharmacology (www.bap.org.uk/onlinecpd.php)—Subscription based modules on the drug treatment of psychiatric disorders including bipolar disorder, delivered by UK experts in the field
- International Society of Bipolar Disorders (www.isbd.org/)—Forum for professional collaboration and education on bipolar disorders

Resources for patients

- NHS Choices (www.nhs.uk/Conditions/Bipolar-disorder/)—An introduction to symptoms, diagnosis, and treatment for bipolar disorder with links to UK resources
- Bipolar UK (www.bipolaruk.org.uk)—Self help organisation for people with bipolar disorder, their families, and carers; provides a range of self help groups and self management courses
- Bipolar Scotland (www.bipolarscotland.org.uk/)—Self help organisation providing services and support in Scotland
- National Institutes of Mental Health (www.nimh.nih.gov/health/publications/bipolar-disorder/complete-index.shtml)—A detailed downloadable booklet on bipolar disorder
- Royal College of Psychiatrists (www.rcpsych.ac.uk/mentalhealthinfo/problems/bipolardisorder.aspx)—Information on a wide range of aspects related to bipolar disorder and the experience of patients.

SOURCES AND SELECTION CRITERIA

As well as searching the Cochrane Library, we searched Medline for reviews, systematic reviews, and meta-analyses published since 2007 using the terms "bipolar disorder", "mania", and "bipolar depression". These references were used to update and supplement those obtained from recent evidence based guidelines on treating bipolar disorder, including ones from the National Institute for Health and Clinical Excellence, the British Association for Psychopharmacology, the Canadian Network for Mood and Anxiety Treatments, and the International Society for Bipolar Disorder. We also used our personal reference libraries. High quality systematic reviews, meta-analyses, and large randomised controlled trials were selected where possible and lower quality evidence and guideline recommendations when these were lacking.

considered for treatment resistant mania and rapid cycling, although evidence is limited.[18]

Consider referral to a tertiary treatment centre for difficult or complex cases.[19]

What is the outlook for patients with bipolar disorder?

Most patients recover from their first episode but about 80% relapse within five to seven years. Most have three or more episodes over 20 years,[13] with the risk of relapse persisting into old age. In longitudinal follow-up studies patients experience moderate to severe impairment for 26-32% of the time. The course of illness and function are worse in patients with severe episodes, an early onset, and cognitive deficits.[43] Treatment is more effective earlier in the course of illness, emphasising the need for early initiation of long term treatment. Nevertheless, many patients have a good outcome and can live a full life, although they need to remain aware of, and manage, the risks and triggers associated with relapse.

Contributors: IMA planned the organisation and structure of the paper and wrote the first draft. PMH contributed to and edited the pharmacological sections and JS contributed to and edited the diagnostic and psychological treatment sections. IMA organised the sections and all authors reviewed and provided final edits. IMA is guarantor.

Competing interests: All authors have completed the ICMJE uniform disclosure form at www.icmje.org/coi_disclosure.pdf (available on request from the corresponding author) and declare: no support from any third party for the submitted work; IMA has received expenses to attend conferences from Servier and a lecture fee from Lundbeck; his supporting institution has received unrestricted grants from Servier and AstraZeneca and consultancy fees from Servier and Alkermes; PMH has received expenses to attend conferences or fees for lecturing and consultancy work (including attending advisory boards) from AstraZeneca, Bristol-Myers Squibb, Eli Lilly, Janssen-Cilag, Lundbeck, Otsuka, and Servier; JS has received expenses to attend conferences and she or her supporting institution have received fees for lecturing from AstraZeneca, Janssen-Cilag, Lundbeck, and Servier; her supporting institution has received an unrestricted grant from AstraZeneca.

Provenance and peer review: Commissioned; externally peer reviewed.

1 Nordentoft M, Mortensen PB, Pedersen CB. Absolute risk of suicide after first hospital contact in mental disorder. *Arch Gen Psychiatry* 2011;68:1058-64.
2 Johnson SL, Morriss R, Scott J, Paykel E, Kinderman P, Kolamunnage-Dona R,et al. Depressive and manic symptoms are not opposite poles in bipolar disorder. *Acta Psychiatr Scand* 2011;123:206-10.
3 Merikangas KR, Jin R, He JP, Kessler RC, Lee S, Sampson NA,et al. Prevalence and correlates of bipolar spectrum disorder in the world mental health survey initiative. *Arch Gen Psychiatry* 2011;68:241-51.
4 Malhi GS, Chengappa KN, Gershon S, Goldberg JF. Hypomania: hype or mania? *Bipolar Disord* 2010;12:758-63.
5 Benazzi F. Is there a continuity between bipolar and depressive disorders? *Psychother Psychosom* 2007;76:70-6.
6 Duffy A, Alda M, Hajek T, Sherry SB, Grof P. Early stages in the development of bipolar disorder. *J Affect Disord* 2010;121:127-35.

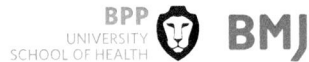

7 Sullivan PF, Daly MJ, O'Donovan M. Genetic architectures of psychiatric disorders: the emerging picture and its implications. *Nat Rev Genet* 2012;13:537-51.

8 Etain B, Henry C, Bellivier F, Mathieu F, Leboyer M. Beyond genetics: childhood affective trauma in bipolar disorder. *Bipolar Disord* 2008;10:867-76.

9 Martinowich K, Schloesser RJ, Manji HK. Bipolar disorder: from genes to behavior pathways. *J Clin Invest* 2009;119:726-36.

10 Latalova K. Insight in bipolar disorder. *Psychiatr Q* 2012;83:293-310.

11 Judd LL, Schettler PJ, Akiskal HS, Maser J, Coryell W, Solomon D,et al. Long-term symptomatic status of bipolar I vs. bipolar II disorders. *Int J Neuropsychopharmacol* 2003;6:127-37.

12 Howes OD, Falkenberg I. Early detection and intervention in bipolar affective disorder: targeting the development of the disorder. *Curr Psychiatry Rep* 2011;13:493-9.

13 Wittchen HU, Mhlig S, Pezawas L. Natural course and burden of bipolar disorders. *Int J Neuropsychopharmacol* 2003;6:145-54.

14 Correa R, Akiskal H, Gilmer W, Nierenberg AA, Trivedi M, Zisook S. Is unrecognized bipolar disorder a frequent contributor to apparent treatment resistant depression? *J Affect Disord* 2010;127:10-8.

15 Bora E, Harrison BJ, Yucel M, Pantelis C. Cognitive impairment in euthymic major depressive disorder: a meta-analysis. *Psychol Med* 2012; published online 26 October.

16 Novick DM, Swartz HA, Frank E. Suicide attempts in bipolar I and bipolar II disorder: a review and meta-analysis of the evidence. *Bipolar Disord* 2010;12:1-9.

17 Roshanaei-Moghaddam B, Katon W. Premature mortality from general medical illnesses among persons with bipolar disorder: a review. *Psychiatr Serv* 2009;60:147-56.

18 Goodwin GM. Evidence-based guidelines for treating bipolar disorder: revised second edition—recommendations from the British Association for Psychopharmacology. *J Psychopharmacol* 2009;23:346-88.

19 National Institute for Health and Clinical Excellence. Bipolar disorder: the management of bipolar disorder in adults, children and adolescents, in primary and secondary care. CG38. 2006. www.nice.org.uk/cg38.

20 Hirschfeld RM, Williams JB, Spitzer RL, Calabrese JR, Flynn L, Keck PE Jr,et al. Development and validation of a screening instrument for bipolar spectrum disorder: the mood disorder questionnaire. *Am J Psychiatry* 2000;157:1873-5.

21 Angst J, Adolfsson R, Benazzi F, Gamma A, Hantouche E, Meyer TD,et al. The HCL-32: towards a self-assessment tool for hypomanic symptoms in outpatients. *J Affect Disord* 2005;88:217-33.

22 Mitchell PB, Goodwin GM, Johnson GF, Hirschfeld RM. Diagnostic guidelines for bipolar depression: a probabilistic approach. *Bipolar Disord* 2008;10:144-52.

23 Cipriani A, Barbui C, Salanti G, Rendell J, Brown R, Stockton S,et al. Comparative efficacy and acceptability of antimanic drugs in acute mania: a multiple-treatments meta-analysis. *Lancet* 2011;378:1306-15.

24 Smith LA, Cornelius V, Warnock A, Tacchi MJ, Taylor D. Acute bipolar mania: a systematic review and meta-analysis of co-therapy vs. monotherapy. *Acta Psychiatr Scand* 2007;115:12-20.

25 Vieta E, Locklear J, Gunther O, Ekman M, Miltenburger C, Chatterton ML,et al. Treatment options for bipolar depression: a systematic review of randomized, controlled trials. *J Clin Psychopharmacol* 2010;30:579-90.

26 Sidor MM, Macqueen GM. Antidepressants for the acute treatment of bipolar depression: a systematic review and meta-analysis. *J Clin Psychiatry* 2011;72:156-67.

27 Vieta E, Gunther O, Locklear J, Ekman M, Miltenburger C, Chatterton ML,et al. Effectiveness of psychotropic medications in the maintenance phase of bipolar disorder: a meta-analysis of randomized controlled trials. *Int J Neuropsychopharmacol* 2011;14:1029-49.

28 Goodwin GM, Bowden CL, Calabrese JR, Grunze H, Kasper S, White R,et al. A pooled analysis of 2 placebo-controlled 18-month trials of lamotrigine and lithium maintenance in bipolar I disorder. *J Clin Psychiatry* 2004;65:432-41.

29 Geddes JR, Goodwin GM, Rendell J, Azorin JM, Cipriani A, Ostacher MJ,et al. Lithium plus valproate combination therapy versus monotherapy for relapse prevention in bipolar I disorder (BALANCE): a randomised open-label trial. *Lancet* 2010;375:385-95.

30 Yatham LN, Kennedy SH, Schaffer A, Parikh SV, Beaulieu S, O'Donovan C,et al. Canadian Network for Mood and Anxiety Treatments (CANMAT) and International Society for Bipolar Disorders (ISBD) collaborative update of CANMAT guidelines for the management of patients with bipolar disorder: update 2009. *Bipolar Disord* 2009;11:225-55.

31 Hollon SD, Ponniah K. A review of empirically supported psychological therapies for mood disorders in adults. *Depress Anxiety* 2010;27:891-932.

32 Anaya C, Martinez AA, Ayuso-Mateos JL, Wykes T, Vieta E, Scott J. A systematic review of cognitive remediation for schizo-affective and affective disorders. *J Affect Disord* 2012;142:13-21.

33 Miklowitz DJ, Scott J. Psychosocial treatments for bipolar disorder: cost-effectiveness, mediating mechanisms, and future directions. *Bipolar Disord* 2009;11(suppl 2):110-22.

34 Tondo L, Vazquez G, Baldessarini RJ. Mania associated with antidepressant treatment: comprehensive meta-analytic review. *Acta Psychiatr Scand* 2010;121:404-14.

35 Muller-Oerlinghausen B, Retzow A, Henn FA, Giedke H, Walden J. Valproate as an adjunct to neuroleptic medication for the treatment of acute episodes of mania: a prospective, randomized, double-blind, placebo-controlled, multicenter study. European Valproate Mania Study Group. *J Clin Psychopharmacol* 2000;20:195-203.

36 Sajatovic M, Valenstein M, Blow F, Ganoczy D, Ignacio R. Treatment adherence with lithium and anticonvulsant medications among patients with bipolar disorder. *Psychiatr Serv* 2007;58:855-63.

37 Weisler RH, Nolen WA, Neijber A, Hellqvist A, Paulsson B. Continuation of quetiapine versus switching to placebo or lithium for maintenance treatment of bipolar I disorder (Trial 144: a randomized controlled study). *J Clin Psychiatry* 2011;72:1452-64.

38 Cipriani A, Pretty H, Hawton K, Geddes JR. Lithium in the prevention of suicidal behavior and all-cause mortality in patients with mood disorders: a systematic review of randomized trials. *Am J Psychiatry* 2005;162:1805-19.

39 National Patient Safety Agency. Safer lithium therapy. Patient safety alert NPSA/2009/PSA005. 2009. www.nrls.npsa.nhs.uk/resources/type/alerts/?entryid45=65426&q=0%c2%aclithium%c2%ac.

40 Goodwin GM. Recurrence of mania after lithium withdrawal. Implications for the use of lithium in the treatment of bipolar affective disorder. *Br J Psychiatry* 1994;164:149-52.

41 Sharma V, Pope CJ. Pregnancy and bipolar disorder: a systematic review. *J Clin Psychiatry* 2012;73:1447-55.

42 Dierckx B, Heijnen WT, van den Broek WW, Birkenhager TK. Efficacy of electroconvulsive therapy in bipolar versus unipolar major depression: a meta-analysis. *Bipolar Disord* 2012;14:146-50.

43 Treuer T, Tohen M. Predicting the course and outcome of bipolar disorder: a review. *Eur Psychiatry* 2010;25:328-33.

Related links

bmj.com
- For all the latest BMJ Group articles on psychiatry visit our specialty portal

bmj.com/archive
- Advances in radiotherapy (2012;345:e7765)
- Diagnosis and management of supraventricular tachycardia (2012;345:e7769)
- Generalized anxiety disorder: diagnosis and treatment (2012;345:e7500)
- Resistant hypertension (2012;345:e7473)
- Preparing young travellers for low resource destinations (2012;345:e7179)
- Childhood constipation (2012;345:e7309)

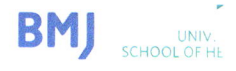

Personality disorder

Linda Gask, professor of primary care psychiatry[1], Mark Evans, consultant psychiatrist in psychotherapy[2], David Kessler, senior lecturer[3]

[1]Centre for Primary Care, Institute of Population Health, University of Manchester, Manchester M13 9PL, UK

[2]Gaskell House, Manchester Mental Health and Social Care NHS Trust, Manchester, UK

[3]School of Social and Community Medicine, University of Bristol, UK

Correspondence to: L Gask Linda. Gask@manchester.ac.uk

Cite this as: BMJ 2013;347:f5276

DOI: 10.1136/bmj.f5276

http://www.bmj.com//content/347/bmj.f5276

Most non-psychiatrists are aware of the diagnosis of personality disorder but rarely make it with confidence. In the past, this diagnosis came with a tacit admission that not much can be done, but there is now increasing evidence that treatment can be effective. Epidemiological studies show that 4-12% of the adult population have a formal diagnosis of personality disorder; if milder degrees of personality difficulty are taken into account this is much higher.[1] People carry the label of personality disorder with them, and this can influence their care when they come into contact with services, including mental health providers. GPs also carry the clinical responsibility for their patients with personality disorder, and this can be challenging over the long term. This article aims to review the current evidence for the diagnosis and treatment of personality disorder.

What is personality disorder?

The exact definition of personality disorder is open to debate and differs between the two main diagnostic systems used for mental health problems, ICD (International Classification of Diseases) and DSM (*Diagnostic and Statistical Manual of Mental Disorders*). Temperamental differences between children can be seen from a very young age and probably have a large inherited component. "Personality" refers to the pattern of thoughts, feelings, and behaviour that makes each of us the individuals that we are. This is flexible and our behaviour differs according to the social situations in which we find ourselves.

People with personality disorder seem to have a persistent pervasive abnormality in social relationships and social functioning in general.[2] More specifically, there seems to be an enduring pattern of perceiving, relating to, and thinking about the outside world and the self that is inflexible, deviates markedly from cultural expectations, and is exhibited in a wide range of social and personal contexts. People with personality disorder have a more limited range of emotions, attitudes, and behaviours with which to cope with the stresses of everyday life.

Personality disorder is viewed as different from mental illness because it is more persistent throughout adult life, whereas mental illness results from a morbid process of some kind and has a more recognisable onset and time course.[3] A cohort study found good rates of remission in people with borderline personality disorder (78-99% at 16 year follow-up), but remission took longer to occur than in people with other personality disorders and recurrence was more common.[4] Evidence from two randomised controlled trials also suggests that most people with this disorder will show persistent impairment of social functioning even after specialist treatment.[5][6]

Why is personality disorder important?

People with personality disorders experience considerable distress, suffering, and stigma. They can also cause distress to others around them.

Epidemiological research has shown that comorbid mental health problems, such as depression, anxiety, and substance misuse, are more common in people with personality disorder,[7] are more difficult to treat, and have worse outcomes. One systematic review found that in depression, personality disorder is an important risk factor for chronicity.[8] Two recent narrative reviews of the epidemiological literature concluded that personality disorder is also associated with higher use of medical services, suicidal behaviour and completed suicide, and excess medical morbidity and mortality, especially in relation to cardiovascular disease.[9][10] One systematic review found an association with violent behaviour.[11]

How is personality disorder diagnosed?

The two major diagnostic systems in psychiatry have taken very different views on how to revise their classification of personality disorder. There has been growing criticism of a purely categorical approach that requires a decision as to whether a person meets criteria for paranoid, borderline, or antisocial personality disorder. Considerable overlap exists between categories, which do not take into account the wide variation in impairment seen in everyday practice, and reinforce the stigma associated with the diagnosis. There has been debate about whether a dimensional approach using scores for personality traits or applying a simple measure of severity of disorder would be an improvement. The recently published fifth edition of DSM (DSM-5) has left the previous categorical classification unchanged,[12] although an alternative, more complex, classification that was rejected before publication is also included in a later section. The eleventh revision of ICD (ICD-11) is still in preparation,[13] but recent publications propose a dimensional approach using five levels of severity. A criticism of this approach has been that the diagnosis of borderline personality disorder, which has considerable clinical utility, is lost. The diagnosis is in some sense a misnomer because the primary category to which the condition was thought to be borderline was schizophrenia, and this is no longer the case. However, it

SUMMARY POINTS

- People with personality disorder have a persistent pervasive abnormality in social relationships and functioning
- Personality disorder is associated with high service use and excess medical morbidity and mortality
- Diagnosis of personality disorder along a single dimension of severity is a major change from traditional categorical approaches
- Depression, anxiety, substance use, suicidal behaviour, and suicide are all more common in these patients; comorbid mental health problems are more difficult to treat and have poorer outcomes
- General principles of management include consistency, reliability, encouraging autonomy, and the sensitive management of change
- Specialist treatments with evidence of effectiveness in borderline personality disorder include dialectical behaviour therapy, mentalisation based treatment, transference focused therapy, cognitive analytic therapy, and schema focused therapy

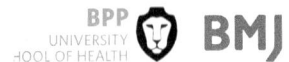

is still possible to describe borderline personality disorder using a combination of traits (figure).

Controversy remains about diagnosing personality disorder in adolescence, not least because of the current pejorative nature of the diagnosis. Referral to a specialist is recommended for suspected cases.

What do we know about the causes of personality disorder?

As with other mental health problems, personality disorders are probably the result of multiple interacting genetic and environmental factors. There is growing evidence for a genetic link, with results from twin studies suggesting heritability of personality traits and personality disorders ranging from 30% to 60%.[14] A narrative review of epidemiological studies also suggests that family and early childhood experiences are important, including experiencing abuse (emotional, physical, and sexual), neglect, and bullying.[10]

How is personality disorder managed and treated?

Across the range of personality disorders, there is still little evidence for what treatments are helpful. An exception to this is borderline personality disorder, for which there is now a growing evidence base, and (to a lesser extent) antisocial personality disorder. National Institute for Health and Care Excellence (NICE) guidelines have now been produced for both of these.[15] Unusually for people with personality disorder, those with a borderline diagnosis tend to seek treatment, whereas those with antisocial personality disorder and other categories tend to be reluctant to commit to treatment. In view of the prevailing evidence, we will focus this section on the general management and specific treatment of these two categories.

What are the basic principles of managing personality disorders?

When working with people with all types of personality disorder, it is important to explore treatment options in an atmosphere of hope and optimism, building a trusting relationship with an open non-judgmental manner. Services should be accessible, consistent, and reliable, bearing in mind that many people will have had previous experiences of trauma and abuse. Consideration should be given to working in partnership, helping people to develop autonomy, and encouraging those in treatment to be actively involved in finding solutions to their problems.

Managing borderline personality disorder

Consider borderline personality disorder in a person presenting to primary care who has repeatedly self harmed and shown persistent risk taking behaviour or marked emotional instability. Primary care doctors should aim to help manage patients' anxiety by enhancing coping skills and helping patients to focus on the current problems. Techniques for doing this include looking at what has worked in the past, helping patients to identify manageable changes that will enable them to deal with the current problems, and offering follow-up appointments at agreed times. When a patient with borderline personality disorder presents to primary care in crisis, it is important to assess the current level of risk to self and others.

People with this disorder require special attention when managing transitions (including changes to and endings of treatment) given the likelihood of intense emotional reactions to any perceived rejection or abandonment.

Referral to specialist mental health services can be useful to establish a diagnosis. Also consider referral when a patient with this disorder is in crisis, when levels of distress and risk of self harm or harm to others are increasing.

Specialist treatment

The past 20 years have seen increased emphasis on understanding the underlying problems, symptoms, and states of mind of people with borderline personality disorder and an accompanying development of specific treatments to target them (box).

Dialectical behaviour therapy is a modified version of cognitive behavioural therapy that also uses the concept of "mindfulness" drawn from Buddhist philosophy. Several randomised controlled trials focusing mainly on women who repeatedly self harm have shown reductions in anger, self harm, and attempts at suicide.[16]

People with borderline personality disorder are less able than the general population to "mentalise;" that is, to understand their own and other people's mental states and intentions. Randomised controlled trials of mentalisation based treatment, which focuses on improving mentalising capacity, have shown reduced suicidal behaviour and

DSM-5	Latest information on proposals for ICD-11
Definition: An enduring pattern of inner experience and behaviour that deviates markedly from the expectations of the individual's culture. This pattern is manifested in two (or more) of the following areas: 1. Cognition (ways of perceiving and interpreting self, other people, and events) 2. Affectivity (range, intensity, lability, and appropriateness of emotional response) 3. Interpersonal functioning 4. Impulse control B. The enduring pattern is inflexible and pervasive across a broad range of personal and social situations C. The enduring pattern leads to clinically significant distress or impairment in social, occupational, or other important areas of functioning D. The pattern is stable and of long duration, and its onset can be traced back at least to adolescence or early adulthood E. The enduring pattern is not better accounted for as a manifestation or consequence of another mental disorder. F. The enduring pattern is not due to the direct physiological effects of a substance (such as drug misuse or a medication) or a general medical condition (such as head trauma) DSM-5 has retained the 10 categories of personality disorder that are briefly summarised below: **Cluster A personality disorders (odd or eccentric disorders)** **Paranoid personality disorder:** by nature patients will experience a distrust of others as well as irrational suspicions **Schizoid personality disorder:** defined by a disinterest in engaging in social relationships and spending time with others. Patients are often unable to find pleasure in enjoyable activities and will spend time contemplating their own mental and emotional state **Schizotypal personality disorder:** typical characteristics include odd behaviour or thinking **Cluster B personality disorders (dramatic, emotional, or erratic disorders)** **Antisocial personality disorder:** characterised by an ignorance of the entitlements of others, the absence of empathy, and (generally) a pattern of consistent criminal activity **Borderline personality disorder:** unstable and intense interpersonal relationships, self perception, and moods. These feelings can lead to both self harm and impulsive behaviour **Histrionic personality disorder:** attention seeking behaviour that often includes inappropriate seductive conduct and superficial or inflated emotions **Narcissistic personality disorder:** characterised by the consistent need for praise and admiration and a belief that they are special and "entitled." Extreme jealousy, arrogance, and a lack of empathy are also usually present **Cluster C personality disorders (anxious or fearful disorders)** **Avoidant personality disorder:** patients commonly feel socially inhibited and inadequate and are extremely sensitive to any form of criticism or evaluation that may be interpreted as negative **Dependent personality disorder:** an extreme psychological dependence on others **Obsessive-compulsive personality disorder:** this is not the same as obsessive-compulsive disorder, and is characterised by conforming to rules and moral codes on a severe and unyielding basis. Excessive orderliness is also usually present	**Is personality disturbance present?** There is a long term pattern of poor interpersonal functioning (a pattern of general impairment in human relationships that prevents mutual understanding) and relationships with others. This can occur at any age, is not part of any other mental disorder, and leads to at least some degree of impairment or distress to self or others **If so, what is the level of severity?** **Personality difficulty:** The problems created by the personality features are closely linked to setting and are only present in some situations in other settings, interpersonal and social functioning is adequate or good. When personality disturbance is present, it may cause distress but does not pose any risk to self or others **Personality disorder:** The problems created by the personality features are well circumscribed but are present all the time and are largely independent of situation. The patient shows a persistent lack of mutual understanding that impairs most relationships. There are continuous difficulties in interpersonal and social functioning, and these may distress the patient but also create problems for others. Occasionally, this may lead to some risk to self or others **Complex personality disorder:** The problems created by the personality disturbance are widespread and affect many different domains of personality. These may fluctuate in terms of behaviour, but they are present in some form continuously and are largely independent of situation. There are persistent difficulties in interpersonal and social functioning, and these may distress the patient but also create problems for others. The lack of mutual understanding leads to overt conflict with others and prevents adjustment at work and at leisure. Occasionally, this may lead to some risk to self or others **Severe personality disorder:** The problems created by the personality disturbance are the same as for complex personality disorder, but in addition the manifestations of the personality disturbance are so disturbing or threatening that they lead to a serious risk to self or others. Action of some sort is necessary if the risk is to be reduced or offset **How can it be described? (more than one may apply especially in severe personality disorder)** **Four domains are currently proposed:** **Detached:** social indifference and impaired capacity to experience pleasure. Traits include aloofness, reduced expression of emotions **Dissocial:** Disregard for social obligations and conventions and the rights of others. "Psychopathy" fails within this domain **Anankastic:** concern over the control and regulation of behaviour. Traits include perfectionism, constraint, stubbornness **Emotional distress or negative emotional:** sensitivity to scrutiny by others, self consciousness, vigilance, fearfulness, pessimism, and emotional dysregulation Description, for example, of someone with borderline personality disorder with a high degree of hostility and punitiveness: General title: Personality disorder Secondary title: Severe personality disorder Full title with domain trait: severe personality change with dissocial and emotional domain traits

Summary of differences between *Diagnostic and Statistical Manual of Mental Disorders*, fifth edition (DSM-5) and latest available information about international classification of diseases, 11th revision (ICD-11) for diagnosis of personality disorder

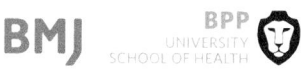

hospital admissions, as well as an improvement in associated symptoms.[6] [17] Other therapies, all with trial evidence of effectiveness in reducing borderline symptoms are schema focused therapy,[18] [19] transference focused therapy,[20] and cognitive analytic therapy.[21] In addition to improving core symptoms, schema focused therapy improved psychological functioning and quality of life; transference focused therapy improved psychosocial functioning and reduced inpatient admissions; and cognitive analytic therapy improved interpersonal functioning and overall wellbeing and led to a reduction in dissociation (splitting of the personality).

A systematic review of randomised trials identified two other treatments with evidence of effectiveness in this group of patients. The first, problem solving for borderline personality disorder, is an integrated treatment that combines cognitive behavioural elements, skills training, and intervention with family members. It can reduce borderline symptoms and improve impulsivity—the tendency to experience negative emotions and global functioning.[22] The second, manual assisted cognitive treatment, aimed at reducing deliberate self harm, was successful in a study of patients with borderline personality disorder who self harm.[23]

Effective management and care coordination
Specialist treatments are not generally available in the community, and it may be difficult to motivate people struggling with chaotic lifestyles and unstable support systems to engage with them. Evidence is emerging that well structured general psychiatric management can be as effective as branded specialised treatments when delivered under research conditions.[5] In this randomised trial, general psychiatric management involved case management and weekly individual sessions using a psychodynamic approach that focused on relationships and management of symptom targeted drugs.

Good care coordination within a community mental health setting is key to stabilising patients, some of whom may later receive more specialist interventions. Indeed, the type of therapy may not be important, but rather that management is consistent, reliable, encourages autonomy, and is sensitive to change. Management should be systematic and preferably manualised (guided by a "manual" for the therapist with a series of prescribed goals and techniques to be used during each session or phase of treatment) to provide a clear model for patient and therapist to work with. This helps the mental health professional to deal with common clinical problems, such as self harm and risk of suicide, by talking with the patient about any precipitants to unmanageable feelings, giving basic psychoeducation about managing mood states, and encouraging problem solving and the sharing of risk and responsibility. In addition, close attention should be paid to any emerging problems in the therapeutic alliance.[24]

Are there any drug treatments available for borderline personality disorder?
There is no clear evidence for the efficacy of drugs for the core borderline symptoms of chronic feelings of emptiness, identity disturbance, and abandonment. Some randomised trials have shown benefits with second generation antipsychotics, mood stabilisers, and dietary supplements of omega-3 fatty acids,[25] but these are mostly based on single studies with small sample sizes and are not recommended by NICE.[15] Antidepressants may be helpful only in the presence of coexisting depression or anxiety.

Managing antisocial personality disorder
The treatment of people with antisocial personality disorder will be facilitated by working within a clearly described care pathway because a diverse range of services are often be involved. The pathways should specify likely helpful interventions at each point and should enable effective communication between clinicians and organisations. Locally agreed criteria should be established to facilitate transfer between services with shared objectives and a comprehensive assessment of risk. Services should consider establishing multiagency antisocial personality disorder networks that actively involve service users. Once established, they can play a central role in training, the provision of support and supervision to staff, and the development and maintenance of standards.[15]

Although it may not be appropriate or possible to provide specific therapeutic interventions for antisocial personality disorder in primary care, GPs still need to offer treatment for patients with comorbid disorders in line with standard care. In doing so, GPs should be aware that the risk of poor adherence, misuse of drugs, and drug interactions with alcohol and illicit drugs is increased in this group. It may be helpful to liaise closely with other agencies involved in the care of these patients, including the criminal justice system and drug support workers. Local schemes are available in primary care in the UK for the management of patients who have been violent or threatening towards their GPs or other primary care staff. Assessment of risk in primary care should include history of violence, its severity, and precipitants; the

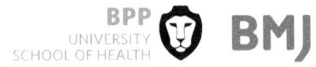

presence of comorbid mental disorders; use of alcohol and illicit drugs and the potential for drug interactions; misuse of prescribed drugs; current life stressors; and accounts from families or carers if available.

Specialist treatments

Robust evidence for the effectiveness of specific psychological interventions in antisocial personality disorder is currently lacking.[26] However, NICE guidelines suggest the use of group based cognitive and behavioural interventions that focus on the reduction of offending and other antisocial behaviour.[15] Particular care is needed in assessing the level of risk and adjusting the duration of programmes accordingly. Participants will need to be supported and encouraged to attend and complete programmes. People with dangerous and severe personality disorder will often come through the criminal justice system and will require forensic psychiatry services. Treatments (including anger management and violence reduction programmes) will essentially be the same as above but will last longer. Staff involved in such programmes will require close support and supervision.

Are there any drug treatments available for antisocial personality disorder?

No specific drugs are recommended for the core symptoms and behaviours of antisocial personality disorder (including aggression, anger, and impulsivity).[27] Drugs may be considered for the treatment of comorbid disorders.

Other treatments

Therapeutic communities, which provide a longer term, group based, and often residential approach to therapy, have a long history in the treatment of personality disorder, but there is no evidence for their effectiveness. In the UK, the Department of Health set up pilot projects for management of personality disorder in 2004-05. One of these, the Service User Network model, offers community based open access support groups for people with personality disorder, with service users engaged in the design and delivery of the service.[28] Analysis of routine data, together with a cross sectional survey, showed that the service attracted a large number of people with serious health and social problems and that use of the service was associated with improved social functioning and reduced use of other services. Nidotherapy (nest therapy) is a new treatment approach for people with mental illness and personality disorder, which involves manipulation of the environment to create a better fit between the person and his or her surroundings, rather than trying to change a person's symptoms or behaviour. Evidence from a systematic review in which only one study met inclusion criteria showed an improvement in social functioning and engagement with non-inpatient services.[29]

What are the problems in everyday practice?

Personality disorder affects the doctor-patient relationship. Misunderstandings and even angry reactions are not uncommon and consistency, clarity, and forward planning are all important in managing the relationship. The diagnosis of personality disorder should never be given to a patient whom the doctor simply finds "difficult." There is evidence of a disparity between a formal diagnosis of personality disorder achieved using a research interview and the diagnoses made by GPs.[30] However, it is important to be aware that a diagnosis of comorbid personality disorder is a possibility in patients who do not respond to

treatment or seem particularly difficult to manage. A simple eight item screening interview (standardised assessment of personality: abbreviated scale) is useful in this respect.[31] It is useful to have clear management plans in place to deal with recurring patterns of crisis, with agreement between GP, specialist mental healthcare, and the service user about potential options for managing likely problems, possible sources of support and advice, and when to urgently refer to specialist care.

Efforts need to be made to challenge stigma and unhelpful attitudes of healthcare professionals,[32] develop professional skills in understanding and managing difficult encounters with challenging patients,[33] [34] and promote engagement in psychological therapy if it is likely to be helpful. However, people with comorbid substance misuse may face problems in accessing psychological therapies (some services do not offer them to these people), specialist therapies may not be locally available, and barriers persist in accessing mental healthcare for people with personality disorder in the UK despite policy guidance to the contrary.[35]

No patient should be excluded from mental health services because he or she has a personality disorder, nor should the incorrect notion that personality disorder is all pervasive and immutable be used to deny people access to valuable therapeutic interventions.

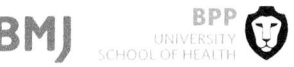
BMJ BPP
UNIVERSITY
SCHOOL OF HEALTH

QUESTIONS FOR FUTURE RESEARCH

- Can early intervention in childhood reduce the risk of developing personality disorders?
- Can we reliably and usefully screen for personality disorder in primary care?
- Would implementation of action plans for crisis management in primary care make a difference?
- How can we improve access to psychological therapy for people with personality disorder?
- What is the optimal length of time that psychological therapy for personality disorder should last?
- Can we reliably and effectively implement general psychiatric management more widely in mental healthcare for people with borderline personality disorder?
- Can we develop more useful generic guidelines for personality disorder?
- Will application of a dimensional approach to diagnosis (as in International Classification of Diseases, eleventh revision) change attitudes to the diagnosis of personality disorder?

SOURCES AND SELECTION CRITERIA

We searched Medline, the Cochrane Database of Systematic Reviews, Clinical Evidence, and the database of the Centre for Reviews and Dissemination using the search term "personality disorder". We focused mainly on systematic reviews, meta-analyses, high quality observational studies, and randomised controlled trials published in the past five years. We also consulted our own reference archives and expert contacts.

Contributors: LG is the lead author and responsible for overall content as guarantor. ME and DK both contributed to the writing of the paper and approved the final version.

Competing interests: We have read and understood the BMJ Group policy on declaration of interests and declare the following interests: None.

Provenance and peer review: Commissioned; externally peer reviewed.

1 Yang M, Coid J, Tyrer P. Personality pathology recorded by severity: national survey. *Br J Psychiatry* 2010;197:193-9.

2 Rutter M. Temperament, personality and personality disorder. *Br J Psychiatry* 1987;150:443-58.

3 Kendell RE. The distinction between personality disorder and mental illness. *Br J Psychiatry* 2002;180:110-5.

4 Zanarini MC, Frankenburg FR, Reich DB, Fitzmaurice G. Attainment and stability of sustained symptomatic remission and recovery among patients with borderline personality disorder and axis II comparison subjects: a 16-year prospective follow-up study. *Am J Psychiatry* 2012;169:476-83.

5 McMain SF, Guimond T, Streiner DL, Cardish RJ, Links PS. Dialectical behavior therapy compared with general psychiatric management for borderline personality disorder: clinical outcomes and functioning over a 2-year follow-up. *Am J Psychiatry* 2012;169:650-61.

6 Bateman A, Fonagy P. 8-year follow-up of patients treated for borderline personality disorder: mentalization-based treatment versus treatment as usual. *Am J Psychiatry* 2008;165:631-8.

7 Jackson HJ, Burgess PM. Personality disorders in the community: results from the Australian national survey of mental health and well-being, part III. Relationships between specific type of personality disorder, axis I mental disorders and physical conditions with disability and health consultations. *Soc Psychiatry Psychiatr Epidemiol* 2004;39:765-7.

8 Hölzel L, Härter M, Reese C, Kriston L. Risk factors for chronic depression—a systematic review. *J Affect Disord* 2010;129:1-13.

9 Athanassios D, Tsopelas C, Tzeferakos G. Medical comorbidity of cluster B personality disorders. *Curr Opin Psychiatry* 2012;25:398-404.

10 Samuels J. Personality disorders: epidemiology and public health issues. *Int Rev Psychiatry* 2011;23:223-33.

11 Yu R, Geddes JR, Fazel S. Personality disorders, violence, and antisocial behavior: a systematic review and meta-regression analysis. *J Personal Disord* 2012;26:775-92.

12 American Psychiatric Association. Diagnostic and statistical manual of mental disorders. 5th ed. American Psychiatric Publishing, 2013.

13 Tyrer P, Crawford M, Mulder R, Blashfield R, Farnam A, Fossati A, et al. The rationale for the reclassification of personality disorder in the 11th revision of the international classification of diseases (ICD-11). *Personal Ment Health* 2011;5:246-59.

14 Reichborn-Kjennerud T. Genetics of personality disorders. *Psychiatr Clin N Am* 2008;31:421-40.

15 Kendall T, Pilling S, Tyrer P, Duggan C, Burbeck R, Meader N, et al. Borderline and antisocial personality disorders: summary of NICE guidance. *BMJ* 2009;338:293-5.

16 Linehan MM, Comtois KA, Murray AM, Brown MZ, Gallop RJ, Heard HL, et al. Two-year randomized controlled trial and follow-up of dialectical behavior therapy vs. therapy by experts for suicidal behaviours and borderline personality disorder. *Arch Gen Psychiatry* 2006;63:757-66.

17 Bateman A, Fonagy P. Randomized controlled trial of outpatient mentalization-based treatment versus structured clinical management for borderline personality disorder. *Am J Psychiatry* 2009;166:1355-64.

18 Young JE, Klosko J, Weishaar ME. Schema therapy: a practioner's guide. Guilford Press, 2003.

19 Giesen-Bloo J, van Dyck R, Spinhoven P, van Tilburg W, Dirksen C, van Asselt T, et al. Outpatient psychotherapy for borderline personality disorder: randomized trial of schema-focused therapy vs. transference-focused psychotherapy. *Arch Gen Psychiatry* 2006;63:649-58.

20 Doering S, Horz S, Rentrop M, Fischer-Kern M, Schuster P, Benecke C, et al. Transference-focused psychotherapy v treatment by community psychotherapists for borderline personality disorder: randomised controlled trial. *Br J Psychiatry* 2010;196:389-95.

21 Clarke S, Thomas P, James K. Cognitive analytic therapy for personality disorder: randomised controlled trial. *Br J Psychiatry* 2013;202:129-34.

22 Blum N, St John D, Pfohl B, Stuart S, McCormick B, Allen J, et al. Systems training for emotional predictability and problem solving (STEPPS) for outpatients with borderline personality disorder: a randomized controlled trial and 1-year follow-up. *Am J Psychiatry* 2008;165:468-78.

23 Weinberg I, Gunderson JG, Hennen J, Cutter CJ Jr. Manual assisted cognitive treatment for deliberate self-harm in borderline personality disorder patients. *J Pers Disord* 2006;20:482-92.

24 Bateman A. Treating borderline personality disorder in clinical practice. *Am J Psychiatry* 2012;169:560-3.

25 Lieb K, Vollm B, Rucker G, Timmer A, Stoffers JM. Pharmacotherapy for borderline personality disorder: Cochrane systematic review of randomised trials. *Br J Psychiatry* 2010;196:4-12.

26 Gibbon S, Duggan C, Stoffers J, Huband N, Vollm BA, Ferriter M, et al. Psychological interventions for antisocial personality disorder. *Cochrane Database Syst Rev* 2010;6:CD007668.

27 Khalifa N, Duggan C, Stoffers J, Huband N, Völlm BA, Ferriter M, et al. Pharmacological interventions for antisocial personality disorder. *Cochrane Database Syst Rev* 2010;8:CD007667.

28 Miller S, Crawford M. Open access community support groups for people with personality disorder: attendance and impact on use of other services. *Psychiatrist* 2010;34:177-81.

29 Chamberlain IJ, Sampson S. Nidotherapy for schizophrenia. *Schizophr Bull* 2013;39:17-21.

30 Moran P, Rendu A, Jenkins R, Tylee A, Mann A. The impact of personality disorder in UK primary care: a 1-year follow-up of attenders. *Psychol Med* 2001;31:1447-54.

31 Moran P, Leese M, Lee T, Walters P, Thornicroft G, Mann A. Standardised assessment of personality-abbreviated scale (SAPAS): preliminary validation of a brief screen for personality disorder. *Br J Psychiatry* 2003;183:228-32.

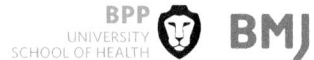

32 Westwood L, Baker J. Attitudes and perceptions of mental health nurses towards borderline personality disorder clients in acute mental health settings: a review of the literature. *J Psychiatr Ment Health Nursing* 2010;17:657-62.

33 Goodrich J. Schwartz centre rounds: evaluation of UK pilots. King's Fund, 2011. www.kingsfund.org.uk/publications/schwartz-center-rounds-pilot-evaluation.

34 Kjeldmand D, Holmstrom I. Balint groups as a means to increase job satisfaction and prevent burnout among general practitioners. *Ann Fam Med* 2008;6:138-45.

35 Department of Health. Personality disorder: no longer a diagnosis of exclusion: policy implementation guidance for the development of services for people with personality disorder. 2003.

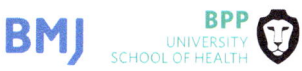

Suicide risk assessment and intervention in people with mental illness

James M Bolton, associate professor[1], David Gunnell, professor of epidemiology[2], Gustavo Turecki, professor of psychiatry[3]

[1]Departments of Psychiatry, Psychology, and Community Health Sciences, University of Manitoba, Winnipeg, MB, R3E 3N4, Canada

[2]School of Social and Community Medicine, University of Bristol, Bristol, UK

[3]Departments of Psychiatry, McGill University, Montreal, QC, Canada

Correspondence to: J M Bolton
jbolton@hsc.mb.ca

Cite this as: *BMJ* 2015;351:h4978

DOI: 10.1136/bmj.h4978

http://www.bmj.com/content/351/bmj.h4978

ABSTRACT

Suicide is the 15th most common cause of death worldwide. Although relatively uncommon in the general population, suicide rates are much higher in people with mental health problems. Clinicians often have to assess and manage suicide risk. Risk assessment is challenging for several reasons, not least because conventional approaches to risk assessment rely on patient self reporting and suicidal patients may wish to conceal their plans. Accurate methods of predicting suicide therefore remain elusive and are actively being studied. Novel approaches to risk assessment have shown promise, including empirically derived tools and implicit association tests. Service provision for suicidal patients is often substandard, particularly at times of highest need, such as after discharge from hospital or the emergency department. Although several drug based and psychotherapy based treatments exist, the best approaches to reducing the risk of suicide are still unclear. Some of the most compelling evidence supports long established treatments such as lithium and cognitive behavioral therapy. Emerging options include ketamine and internet based psychotherapies. This review summarizes the current science in suicide risk assessment and provides an overview of the interventions shown to reduce the risk of suicide, with a focus on the clinical management of people with mental disorders.

Introduction

Suicide is a major international public health problem, claiming one life every 40 seconds.[1] It is the second leading cause of death in people aged 15-29 years and was responsible for 39 million disability adjusted life years in 2012.[2] At least six close relatives or friends are bereaved by every suicide, and these people also have an increased risk of depression and suicide.[3][4][5] For every death from suicide, 30 people attempt suicide; in the United States, this amounts to one million people each year.[6] The economic cost of suicide and self harm is considerable, with estimated annual costs (direct and indirect) of $41bn (£27bn; €36bn) in the US.[7] Improved understanding of who is at risk of suicide and the development of interventions to reduce suicide in key high risk groups are priority targets of national research agendas and government suicide prevention strategies.[8]

Several reviews have examined the prevention and epidemiology of suicide, as well as the risk factors.[9][10][11][12] This review will complement these by examining two facets of the clinical care of people at risk of suicide—the assessment of suicide risk and interventions that can reduce that risk. We will focus on people with mental health problems and will not deal with broader public health strategies to prevent suicide. We will begin by describing the epidemiology of suicide and suicidal behavior in clinical populations, highlighting specific patient subgroups that are at higher risk. Risk assessment approaches will be discussed in detail, with a review of specific assessment tools and how the science of risk assessment is evolving. Interventions that have been shown to reduce suicidal behavior or prevent suicide, such as pharmacotherapy,

psychotherapy, and follow-up care, will be reviewed. Given the prominence of suicide as a health problem and the demands on clinicians to manage this challenging condition, this review will provide an overview of evidence based assessment and treatment approaches to help guide clinical work with this at risk population.

Epidemiology

Suicide is currently the 15th most common cause of death worldwide. In 2012, 804 000 people died by suicide, accounting for 1.4% of deaths worldwide and an average population rate of 11.4 per 100 000.[1] In high income countries suicide rates are around three times higher in males than in females, and key risk factors include previous self harm, depression, alcohol misuse, physical illness, low socioeconomic position, and relationship breakdown.[10][11]

People with mental health problems have a substantially higher risk of suicide and self harm than that found in the general population (fig 1).[13][14] In a 36 year observational follow-up study of the Danish population, the cumulative risk of suicide in people who had inpatient or outpatient clinical contact with specialized mental health services was 4% in men and 2% in women.[15] The rate varied across disorders and was highest in people with comorbidity and a history of self harm. This risk varies across different clinical populations, with psychiatric inpatients showing the highest risk of suicide within the next year.[13] The risk of suicide seems to be greatest during the first few months after diagnosis across all mental disorders.[16][17][18] The risk of suicide is also influenced by treatment factors, which will be described later in the review.

Inpatients and recent discharge

Although admission to hospital is often intended to provide a safe environment for the suicidal patient, the risk of suicide while an inpatient is high. The rate of suicide has been reported at five per 1000 occupied beds each year.[19] A meta-analysis of 27 studies reported a rate of 147 suicides per 100 000 inpatient years, with individual studies reporting figures as high as 860 suicides per 100 000 inpatient years.[20] Suicide tends to occur early during the course of an admission, with 40% occurring within the first three days.[21] A suicide attempt preceding the admission significantly increases the risk of suicide while an inpatient.

The risk of suicide is high in the first week after discharge from a psychiatric hospital admission, remains high for the first few months after discharge, and then slowly decreases (fig 2).[22][23][24] In a UK national study of suicide among psychiatric patients, a quarter of suicides occurred within three months of discharge.[25] Almost half of patients who die by suicide within three months of discharge die within the first month, often before their first follow-up contact.[26] The risk of suicide after discharge is especially high for psychiatric patients who were admitted to hospital with a suicide attempt. In a Swedish observational study, about a

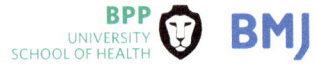

fifth of men with schizophrenia or bipolar disorder died by suicide within one year of admission for a suicide attempt.[27]

The emergency department

The emergency department is a common point of contact between suicidal people and treatment providers. Rates of future suicide among people presenting to the emergency department with self harm are high: 2% of these people will kill themselves within one year, and the five year estimate of suicide is 4%.[28] This risk is more than 50 times greater than that seen in the general population and is associated with a 40 year reduction in average life expectancy.[29][30] Rates of repeat self harm after contact with the emergency department are 10% at one month and as high as 27% at six months.[31][32]

Higher suicide risk shortly after clinical contact

Recent discussions have cited the need to improve the prediction of suicide in much shorter time intervals (hours, days, and weeks).[33][34] This is especially important in the emergency department and other acute care settings. This line of reasoning corresponds with current dialogue on targeting prevention efforts in high risk periods,

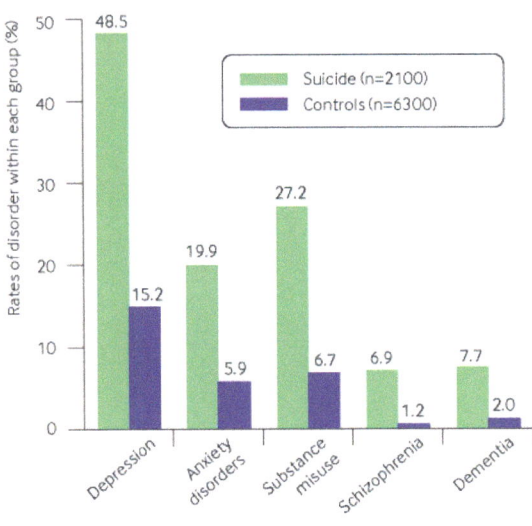

Fig 1 Rates of selected physician diagnosed mental disorders in people who died by suicide in Manitoba, Canada, 1996-2009 compared with score matched living controls from the general population (matched 3:1). Propensity score matching was based on age, sex, income, region of residence, and marital status[16]

particularly after clinical contact.[35] This places clinicians in a difficult position because patients are arguably most vulnerable in the phase after the interaction has ended. Future research is needed to develop methods of more accurately assessing suicide risk within hours or days; this will allow informed delivery of treatment services to those at highest risk.[35]

Suicide risk assessment

The concept of suicide risk assessment is controversial and much debated in suicide research. National guidelines provide recommendations for risk assessment yet there is no widely accepted standard of care. What constitutes a risk assessment is also an important question. While risk assessment is often synonymous with risk assessment tools or scales, at its most basic it represents a clinical encounter where a patient is asked about suicidal thoughts and plans. Although risk assessments are often conducted in emergency departments and specialty mental health settings, many occur in primary care—30% of American adults who die by suicide have seen their primary care provider in the month before suicide.[36] Frameworks for approaches to suicide assessment are generally consistent; they suggest collecting information on previous suicidal behavior, current suicidal thoughts and plans, hopelessness, stressors, the presence of mental disorder symptoms, themes of impulsivity and self control, ready access to highly lethal methods (such as firearms), and protective factors.[37][38][39]

A collaborative, therapeutic alliance between clinician and patient is important when conducting the assessment.[40] Even a single mental health assessment in the emergency department has been associated with a reduced risk of repeat suicidal behavior that may be as high as 40% in the short term.[41] The Collaborative Assessment and Management of Suicidality (CAMS) is one such therapeutic relationship approach that has been shown to enhance treatment retention and reduce suicidal ideation initially and at one year follow-up.[42] This approach involves a range of four to 12 sessions during which the clinician and patient collaboratively engage in a structured assessment of the patient's suicidal thoughts and treatment planning.

Does asking about suicide make a patient more likely to act on it?

Patients and general practitioners think that patients with depression should be asked about suicidal thoughts, yet many GPs have received no formal training in suicide assessment.[43] A further barrier to assessment is the belief held by some clinicians that asking about suicidal thoughts will induce such thoughts in patients. A non-systematic review published in 2014 examined 13 studies published between 2001 and 2013 that investigated this question and found that none reported a significant increase in suicidal ideation in patients who were asked about suicide.[44] This review included studies of adults and adolescents, with methodologies ranging from small cohort studies to larger randomized controlled trials (RCTs). Of note, one RCT showed that asking about suicide did not increase distress or suicidal thoughts, in both a general group of students and those with depression or previous self harm.[45]

Challenges in risk assessment

There are considerable difficulties in obtaining an accurate suicide risk assessment. A fundamental challenge is determining which people determined to be "high risk"

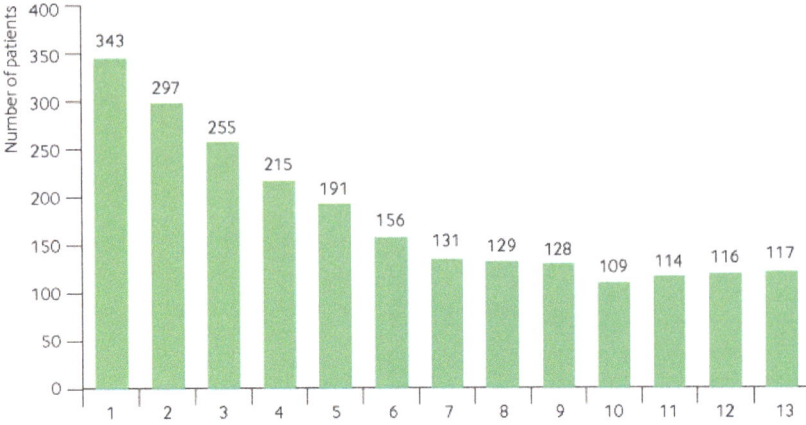

Fig 2 Number of suicides a week in patients with mental illness recently discharged from inpatient hospital wards in England during 2003 to 2013[22]

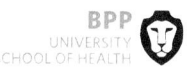

will later die by suicide ("true positives"). The positive predictive value (PPV) of any risk tool that assesses an event with a low base rate in the population, such as suicide, is likely to be low even when sensitivity and specificity values are high (see box 1 for definitions of statistical tests).[46] As such, many people will be inappropriately labeled "high risk" and provided with resources that they may not have needed (such as inpatient admission). Another challenge is the traditional reliance on subjectively reported information, which can be misleading when assessing the risk of suicide. One study found that almost 80% of people who eventually died by suicide denied suicidal thoughts in their last verbal communication.[47] This has prompted the search for alternative measures of assessment, including computer based implicit association tests that are more sensitive than both patient self report and clinician opinion.[48]

Shifts in the science of risk assessment scales
Traditional suicide risk scales were not developed using empirical evidence. Numerous scales and tools have been created over several decades, but unfortunately few were tested statistically,[49] and several scales have never been tested on their predictive ability for suicidal behavior. Consequently, a systematic review of risk assessment tools in the emergency department found that only 12 studies qualified for inclusion.[50] Current research has therefore shifted to statistical derivation and evaluation of risk assessment tools. Another important shift in the science underlying risk assessment scales has been the move from interview dependent tools to interview independent tools. The table lists risk scales that have been evaluated in their ability to predict suicide together with published psychometrics (specifically sensitivity, specificity, PPVs, negative predictive values (NPVs)).

Conventional risk assessment scales
A conventional approach to the development of suicide risk assessment scales has been to collate likely risk factors for suicide based on concepts of face validity or content validity. The most commonly studied risk scales include the Beck hopelessness scale (BHS), the Beck depression inventory (BDI), the Beck scale for suicide ideation (BSS), the suicide intent scale (SIS), and the SAD PERSONS scale.

Beck hopelessness scale (BHS)
The BHS has been studied in psychiatric inpatients and outpatients, and these studies examined its ability to predict suicide over long follow-up periods (5-20 years).[51] [52] [54] [63] BHS scores differentiated those who died by suicide from those who did not, so the BHS was deemed to be a successful prediction tool in some studies; however, specificity was low and one American study reported a PPV of 1%.[54] A subsequent meta-analysis of 10 BHS studies, four of which investigated suicide and six non-fatal self harm, found similar results for suicide and self harm—the BHS had a sensitivity of 78-80% but a specificity of 42%.[56]

Beck depression inventory (BDI) and the Beck scale for suicide ideation (BSS)
The BDI and BSS also performed with low precision in the American study mentioned above, with PPVs of 2% and 3%, respectively,[54] for predicting future suicide.

Suicide intent scale (SIS)
A review of the SIS found that it has been assessed in 158 studies.[64] Of these, 13 assessed its ability to predict suicide and 17 studied its ability to predict self harm. Regarding suicide prediction, most studies reported no significant associations between scale scores and later suicide, and only two reported predictive statistics.[57] [58] PPV values were low in both studies (4% and 10%) but higher in the study that performed a secondary analysis on the subset of people aged over 55 years (23%).[57] In a subsequent Swedish study that assessed the ability of the SIS to predict suicide over 10-15 years in outpatients with a history of suicide attempts, specificity was 52% and the PPV was 17%.[59] Together, these studies illustrate the tendency for scales to have low predictive accuracy, as well as how the duration of follow-up (more time at risk) and more suicidal case mix (higher risk people) can influence PPV.

SAD PERSONS scale
The SAD PERSONS scale is a mnemonic of 10 items where each letter corresponds to a potential risk factor for suicide.[65] It is one of the most widely used tools for suicide assessment even though it was never formally tested during its development. In a representative sample of hospitals in England, it was the most commonly used scale.[66] A recent systematic review showed that only three studies have examined its ability to predict suicide outcomes, and none of these found it to be predictive.[67] The PPV of the SAD PERSONS scale to predict repeat self harm in emergency department patients at six months was 5%, and its sensitivity for predicting suicide at one year follow-up was 23%.[60] [68]

Suicide assessment scale (SUAS) and Karolinska interpersonal violence scale (KIVS)
These two scales have also been used to assess suicidal intent.[62] [69] The 20 item SUAS assesses a range of emotions, personal characteristics, and suicidal thoughts and behaviors. In the one study that used it to predict suicide over one year, it showed 75% sensitivity and 86% specificity, but the PPV was 19%.[61]

The KIVS features two subscales that assess exposure to, and expression of, violence in childhood and adulthood.

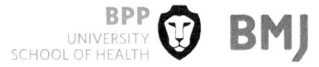

Its use as a risk assessment tool is based on observations that people attempting suicide often have higher levels of aggression and impulsivity. When administered to people who had attempted suicide, both subscales predicted suicide within four years with 80-88% sensitivity but lower specificity (60-65%) and a low PPV (range 7-14%).[62]

Newer suicide risk scales
The Columbia-suicide severity rating scale (C-SSRS), the suicide trigger scale (STS), and the suicide probability scale (SPS) are based on conventional approaches.

The C-SSRS measures four domains of suicidal thoughts and behavior including the severity of ideation, intensity of ideation, type of suicidal behavior, and lethality of suicide attempts.[70] One study has shown that it predicts future suicidal behavior with sensitivity and specificity of 67% and 76%, respectively.[71] In this mixed sample of 3776 people (some with major depression and post-traumatic stress disorder and others with epilepsy and fibromyalgia), 201 (5.3%) reported suicidal behavior during the follow-up period. A positive baseline test had a PPV of 14% and NPV of 98% of predicting future suicidal behavior during a mean follow-up of nine weeks.

The STS scale is based on five areas linked to suicide: suicidality, mood symptoms, trauma, impulsivity, and

Studies evaluating risk assessment tools in the prediction of suicide

First author	Population sample (n)	No (%) of suicides	Scale cut-off score	Relevant statistics	Follow-up
Beck's hopelessness scale (BHS)					
Beck (1985)[51]	Psychiatric inpatients with suicidal ideation (207)	11 (6.7)	9	Sensitivity 91%	10 years
				Specificity 51%	
Beck (1990)[52]	Psychiatric outpatients (1958)	17 (0.9)	8	Sensitivity 94%	7.5 years
				Specificity 41%	
Nimeus (1997)[53]	Psychiatric inpatients with suicide attempts (212)	13 (6.1)	13	Sensitivity 77%	8 years
				Specificity 61%	
				PPV 13%	
Brown (2000)[54]	Psychiatric outpatients (6891)	49 (0.7)	8	PPV 1%	20 years
				NPV 100%	
Suominen (2004)[55]	Patients with suicide attempts (212)	17 (7.6)	Not available	Sensitivity 60%	12 years
				Specificity 52%	
McMillan (2007)[56]	Meta-analysis	Not applicable	9	Sensitivity 80%	5-12 years
				Specificity 42%	
Beck's depression inventory (BDI)					
Beck (1990)[52]	Psychiatric outpatients (1958)	17 (0.9)	22	Sensitivity 77%	7.5 years
				Specificity 64%	
Brown (2000)[54]	Psychiatric outpatients (6891)	49 (0.7)	22	PPV 2%	20 years
				NPV 100%	
Beck's scale for suicide ideation (BSS)					
Brown (2000)[54]	Psychiatric outpatients (6891)	49 (0.7)	2	PPV 3%	20 years
				NPV 100%	
Suicide intent scale (SIS)					
Nimeus (2002)[57]	Patients presenting with self harm (555)	22 (4.0)	19	Sensitivity 59%	4.5 years
				Specificity 77%	
				PPV 10%	
Harriss (2005)[58]	Patients presenting with self harm (2489)	54 (2.2)	10 (men)	Sensitivity 77%	5.2 years
				Specificity 49%	
				PPV 4%	
			14 (women)	Sensitivity 67%	
				Specificity 75%	
				PPV 4%	
Stefansson (2012)[59]	Psychiatric outpatients with suicide attempts (81)	7 (8.6)	16	Sensitivity 100%	10-15 years
				Specificity 52%	
				PPV 17%	
SAD PERSONS scale					
Kurz (1988)[60]	Inpatients with self harm (485)	13 (2.7)	5	Sensitivity 23%	1 year
				Specificity 89%	
Suicide assessment scale (SUAS)					
Nimeus (2000)[61]	Inpatients with suicide attempts (191)	8 (4.2)	39	Sensitivity 75%	1 year
				Specificity 86%	
				PPV 19%	
Karolinska interpersonal violence scale (KIVS)					
Jokinen (2010)[62]	Patients with suicide attempts (161)	5 (3.1)	Childhood violence subscale: 3	Sensitivity 80%	4 years
				Specificity 65%	
				PPV 7%	
			Adult violence subscale: 3	Sensitivity 88%	
				Specificity 60%	
				PPV 14%	
ReACT self-harm rule					
Steeg (2012)[32]	Emergency department patients with self harm (18 680)	92 (0.49)	1	Sensitivity 88-91%	6 months
				Specificity 15-24%	
				PPV 0.4-0.5%	
				NPV 100%	

PPV=positive predictive value; NPV=negative predictive value.

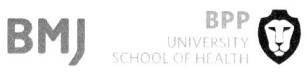

attachment style. In a study of psychiatric inpatients that compared the STS with the C-SSRS and BSS, only the STS was predictive of future suicide attempts within six months.[72] This study is one example of a limited number of studies directly comparing performance of risk assessment scales.

Empirically derived tools

Several newer studies have used the more robust methodology of empirically deriving a prediction tool using a development dataset and then testing it in a separate validation dataset.

Manchester self-harm rule

This tool was the end result of statistical selection from a list of 50 candidate variables assessed in almost 10000 people presenting to the emergency department with self harm.[73] The assessment of four clinical variables (with endorsement of one or more being classified as moderate-high risk) yielded high sensitivity (97%) for self harm or suicide within six months. The rate of repeat self harm (including suicide) in this population was 17%. The four variables, which have the advantage of being interview independent, were: history of self harm, previous psychiatric treatment, presents with a benzodiazepine overdose, and current psychiatric treatment. Specificity was low (26%), as was the PPV (22%). This rule was also tested in a Swedish population and predicted repeat self harm with similar psychometric scores.[74]

ReACT self-harm rule

A subsequent study from the same UK study group and dataset yielded a slightly different predictive model named the ReACT self-harm rule.[32] It was based on a larger number of presentations (almost 30000), using the same list of candidate variables and using a derivation and validation dataset. Statistical based selection of predictor variables identified four: recent self harm, living alone or homeless, cutting as a method of self harm, and treatment for a current psychiatric disorder. High risk classification (based on presence of one or more of these four variables) predicted suicide within six months with high sensitivity (88%) and NPV (almost 100%), but low specificity (24%) and PPV (0.5%).

Repeated episodes of self-harm (RESH) score

This statistically derived tool was developed in Australia using administrative databases.[75] The authors investigated the risk of repeat self harm (including suicide) within six months in all people admitted to hospital with a baseline self harm episode in two states. As opposed to the UK studies, which involved emergency department presentations, this study looked only at self harm incidents that involved admission to hospital. Using separate development and validation samples, a tool measuring four variables (number of previous self harm episodes, time between episodes, diagnosis of a mental disorder in the past year, psychiatric admission in the past year) showed fair prediction. Sensitivity was lower than that seen for the UK tools, but at higher scores (>16) it showed high specificity (98%) and PPV (82%).

A statistically derived tool also examining the prediction of future suicide attempt in the emergency setting was developed from a Canadian sample.[76] It used a baseline sample of all people who presented to the emergency departments of two hospitals over four years (for self harm and non-self harm) who received a psychiatric consultation. The tool was developed on the basis of the outcome of suicide attempts within six months. Of 16 candidate variables, only two significantly accounted for variance in future suicide attempts: suicidal ideation at presentation and history of psychiatric care or suicide attempts. The presence of at least one of these variables showed high sensitivity (91%) and NPV (99%) but low specificity (24%) and PPV (3%) for future attempts. An important consideration when interpreting the results of assessment tools completed in clinical situations is that the psychometric performance of the tools probably varies according to the availability and effectiveness of local mental health services and the response of clinicians to the assessment results.

Novel methods of risk assessment

Advances in suicide risk assessment include forays into the use of implicit thoughts and neurocognitive functioning. Implicit thoughts of suicide represent an appealing substrate for risk modeling because they overcome the inherent challenge of patients denying (or even being unaware of) their true suicide intent.

The implicit association test (IAT) is an established psychological test that measures a person's unconscious beliefs on a subject or motivations towards a specific behavior. A computer displays an image (in this case relative to suicidal behavior) or a neutral image, and the subject presses a key to indicate whether or not they view the image as related to self. The reaction time in this task provides the measure of their propensity for suicidal behavior. A cohort study of 157 patients in a psychiatric emergency department showed that a specific death-life IAT test predicted future suicidal behavior within six months, independently of the person's voiced intention and the clinician's belief of future suicidal behavior (sensitivity 50%, specificity 81%, PPV 32%, NPV 90%).[48] This finding was replicated in a Canadian emergency department cohort study of 107 patients, which showed that the death-life IAT independently predicted suicidal behavior within three months (sensitivity 43%, specificity 79%).[77] Of note, the accuracy of the IAT was improved when used with other variables (previous self harm, education level, depression with psychosis, and non-poisoning self harm).

Several neurocognitive tests have been examined for their ability to detect suicidal behavior. A recent meta-analysis showed that only three of these tests significantly correlate with a history of suicidal behavior: the Stroop test, the verbal fluency test, and the Iowa gambling task.[78] Conceptually, these results match with observations that suicidal people tend to fixate on suicidal thoughts (deficits in attentional shifting), they have difficulty communicating a need for help (deficits in verbal fluency), and they are prone to impulsive and risky behavior (poor decision making). However, almost all studies in this area have tested people in cross section, so the predictive accuracy for future suicidal behavior is currently unknown. The one exception is a prospective US study that administered the Stroop test to 124 people in a psychiatric emergency department.[79] Attentional bias towards suicidal themes independently predicted suicide attempts within six months even after controlling for a variety of factors including

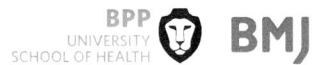

history of suicidal behavior, severity of suicidal ideation, and prediction of suicidal behaviour by both clinicians and patients.

Is suicide risk assessment worth while?

The World Health Organization recommends that all people over the age of 10 years with a mental disorder or other risk factor should be asked about thoughts or plans of self harm within the past month.[1] The use of scales or tools is more controversial. National Institute for Health and Care Excellence guidelines encourage risk assessment and needs assessment of patients but oppose the use of risk assessment tools to determine patient disposition and treatment.[80] Similarly, a review for the US Preventative Services Task Force found insufficient evidence to support screening tools in primary care.[81] Opponents of tools argue that the low precision of assessment tools renders them useless. They are consistent in their low specificity and PPV, which limits their predictive utility and can result in the inappropriate allocation of sparse resources.[82]

Furthermore, one of the most consistent predictive variables for future self harm is a history of previous self harm, and this subgroup may already be in treatment. The prediction of incident self harm is a high clinical priority but extremely challenging given its relatively low incidence. It may be a worthwhile approach to optimize NPV in risk assessment because the identification of true negatives could help preserve health resources. One observational UK study found that the process of assessment itself correlated with a lower likelihood of future suicidal behavior.[83] This speaks to an often overlooked aspect in risk assessment: that doctor-patient contact can provide an important therapeutic effect. Education of trainees in the assessment of suicidal risk is needed yet difficult to achieve when assessment practices are highly variable. It is imperative that standards of care are consistent across and within

regions, and in an effort to achieve this the National Action Alliance for Suicide Prevention recently published training guidelines for clinicians.[84]

Guidelines for risk assessment

Several organizations have published clinical practice guidelines for assessing and preventing suicide. These include national guidelines from various countries and practice guidelines from specific organizations. Box 2 details a selected list of guidelines available online. A review published in 2014 noted that although some components are similar across most guidelines, inconsistencies include how to stratify risk, recommendations for outpatient management and means restriction, and guidelines for training.[85] Consistent aspects of suicide prevention guidelines include the importance of assessing risk and protective factors and of clarifying the degree of suicidal intent, as well as recommendations regarding interventions.

Interventions to reduce suicide in people with mental health problems

Mental healthcare can reduce suicide rates,[86] yet most suicidal people receive no treatment.[87] Studies from the UK and US show that only 60% of people presenting with self harm receive a mental health assessment in the emergency department.[88] [89] This section will highlight specific areas of clinical interventions for suicide. Although it is not a comprehensive review, it will complement other reviews that have examined interventions to prevent suicidal behavior.[90] [91] [92] [93]

Pharmacotherapy

Evidence supports specific psychotropic drugs to reduce the risk of suicide.[94] However, research in this area has not rigorously pursued RCTs that aim to prevent death by suicide associated with psychiatric illness. Psychological autopsy studies in high income countries suggest that more than 90% of people who have died by suicide had a mental disorder at the time of their death,[95] implicating mental illness as an important and potentially modifiable risk factor. This implies that drug treatment of mental disorders is an important approach to preventing suicide.

Antidepressants

Identification and treatment of depression is a key aspect of suicide prevention.[10] Several studies have shown that antidepressants reduce suicidal thoughts and behavior, although evidence for their effect on suicide is controversial and may vary with age (see below). A non-systematic review described a series of clinical cohort studies showing risk reductions of between 40% and 81% in suicide attempts and suicide among depressed patients taking antidepressants.[96] One meta-analysis of randomized placebo controlled trials of antidepressants found an increased risk of suicidal thoughts and behavior in participants aged less than 25 (odds ratio 1.62, 95% confidence interval 0.97 to 2.71), but a protective effect in those aged 25-64 years (0.79, 0.64 to 0.98) and those over 65 years (0.37, 0.18 to 0.76).[97] An observational study from Finland showed that current use of antidepressants was associated with a 39% increased risk

---

BOX 2 SELECTED CLINICAL GUIDELINES FOR SUICIDE PREVENTION AVAILABLE ONLINE

WHO

- Self harm and suicide. 2015. www.who.int/mental_health/mhgap/evidence/suicide/en/

International Association for Suicide Prevention (IASP)

- IASP guidelines for suicide prevention. 2015. www.iasp.info/suicide_guidelines.php

National Institute for Health and Care Excellence (NICE)

- Self-harm: the short-term physical and psychological management and secondary prevention of self-harm in primary and secondary care. 2004. www.nice.org.uk/guidance/cg16/chapter/1-recommendations

- New NICE guidance for the longer-term management of self-harm. 2011. www.nice.org.uk/guidance/cg133/resources/new-nice-guidance-for-the-longerterm-management-of-selfharm

American Psychiatric Association (APA)

- Practice guideline for the assessment and treatment of patients with suicidal behaviors. 2010. http://psychiatryonline.org/pb/assets/raw/sitewide/practice_guidelines/guidelines/suicide.pdf

Royal Australian and New Zealand College of Psychiatrists (RANZCP)

- Australian and New Zealand clinical practice guidelines for the management of adult deliberate self-harm. 2004. www.ranzcp.org/Files/Resources/Publications/CPG/Clinician/CPG_Clinician_Full_DSH-pdf.aspx

Substance Abuse and Mental Health Services Administration (SAMHSA)

- SuicideAssessment Five-step Evaluation and Triage. 2009. www.integration.samhsa.gov/clinical-practice/safe-t_card.pdf

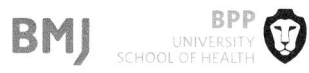

of suicide attempts but a 32% reduced rate of completed suicide compared with periods without antidepressant use.[98] The risk of attempted suicide is 2.5 times higher in the month before starting an antidepressant compared with the period of antidepressant use.[99] When interpreting these findings it is important to consider regression to the mean as an explanatory mechanism because the natural course of depression may result in its improvement (and consequent decrease in suicidal behavior), irrespective of the effects of treatment.

Self poisoning

A challenge when using psychotropic drugs is that self poisoning is a common method of suicide and the agents used to self harm are often the same ones prescribed with therapeutic intent. Antidepressant drugs are involved in 20% of self poisoning suicides in the UK,[100] and tricyclic antidepressants are the most lethal. A UK study found that tricyclic antidepressants have more than a 20 times greater case fatality in overdose than the selective serotonin reuptake inhibitors (SSRIs).[101] In that study, 1088 suicide deaths in England and Wales involved tricyclic antidepressants, whereas 85 deaths involved an SSRI.

Venlafaxine has an intermediate risk in overdose, and among selective serotonin reuptake inhibitors the risk of poisoning death seems to be greatest with citalopram. Clinicians can try to mitigate this risk by choosing less toxic agents when treating patients potentially at higher risk (those with repeated self poisonings) and by prescribing limited supplies of the drug on a single prescription, at least in the early stages of treatment when risk is greatest.

Link with suicidal behavior

The problem is even more complex when considering the major controversy over the past 12 years regarding the Food and Drug Administration imposed black box warnings about suicidal behavior and antidepressants. The controversy persists today, with opponents highlighting reduced rates of antidepressant use, a reluctance of physicians in the US to diagnose depression, and increased rates of suicides in young people in regions with lower rates of antidepressant prescription.[102] [103] An analysis of four RCTs that examined the use of fluoxetine for major depression in young people (708 treated) found no increase in suicidal behavior,[104] whereas a meta-analysis of antidepressant drug use for all categories of depression (4780 young people treated) showed a 2.3 increased odds of suicidal behaviour (1.04 to 5.09). This last finding corresponded to an absolute risk increase of 3.6 suicidal behaviour events per 1000 people when antidepressant treatment was compared with placebo.[97] However, older adults who take antidepressants consistently have a reduced risk of suicidal behavior. Active monitoring of suicidal thoughts in people taking antidepressants, particularly young patients, and frequent follow-up in the short term are sound clinical decisions that may help to mitigate the risk of suicide during early phases of treatment.

Other psychotropic drugs

Lithium

There is good evidence for the antisuicidal properties of lithium.[96] Meta-analyses of RCTs in unipolar and bipolar disorders show that lithium significantly reduces suicide compared with placebo (odds ratio 0.13, 0.03 to 0.66).[105]

[106] Interestingly, observational studies of naturally occurring lithium in drinking water show an inverse association with suicide; regions with higher concentrations (albeit subtherapeutic) have lower rates of suicide.[107] [108] [109] In a Danish observational study, outpatients who continued to fill prescriptions for lithium had a lower risk of suicide than did those who filled only one script (relative risk 0.43, 0.2 to 0.69).[110] Taken together, this consistent line of evidence underscores lithium as an important intervention for preventing suicide in patients with mood disorders.

Antiepileptic drugs

Evidence also suggests that other mood stabilizers may reduce suicide risk, although most data come from observational studies.[111] In a cohort study of patients with bipolar disorder, antiepileptic drugs as a class reduced suicide attempts by 81% when compared with patients with bipolar disorder not receiving psychotropic drugs.[112] This protective effect was also seen when compared with the patient's own history before starting the drug. An observational study in Denmark showed that, similar to lithium, continuous use of antiepileptic drugs correlated with lower suicide rates compared with a single prescription.[113] However, a large US cohort study found that the risk of suicide was 2.7 times higher with divalproex treatment than with lithium.[114]

Clozapine

Clozapine has an approved indication for the reduction of suicidal behavior in patients with schizophrenia,[115] but it tends to be reserved as a late option in the treatment algorithm.[116] A meta-analysis of observational studies and randomized trials showed that compared with other antipsychotic drugs, people prescribed clozapine had a reduced incidence of suicidal behavior (risk ratio 3.3, 1.7 to 6.3).[117]

Ketamine: an emerging drug treatment

Early evidence suggests that ketamine may be an effective intervention for preventing suicide.[118] Ketamine seems to possess unique antidepressant effects that are rapid in onset (hours) with consequent neurogenesis mediated through the NMDA (N-methyl-D-aspartate) neurotransmitter system.[119] It also reduces suicidal thoughts within hours, mostly but not entirely due to reductions in depressive symptoms.[120] One RCT using an active placebo (midazolam) showed that 53% of patients treated with ketamine scored 0 on three different measures of suicidal ideation 24 hours after infusion compared with 24% of those treated with midazolam (P=0.03).[121] The reductions in conscious suicidal thoughts were also observed unconsciously through IAT testing. Interestingly, the anti-suicidal effect gained from a single dose of ketamine can be sustained for several days.[122]

Despite these compelling findings, data on ketamine in suicide are limited and no studies have examined its effect on suicidal behavior and suicide. Future research will hopefully answer important questions regarding optimal dosing, frequency of administration, safety, and long term effects. Until then, ketamine remains investigational (and unapproved for this indication) but is nevertheless a potential option for suicidal people.

Electroconvulsive therapy (ECT)

Electroconvulsive therapy has long been recognized as a highly efficacious treatment for people with depression. It is often used in severe and treatment resistant cases

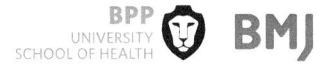

and is recommended for patients with intractable suicidal thoughts.[123] ECT rapidly relieves suicidal thoughts in depressed patients, with one cohort study showing resolution of suicidal thoughts in 38% of patients after three treatments, and 62% after six treatments.[124 125 126] A population based study of all suicides in Finland showed that the rate of ECT use within three months of suicide was extremely low, which could indirectly infer a protective effect or conversely low utilization of ECT.[127] Although ECT seems to reduce suicidal thoughts and behavior in the short term, the limited number of available studies show that ECT treatment does not confer long term protection against suicide. However, it is important to consider the potentially higher risk of patients selected to receive ECT, and that most longer term follow-up studies have methodological limitations and were not designed to examine the effect of ECT on suicide.[128 129]

Psychotherapy

A non-systematic review published in 2014 summarized psychotherapies with evidence of efficacy in reducing suicidal behavior, focusing on those with evidence from RCTs.[130] Participants in these studies were largely people who had self harmed. Meta-analysis of these trials yielded a pooled effect of 32% reduction in likelihood of future self harm when compared with usual care.[81] However, this pooled effect was based on RCTs evaluating a range of different psychotherapies including cognitive behavioral therapy (CBT), dialectical behavioral therapy (DBT), and problem solving therapy in different patient populations; larger trials are needed to identify the most effective approaches to managing people who self harm.

Some individual RCTs have shown that CBT reduces future suicide attempts in people with recent self harm and in patients who present to the emergency department after a suicide attempt; this last study found that people in the CBT group were 50% less likely to reattempt compared with the usual care group.[131 132] Patients with borderline personality disorder who were treated with DBT were half as likely as the control treatment group to attempt suicide,[133] and the mean number of suicidal acts was reduced by 0.91 in those treated with CBT compared with those receiving usual treatment.[134] In a large New Zealand follow-up study over one year, problem solving therapy reduced the risk of repeat episodes of self harm in people with a history of repeated self harm by 61%, but not in those who entered the study with only a single episode of self harm.[135] The knowledge base for this intervention is limited. Specifically, no RCTs of psychotherapy have demonstrated a reduction in suicide, probably because of a lack of statistical power. In a large observational study in Denmark, psychosocial therapy after self harm reduced suicide over longer time frames, with an absolute risk reduction of 0.5%.[136] In addition, the length of follow-up in psychotherapy trials is of short duration; a meta-analysis focusing on interventions in the emergency department found only two trials that examined repeat suicidal behavior over 12 months and the pooled results were non-significant.[137]

Online methods

Online methods of delivering psychotherapy to suicidal people are an appealing option for several reasons, including access, healthcare system costs, and stigma. A Dutch RCT of an online suicide specific intervention that featured an unguided self help approach based in CBT, DBT, mindfulness, and problem solving therapy found a small but significant reduction in suicidal thinking (effect size d=0.28, 0.03 to 0.54).[138] This finding was more pronounced in people with a history of suicidal behavior. However, among people calling a suicide helpline, augmentation of treatment with internet CBT directed at depression did not reduce suicidal ideation compared with usual treatment.[139] This raises an interesting question of whether psychotherapy directed towards the underlying mental disorder is sufficient to reduce suicidal ideation in the individual. A meta-analysis showed that psychotherapy for depressive symptoms did not significantly reduce suicidal thoughts,[140] suggesting that psychotherapeutic approaches specifically directed at suicidal symptoms may be needed. This analysis was limited to only three studies and it again noted that many trials of treatment for depression exclude suicidal participants.

Follow-up care

Follow-up care for suicidal people includes a variety of approaches such as telephone calls, repeat assessments, case management, and caring letters or postcards.[141] Patients themselves often request a need for care in the period after contact with mental health services, preferring telephone contact initially and letters later on.[142] A non-systematic review found that five trials of follow-up care reduced future suicidal behavior, whereas four had mixed results and two did not show a reduction.[92] However a meta-analysis of enhanced usual care (defined as augmenting treatment or adherence with little or no direct therapeutic contact) that included many of the same studies found no significant reduction in suicide attempts (adults: relative risk 0.90, 0.80 to 1.02; adolescents: 1.44, 0.36 to 5.76).[81]

Community mental healthcare has been shown in many countries to be important in preventing suicide. In a national study that examined suicide rates after guideline implementations in the UK, several forms of community care, including follow-up appointments within seven days of discharge, and assertive outreach for people who missed healthcare appointments, significantly reduced absolute suicide rates by 0.53/10 000 person years and 0.34/10 000 person years, respectively.[86] National policy changes that have enhanced care during the 12 weeks after discharge have resulted in significant reductions in non-fatal self harm—14% within one week of discharge and 11% within one month of discharge.[143] In Finland, an ecological study showed lower suicide rates in municipalities that had a higher outpatient to inpatient service type ratio (relative risk 0.93, 0.89 to 0.97).[144]

In another meta-analysis that pooled several methods of follow-up care (phone calls, postcards, letters, and green cards), the number of repeat episodes of self harm per person was reduced (incidence rate ratio 0.66, 0.54 to 0.80) but not the likelihood of any future self harm.[145] The review also specifically examined suicide as an outcome, and although there was a trend towards a reduction in suicide, the finding was not significant. One study included in the meta-analysis was a multi-country RCT of almost 2000 people who had presented to the emergency department with a suicide attempt. It compared treatment as usual with an intervention that included a one hour information session and then nine follow-up contacts over 18 months (telephone calls or personal visits).[146] The intervention group had significantly fewer suicides at the end of the study compared with the usual treatment group (0.2% v 2.2%; P<0.001), but there was no difference in the proportion of participants who had a repeat suicide attempt (7.6% v 7.5%;

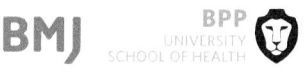

P=0.909).[147] A Swedish RCT (included in the meta-analysis) of two telephone calls over one year to people after a suicide attempt showed no difference in repeat attempts compared with no intervention.[148] In a controlled study in Spain of emergency department patients presenting with a suicide attempt, six calls over the next year reduced rates of a repeat attempt compared with controls (6% v 14%) and delayed the time to the next attempt.[149]

A Danish RCT examined the effect of assertive outreach for people discharged from hospital after a suicide attempt using a case management approach that featured eight to 20 follow-up meetings, telephone calls, and text messages, as well as meetings outside the hospital.[150] The findings did not support the outreach approach over usual treatment—16% of patients in the intervention group were admitted to hospital for repeat suicide attempts compared with 11% in the control group.

It is cheap and intrinsically feasible to mail postcards or letters to people after they present to hospital with self harm, but the results of such an approach are mixed. In an Australian RCT, mailing postcards for a 12 month period after deliberate self poisoning did not reduce the likelihood of any repeat self harm, but it did reduce the number of self harm events (incidence risk ratio 0.55, 0.35 to 0.87; P=0.01).[151] Findings were similar after 24 months and five years (at five years: 0.54, 0.37 to 0.81; P<0.01).[152] [153] Importantly, these results suggested that the postcards had a sustained effect beyond the end of the intervention. An RCT of postcards mailed over 12 months in Iran showed significant reductions in suicidal ideation, any suicide attempt, and number of attempts at one year.[154] The findings were sustained at 24 months, with an 80% reduced risk of suicidal ideation (P<0.001) and 69% reduced risk of suicide attempt compared with controls (P=0.02).[155] Another RCT showed that among people who initially refused psychiatric follow-up, those who received letters regularly over five years had lower suicide rates than those who did not (3.9% v 4.6%), although the difference was significant only during the first two years of the study (P=0.043).[156] By contrast, postcard studies in New Zealand, Taiwan, and England showed no reduction in self harm or number of self harm events.[157] [158] [159]

Conclusions

The assessment and management of suicidal patients is challenging and further complicated by a limited number of efficacious approaches. It is hoped that management will improve as the science of suicide prevention progresses and the number and quality of studies increases. Nevertheless, current evidence shows that several clinical practices can improve the management of suicidal people. Given that risk assessment tools to date are limited in their predictive ability, it might be best to focus efforts on developing effective low resource intensity interventions that acknowledge a high false positive rate. An important first step is to appreciate the heightened risk in specific clinical populations and the temporal association between suicide and service discharge. It is also crucial to recognise the established risk factors such as a history of self harm. Finally, when determining a treatment approach, clinicians should consider suicidal thoughts and behavior as an important therapeutic target.

The authors would like to acknowledge Hayley Chartrand, Yunqiao Wang, and Joanna Bhaskaran for their help with the literature search and manuscript preparation.

Competing interests: We have read and understood BMJ policy on declaration of interests and declare the following interests: none.

Contributors: All authors helped plan and prepare the manuscript and they meet all four ICMJE authorship criteria. Hayley Chartrand, Yunqiao Wang, and Joanna Bhaskaran contributed to the manuscript by performing literature searches and helping with manuscript preparation. JMB wrote the manuscript and is responsible for the overall content as guarantor. The guarantor accepts full responsibility for the work and/or the conduct of the study, had access to the data, and controlled the decision to publish.

Funding: JMB is supported by a Canadian Institutes of Health Research new investigator award (113589) and a Brain and Behavior Research Foundation NARSAD young investigator grant. DG is a National Institute for Health Research senior investigator. GT is supported by grants from the Canadian Institute of Health Research MOP93775, MOP11260, MOP119429, and MOP119430; from the National Institutes of Health 1R01DA033684-01; and by the Fonds de Recherche du Québec-Santé through a Chercheur National salary award and through the Quebec Network on Suicide, Mood Disorders, and Related Disorders.

1   WHO. Preventing suicide—a global imperative. 2014. http://apps.who.int/iris/bitstream/10665/131056/1/9789241564779_eng.pdf?ua=1.
2   WHO. Global Health Estimates. 2014. www.who.int/healthinfo/global_burden_disease/estimates/en/index2.html.
3   Berman AL. Estimating the population of survivors of suicide: seeking an evidence base. Suicide Life Threat Behav2011;41:110-6.
4   Bolton JM, Au W, Leslie WD, et al. Parents bereaved by offspring suicide: a population-based longitudinal case-control study. JAMA Psychiatry2013;70:158-67.
5   Rostila M, Saarela J, Kawachi I. Suicide following the death of a sibling: a nationwide follow-up study from Sweden. BMJ Open2013;3:e002618.
6   Crosby AE, Han B, Ortega LA, et al. Suicidal thoughts and behaviors among adults aged .18 years—United States, 2008-2009. MMWR Surveill Summ2011;63:1-22.
7   CrosbyAE, Ortega L, Stevens MR, et al. Suicides—United States, 2005-2009. MMWR Surveill Summ2013;62(suppl 3):179-83.

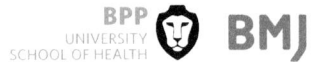

8   US Surgeon General and National Action Alliance for Suicide Prevention. National strategy for suicide prevention: goals and objectives for action. 2012. www.surgeongeneral.gov/library/reports/national-strategy-suicide-prevention/full_report-rev.pdf.

9   Nock MK, Borges G, Bromet EJ, et al. Suicide and suicidal behavior. Epidemiol Rev2008;30:133-54.

10   Mann JJ, Apter A, Bertolote J, et al. Suicide prevention strategies: a systematic review. JAMA2005;294:2064-74.

11   Hawton K, van Heeringen K. Suicide. Lancet2009;373:1372-81.

12   Maris RW. Suicide. Lancet2002;360:319-26.

13   Hjorthoj CR, Madsen T, Agerbo E, et al. Risk of suicide according to level of psychiatric treatment: a nationwide nested case-control study. Soc Psychiatry Psychiatr Epidemiol2014;49:1357-65.

14   Larkin C, Di Blasi Z, Arensman E. Risk factors for repetition of self-harm: a systematic review of prospective hospital-based studies. PLoS One2014;9:e84282.

15   Nordentoft M, Mortensen PB, Pedersen CB. Absolute risk of suicide after first hospital contact in mental disorder. Arch Gen Psychiatry2011;68:1058-64.

16   Randall JR, Walld R, Finlayson G, et al. Acute risk of suicide and suicide attempts associated with recent diagnosis of mental disorders: a population-based, propensity score-matched analysis. Can J Psychiatry2014;59:531-8.

17   Angst F, Stassen HH, Clayton PJ, Angst J. Mortality of patients with mood disorders: follow-up over 34-38 years. J Affect Disord2002;68:167-81.

18   McGirr A, Renaud J, Seguin M, et al. Course of major depressive disorder and suicide outcome: a psychological autopsy study. J Clin Psychiatry2008;69:966-70.

19   Kapur N, Hunt IM, Windfuhr K, et al. Psychiatric in-patient care and suicide in England, 1997-2008: a longitudinal study. Psychol Med2013;43:61-71.

20   Madsen T, Agerbo E, Mortensen PB, et al. Predictors of psychiatric inpatient suicide: a national prospective register-based study. J Clin Psychiatry2012;73:144-51.

21   Hunt IM, Bickley H, Windfuhr K, et al. Suicide in recently admitted psychiatric in-patients: a case-control study. J Affect Disord2013;144:123-8.

22   National Confidential Inquiry into Suicide and Homicide by People with Mental Illness Annual Report 2015: England, Northern Ireland, Scotland and Wales. University of Manchester, 2015.

23   Qin P, Nordentoft M. Suicide risk in relation to psychiatric hospitalization: evidence based on longitudinal registers. Arch Gen Psychiatry2005;62:427-32.

24   Goldacre M, Seagroatt V, Hawton K. Suicide after discharge from psychiatric inpatient care. Lancet1993;342:283-6.

25   Appleby L, Shaw J, Amos T, et al. Suicide within 12 months of contact with mental health services: national clinical survey. BMJ 1999;318:1235-9.

26   Hunt IM, Kapur N, Webb R, et al. Suicide in recently discharged psychiatric patients: a case-control study. Psychol Med2009;39:443-9.

27   Tidemalm D, Langstrom N, Lichtenstein P, et al. Risk of suicide after suicide attempt according to coexisting psychiatric disorder: Swedish cohort study with long term follow-up. BMJ 2008;337:a2205.

28   Carroll R, Metcalf C, Gunnell D. Hospital presenting self-harm and risk of fatal and non-fatal repetition: systematic review and meta-analysis. PLoS One2014;9:389944.

29   Hawton K, Bergen H, Cooper J, et al. Suicide following self-harm: findings from the multicentre study of self-harm in England, 2000-2012. J Affect Disord2015;175:147-51.

30   Bergen H, Hawton K, Waters K, et al. Premature death after self-harm: a multicenter cohort study. Lancet2012;380:1568-74.

31   Olfson M, Marcus SC, Bridge JA. Emergency department recognition of mental disorders and short-term outcome of deliberate self-harm. Am J Psychiatry2013;170:1142-50.

32   Steeg S, Kapur N, Webb R, et al. The development of a population-level clinical screening tool for self-harm repetition and suicide: the ReACT self-harm rule. Psychol Med2012;42:2383-94.

33   Glenn CR, Nock MK. Improving the short-term prediction of suicidal behavior. Am J Prev Med 2014;47:S176-80.

34   Bolton JM. Suicide risk assessment in the emergency department: out of the darkness. Depress Anxiety2015;32:73-5.

35   Olfson M, Marcus SC, Bridge JA. Focusing suicide prevention on periods of high risk. JAMA2014;311:1107-8.

36   Ahmedani BK, Simon GE, Stewart C, et al. Health care contacts in the year before suicide death. J Gen Intern Med2014;29:870-7.

37   Joiner TE, Walker RL, Rudd MD, et al. Scientizing and routinizing the assessment of suicidality in outpatient practice. Prof Psychol Res Pract1999;30:447-53.

38   Bryan CJ, Rudd MD. Advances in the assessment of suicide risk. J Clin Psychol2006;62:185-200.

39   Thienhaus OJ, Piasecki M. Assessment of suicide risk. Psychiatr Serv1997;48:293-4.

40   Fowler JC. Suicide risk assessment in clinical practice: pragmatic guidelines for imperfect assessments. Psychotherapy (Chic)2012;49:81-90.

41   Kapur N, Steeg S, Webb R, et al. Does clinical management improve outcomes following self-harm? Results from the multicenter study of self-harm in England. PLoS One2013;8:e70434.

42   Comtois KA, Jobes DA, O'Conner S, et al. Collaborative assessment and management of suicidality (CAMS): feasibility trial for next-day appointment services. Depress Anxiety2011;28:936-72.

43   Bajaj P, Borreani E, Ghosh P, et al. Screening for suicidal thoughts in primary care: the views of patient and general practitioners. Ment Health Fam Med 2008;5:229-35.

44   Dazzi T, Gribble R, Wessely S, et al. Does asking about suicide and related behaviours induce suicidal ideation? What is the evidence? Psychol Med2014;44:3361-3.

45   Gould MS, Marrocco FA, Kleinman M, et al. Evaluating iatrogenic risk of youth suicide screening programs: a randomized controlled trial. JAMA2005;293:1635-43.

46   Glaros AG, Kline RB. Understanding the accuracy of tests with cutting scores: the sensitivity, specificity, and predictive value. J Clin Psychol1988;44:1013-23.

47   Busch KA, Fawcett J, Jacobs DG. Clinical correlates of inpatient suicide. J Clin Psychiatry 2003;64:14-9.

48   Nock MK, Park JM, Finn CT, et al. Measuring the suicidal mind: implicit cognition predicts suicidal behavior. Psychol Sci2010;21:511-7.

49   Roos L, Sareen J, Bolton JM. Suicide risk assessment tools, predictive validity findings and utility today: time for a revamp? Neuropsychiatry2013;3:483-95.

50   Randall JR, Colman I, Rowe BH. A systematic review of psychometric assessment of self-harm risk in the emergency department. J Affect Disord2011;132:348-55.

51   Beck AT, Steer RA, Kovacs M, et al. Hopelessness and eventual suicide: a 10-year prospective study of patients hospitalized with suicidal ideation. Am J Psychiatry1985;142:559-63.

52   Beck AT, Brown G, Berchick RJ, et al. Relationship between hopelessness and ultimate suicide: a replication with psychiatric outpatients. Am J Psychiatry1990;147:190-5.

53   Nimeus A, Traskman-Bendz L, Alsen M. Hopelessness and suicidal behavior. J Affect Disord 1997;42:137-44.

54   Brown GK, Beck AT, Steer RA, et al. Risk factors for suicide in psychiatric outpatients: a 20-year prospective study. J Consult Clin Psychol2000;68:371-7.

55   Suominen K, Isometsa E, Ostamo A, et al. Level of suicidal intent predicts overall mortality and suicide after attempted suicide: a 12-year follow-up study. BMC Psychiatry 2004;4:11.

56   McMillan D, Gilbody S, Beresford E, et al. Can we predict suicide and non-fatal self-harm with the Beck hopelessness scale? A meta-analysis. Psychol Med2007;37:769-78.

57   Nimeus A, Alsen M, Traskman-Bendz L. High suicide intent scores indicate future suicide. Arch Suicide Res 2002;6:211-9.

58   Harriss L, Hawton K. Suicide intent in deliberate self-harm and the risk of suicide: the predictive power of the suicide intent scale. J Affect Disord2005;86:225-33.

59   Stefansson J, Nordstrom P, Jokinen J. Suicide intent scale in the prediction of suicide. J Affect Disord2012;136:167-71.

60   Kurz A, Moller H, Torhorst A, et al. Validation of six risk scales for suicide attempters. In: Current issues of suicidology1988:174-8.

61   Nimeus A, Alsen M, Traskman-Bendz L. The suicide assessment scale: an instrument assessing suicide risk of suicide attempters. Eur Psychiatry2000;15:416-23.

62   Jokinen J, Forslund K, Ahnemark E, et al. Karolinska interpersonal violence scale predicts suicide in suicide attempters. J Clin Psychiatry2010;71:1025-32.

63   Beck AT, Steer RA. Clinical predictors of eventual suicide: a 5- to 10-year prospective study of suicide attempters. J Affect Disord1989;17:203-9.

64   Freedenthal S. Assessing the wish to die: a 30-year review of the suicide intent scale. Arch Suicide Res2008;12:277-98.

65   Patterson WM, Dohn HH, Bird J, et al. Evaluation of suicidal patients: the SAD PERSONS scale. Psychosomatic1983;24:343-5, 348-9.

66   Quinlivan L, Cooper J, Steeg S, et al. Scales for predicting risk following self-harm: an observational study in 32 hospitals in England. BMJ Open2014;4:e004732.

67   Warden S, Spiwak R, Sareen J, et al. The SAD PERSONS scale for suicide risk assessment: a systematic review. Arch Suicide Res2014;18:313-26.

68   Bolton JM, Spiwak R, Sareen J. Predicting suicide attempts with the SAD PERSONS scale: a longitudinal analysis. J Clin Psychiatry2012;73:3-735-41.

69   Stanley B, Traskman-Bendz L, Stanley M. The suicide assessment scale: a scale evaluating change in suicidal behavior. Psychopharmacol Bull 1986;22:200-5.

70   Posner K, Brown GK, Stanley B, et al. The Columbia-suicide severity rating scale; initial validity and internal consistency findings from three multisite studies with adolescents and adults. Am J Psychiatry2011;168:1266-77.

71   Mundt JC, Greist JH, Jefferson JW, et al. Prediction of suicidal behavior in clinical research by lifetime suicidal ideation and behavior ascertained by the electronic Columbia-suicide severity rating scale. J Clin Psychiatry2013;74:887-93.

72   Yaseen ZS, Kopeykina I, Gutkovich Z, et al. Predictive validity of the suicide trigger scale (STS-3) for post-discharge suicide attempt in high-risk psychiatric inpatients. PLoS One2014;21:e86768.

73   Cooper J, Kapur N, Dunning J, et al. A clinical tool for assessing risk after self-harm. Ann Emerg Med 2006;48:459-66.

74   Bilen K, Ponzer, S, Ottosson C, et al. Deliberate self-harm patients in the emergency department: who will repeat and who will not? Validation and development of clinical decision rules. Emerg Med J 2013;30:650-6.

75   Spittal MJ, Pirkis J, Miller M, et al. The repeated episodes of self-harm (RESH) score: a tool for predicting risk of future episodes of self-harm by hospital patients. J Affect Disord2014;161:36-42.

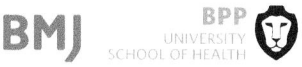

76 Wang Y, Bhaskaran J, Sareen J, et al. Predictors of future suicide attempts among individuals presenting to psychiatric services in the emergency department: a longitudinal study. J Nerv Ment Dis2015;203:507-13.

77 Randall JR, Bowe BH, Dong KA, et al. Assessment of self-harm risk using implicit thoughts. Psychol Assess2013;25:714-21.

78 Richard-Devantory S, Berlim MT, Jollant F. A meta-analysis of neuropsychological markers of vulnerability to suicidal behavior in mood disorders. Psychol Med2014;44:1663-73.

79 Cha CB, Najmi S, Park JM, et al. Attentional bias toward suicide-related stimuli predicts suicidal behavior. J Abnorm Psychol2010;119:616-22.

80 National Institute for Health and Care Excellence. Self-harm: longer-term management. 2014. www.nice.org.uk/guidance/cg133/resources/new-nice-guidance-for-the-longerterm-management-of-selfharm.

81 O'Connor E, Gaynes BN, Burda BU, et al. Screening for and treatment of suicide risk relevant to primary care: a systematic review for the US Preventative Services Task Force. Ann Intern Med 2013;158:741-54.

82 Hatcher S. The Manchester self harm rule had good sensitivity but poor specificity for predicting repeat self harm or suicide. Evid Based Med2007;12:89.

83 Bergen H, Hawton K, Waters K, et al. Psychosocial assessment and repetition of self-harm: the significance of single and multiple repeat episode analyses. J Affect Disord2010;127:257-65.

84 National Action Alliance for Suicide Prevention: Clinical Workforce Preparedness Task Force. Suicide prevention and the clinical workforce: guidelines for training. 2014. http://actionallianceforsuicideprevention.org/sites/actionallianceforsuicideprevention.org/files/Guidelines.pdf.

85 Bernert RA, Hom MA, Roberts LW. A review of multidisciplinary clinical practice guidelines in suicide prevention: toward an emerging standard in suicide risk assessment and management, training and practice. Acad Psychiatry2014;38:585-92.

86 While D, Bickley H, Roscoe A, et al. Implementation of mental health service recommendations in England and Wales and suicide rates, 1997-2006: a cross-sectional and before-and-after observational study. Lancet2012;379:1005-12.

87 Bruffaerts R, Demyttenaere K, Hwang I, et al. Treatment of suicidal people around the world. Br J Psychiatry 2011;199:64-70.

88 Kapur N, Murphy E, Cooper J, et al. Psychosocial assessment following self-harm: results from the multi-centre monitoring of self-harm project. J Affect Disord2008;106:285-93.

89 Olfson M, Marcus SC, Bridge JA. Emergency treatment of deliberate self-harm. Arch Gen Psychiatry 2012;69:80-8.

90 Hawton K, Arensman E, Townsend E, et al. Deliberate self harm: systematic review of efficacy of psychosocial and pharmacological treatments in preventing repetition. BMJ1998;317:441-7.

91 Hepp U, Wittmann L, Schnyder U, et al. Psychological and psychosocial interventions after attempted suicide: an overview of treatment studies. Crisis2004;25:108-17.

92 Luxton DD, June JD, Comtois KA. Can postdischarge follow-up contacts prevent suicide and suicidal behavior? A review of the evidence. Crisis 2013;34:32-41.

93 National Institute for Health and Care Excellence. Review of Clinical Guidelines (CG16)—Self-harm: the short-term physical and psychological management and secondary prevention of self-harm in primary and secondary care. 2012. www.nice.org.uk/guidance/cg16/documents/self-harm-review-decision-february-20122.

94 Griffiths JJ, Zarate CA Jr, Rasimas JJ. Existing and novel biological therapeutics in suicide prevention. Am J Prev Med2014;47:S195-203.

95 Cavanagh JT, Carson AJ, Sharpe M, et al. Psychological autopsy studies of suicide: a systematic review. Psychol Med2003;33:395-405.

96 Rihmer Z, Gonda X. Pharmacological prevention of suicide in patients with major mood disorder. Neurosci Biobehav Rev2013;37:2398-403.

97 Stone M, Laughren T, Jones ML, et al. Risk of suicidality in clinical trials of antidepressants in adults: analysis of propriety data submitted to US Food and Drug Administration. BMJ2009;339:b2880.

98 Tiihonen J, Lonngvist J, Wahlbeck K, et al. Antidepressants and the risk of suicide, attempted suicide, and overall mortality in a nationwide cohort. Arch Gen Psychiatry2006;63:1358-67.

99 Simon GE. How can we know whether antidepressants increase suicide risk? Am J Psychiatry2006;163:1861-3.

100 National Statistics. Deaths related to drug poisoning in England and Wales, 2002-06. Health Stat Q 2007;Winter:66-72.

101 Hawton K, Bergen H, Simkin S et al. Toxicity of antidepressants: rates of suicide relative to prescribing and non-fatal overdose. Br J Psychiatry2010;196:354-8.

102 Friedman RA. Antidepressants' black-box warning—10 years later. N Engl J Med2014;37:1666-8.

103 Katz LY, Kozyrskyj AL, Prior HJ, et al. Effect of regulatory warning on antidepressant prescription rates, use of health services and outcomes among children, adolescents and young adults. CMAJ2008;178:1005-11.

104 Gibbons RD, Brown CH, Hur K, et al. Suicidal thoughts and behavior with antidepressant treatment: reanalysis of the randomized placebo-controlled studies of fluoxetine and venlafaxine. Arch Gen Psychiatry2012;69:580-7.

105 Cipriani A, Hawton K, Stockton S, et al. Lithium in the prevention of suicide in mood disorders: updated systematic review and meta-analysis. BMJ 2013;346:f3646.

106 Baldessarini RJ, Tondo L, Davis P, et al. Decreased risk of suicides and attempts during long-term lithium treatment: a meta-analytic review. Bipolar Disord2006;8:625-39.

107 Ohgami H, Terao T, Shiotsuki I, et al. Lithium levels in drinking water and risk of suicide. Br J Psychiatry2009;195:464-5.

108 Kapusta ND, Mossaheb N, Etzersdorfer E, et al. Lithium in drinking water and suicide mortality. Br J Psychiatry2011;195:346-50.

109 Bluml V, Regier MD, Hlavin G, et al. Lithium in the public water supply and suicide mortality in Texas. J Psychiatr Res2013;47:407-11.

110 Kessing LV, Sondergrad L, Kvist K, et al. Suicide risk in patients treated with lithium. Arch Gen Psychiatry2005;62:860-6.

111 Rihmer Z, Gonda X. The effect of pharmacotherapy on suicide rates in bipolar patients. CNS Neurosci Ther2012;18:238-42.

112 Gibbons RD, Hur K, Brown CH, et al. Relationship between antiepileptic drugs and suicide attempts in patients with bipolar disorder. Arch Gen Psychiatry2009;66:1354-60.

113 Sondergard L, Lopez AG, Andersen PK, et al. Mood-stabilizing pharmacological treatment in bipolar disorders and risk of suicide. Bipolar Disord2008;10:87-94.

114 Goodwin FK, Fireman B, Simon GE, et al. Suicide risk in bipolar disorder during treatment with lithium and divalproex. JAMA2003;290:1467-73.

115 Kasckow J, Felmet K, Zisook S. Managing suicide risk in patients with schizophrenia. CNS Drugs 2011;25:129-43.

116 Agid O, Foussias G, Singh S, et al. Where to position clozapine: re-examining the evidence. Can J Psychiatry2010;55:677-84.

117 Hennen J, Baldessarini RJ. Suicidal risk during treatment with clozapine: a meta-analysis. Schizophr Res2005;73:139-45.

118 DiazGranados N, Ibrahim LA, Brutsche NE, et al. Rapid resolution of suicidal ideation after a single infusion of an N-methyl-D-aspartate antagonist in patients with treatment-resistant major depressive disorder. J Clin Psychiatry2010;71:1605-11.

119 Duman RS, Aghajanian GK. Synaptic dysfunction in depression: potential therapeutic targets. Science2012;338:68-72.

120 Ballard ED, Ionescu DF, Vande Voort JL, et al. Improvement in suicidal ideation after ketamine infusion: relationship to reductions in depression and anxiety. J Psychiatr Res2014;58:161-6.

121 Price RB, Iosifescu DV, Murrough JW, et al. Effects of ketamine on explicit and implicit suicidal cognition: a randomized controlled trial in treatment resistant depression. Depress Anxiety2014;31:335-43.

122 Larkin GL, Beautrais AL. A preliminary naturalistic study of low-dose ketamine for depression and suicide ideation in the emergency department. Int J Neuropsychopharmacol2011;14:1127-31.

123 Kennedy SH, Milev R, Giacobbe P, et al. Canadian Network for Mood and Anxiety Treatments (CANMAT) clinical guidelines for the management of major depressive disorder in adults. IV. Neurostimulation therapies. J Affect Disord2009;117(suppl 1):S44-53.

124 Kellner CH, Fink M, Knapp R, et al. Relief of expressed suicidal intent by ECT: a consortium for research in ECT study. Am J Psychiatry2005;162:977-82.

125 Patel M, Patel S, Hardy DW, et al. Should electroconvulsive therapy be an early consideration for suicidal patients? J ECT2006;22:113-5.

126 Fink M, Kellner CH, McCall WV. The role of ECT in suicide prevention. J ECT2014;30:5-9.

127 Isometsa ET, Henriksson MM, Keikkinen ME. Completed suicide and recent electroconvulsive therapy in Finland. Convuls Ther1996;12:152-5.

128 Sharma V. The effect of electroconvulsive therapy on suicide risk in patients with mood disorders. Can J Psychiatry2001;46:704-9.

129 Prudic J, Sackeim HA. Electroconvulsive therapy and suicide risk. J Clin Psychiatry1999;60:104-10.

130 Brown GK, Jager-Hyman S. Evidence-based psychotherapies for suicide prevention: future directions. Am J Prev Med2014;47:S186-94.

131 Slee N, Garnefski N, van der Leeden R, et al. Cognitive-behavioural intervention for self-harm: randomized controlled trial. Br J Psychiatry2008;192:202-11.

132 Brown GK, Ten Have T, Henriques GR, et al. Cognitive therapy for the prevention of suicide attempts: a randomized controlled trial. JAMA2005;294:563-70.

133 Linehan MM, Comtois KA, Murray AM, et al. Two-year randomized controlled trial and follow-up of dialectical behavior therapy vs therapy by experts for suicidal behaviors and borderline personality disorder. Arch Gen Psychiatry2006;63:757-66.

134 Davidson K, Norrie J, Tyrer P, et al. The effectiveness of cognitive behavior therapy for borderline personality disorder: results from the borderline personality disorder study of cognitive therapy (BOSCOT) trial. J Pers Disord 2006;20:450-65.

135 Hatcher S, Sharon C, Parag V, et al. Problem-solving therapy for people who present to hospital with self-harm: Zelen randomised controlled trial. Br J Psychiatry2011;199:310-6.

136 Erlangsen A, Lind BD, Stuart EA, et al. Short-term and long-term effects of psychosocial therapy for people after deliberate self-harm: a register-based, nationwide multicenter study using propensity score matching. Lancet Psychiatry2014;2:49-58.

137 Inagaki M, Kawashima Y, Kawanishi C, et al. Interventions to prevent repeat suicidal behavior in patients admitted to an emergency department for a suicide attempt: a meta-analysis. J Affect Disord2015;175C:66-78.

138 Van Spijker BA, van Straten A, Kerkhof AJ. Effectiveness of online self-help for suicidal thoughts: results of a randomized controlled trial. PLoS One2014;9:e90118.

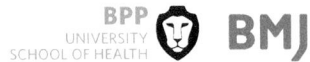

139 Christensen H, Farrer L, Batterham PJ, et al. The effect of a web-based depression intervention on suicide ideation: secondary outcome from a randomized controlled trial in a helpline. BMJ Open2013;3:e002886.

140 Cuijpers P, de Beurs DP, van Spijker BA, et al. The effects of psychotherapy for adult depression on suicidality and hopelessness: a systematic review and meta-analysis. J Affect Disord2013;144:183-90.

141 Brown GK, Green KL. A review of evidence-based follow-up care for suicide prevention: where do we go from here? Am J Prev Med2014;47:S209-15.

142 Cooper J, Hunter C, Owen-Smith A, et al. "Well it's like someone at the other end cares about you." A qualitative study exploring the views of users and providers of care of contact-based interventions following self-harm. Gen Hosp Psychiatry2011;33:166-76.

143 Gunnell D, Metcalfe C, While D, et al. Impact of national policy initiatives on fatal and non-fatal self-harm after psychiatric hospital discharge: time series analysis. Br J Psychiatry2012;201:233-8.

144 Pirkola S, Sund R, Sallas E, et al. Community mental-health services and suicide rate in Finland: a nationwide small-area analysis. Lancet 2009;373:147-53.

145 Milner AJ, Carter G, Pirkis J, et al. Letters, green cards, telephone calls and postcards: systematic and meta-analytic review of brief contact interventions for reducing self-harm, suicide attempts and suicide. Br J Psychiatry2015;206:184-90.

146 Fleischmann A, Bertolote JM, Wasserman D, et al. Effectiveness of brief intervention and contact for suicide attempters: a randomized controlled trial in five countries. Bull World Health Organ2008;86:703-9.

147 Bertolote JM, Fleischmann A, De Leo D, et al. Repetition of suicide attempts: data from emergency care settings in five culturally different low- and middle-income countries participating in the WHO SUPRE-MISS Study. Crisis2010;31:194-201.

148 Cedereke M, Monti K, Ojehagen A. Telephone contact with patients in the year after a suicide attempt: does it affect treatment attendance and outcome? A randomised controlled study. Eur Psychiatry2002;17:82-91.

149 Cebria AI, Parra I, Pamias M, et al. Effectiveness of a telephone management programme for patients discharged from an emergency department after a suicide attempt: controlled study in a Spanish population. J Affect Disord2013;147:269-76.

150 Morthorst B, Krogh J, Eriangsen A, et al. Effect of assertive outreach after suicide attempt in the AID (assertive intervention for deliberate self-harm) trial: randomised controlled trial. BMJ2012;351:34972.

151 Carter GL, Clover K, Whyte IM, et al. Postcards from the EDge project: randomised controlled trial of an intervention using postcards to reduce repetition of hospital treated deliberate self-poisoning. BMJ2005;331:805.

152 Carter GL, Clover K, Whyte IM, et al. Postcards from the EDge: 24-month outcomes of a randomised controlled trial for hospital-treated self-poisoning. Br J Psychiatry2007;191:548-53.

153 Carter GL, Clover K, Whyte IM, et al. Postcards from the EDge: 5-year outcomes of a randomised controlled trial for hospital-treated self-poisoning. Br J Psychiatry2013;202:372-80.

154 Hassanian-Moghaddam H, Sarjami S, Kolahi AA, et al. Postcards in Persia: randomised controlled trial to reduce suicidal behaviours 12 months after hospital-treated self-poisoning. Br J Psychiatry2011;198:309-16.

155 Hassanian-Moghaddam H, Sarjami S, Kolahi AA, et al. Postcards in Persia: a 12-24 month follow-up of a randomised controlled trial for hospital treated deliberate self-poisoning. Arch Suicide Res2015; doi:10.1080/13811118.2015.1004473; published online 16 March.

156 Motto JA, Bostrom AG. A randomized controlled trial of postcrisis suicide prevention. Psychiatr Serv2001;52:828-33.

157 Beautrais AL, Gibb SJ, Faulkner A, et al. Postcard intervention for repeat self-harm: randomised controlled trial. Br J Psychiatry2010;197:55-60.

158 Kapur N, Gunnell D, Hawton K, et al. Messages from Manchester: pilot randomised controlled trial following self-harm. Br J Psychiatry2013;203:73-4.

159 Chen WJ, Ho CK, Shyu SS, et al. Employing crisis postcards with case management in Kaohsiung, Taiwan: 6-month outcomes of a randomised controlled trial for suicide attempters. BMC Psychiatry2013;131:191.

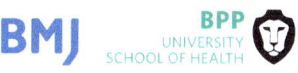

Smoking cessation and reduction in people with chronic mental illness

Jennifer W Tidey, associate professor (research), Mollie E Miller, postdoctoral research associate

Center for Alcohol and Addiction Studies, Brown University, Providence, RI 02912, USA

Correspondence to: J Tidey Jennifer_Tidey@brown.edu

Cite this as: *BMJ* 2015;351:h4065

DOI: 10.1136/bmj.h4065

http://www.bmj.com/content/351/bmj.h4065

ABSTRACT

The high prevalence of cigarette smoking and tobacco related morbidity and mortality in people with chronic mental illness is well documented. This review summarizes results from studies of smoking cessation treatments in people with schizophrenia, depression, anxiety disorders, and post-traumatic stress disorder. It also summarizes experimental studies aimed at identifying biopsychosocial mechanisms that underlie the high smoking rates seen in people with these disorders. Research indicates that smokers with chronic mental illness can quit with standard cessation approaches with minimal effects on psychiatric symptoms. Although some studies have noted high relapse rates, longer maintenance on pharmacotherapy reduces rates of relapse without untoward effects on psychiatric symptoms. Similar biopsychosocial mechanisms are thought to be involved in the initiation and persistence of smoking in patients with different disorders. An appreciation of these common factors may aid the development of novel tobacco treatments for people with chronic mental illness. Novel nicotine and tobacco products such as electronic cigarettes and very low nicotine content cigarettes may also be used to improve smoking cessation rates in people with chronic mental illness.

Introduction

Rates of cigarette smoking among adults in the United States and United Kingdom are two to four times higher in people with current mood, anxiety, and psychotic disorders than in those without mental illness.[1][2] For example, a recent study in more than 9000 people with severe psychotic disorders found that these people had a higher risk of having ever smoked 100 cigarettes (odds ratios 4.61, 95% confidence interval 4.3 to 4.9) relative to the general population after controlling for sex, race, age, and geographical region.[3]

Smokers with chronic mental illness are also more dependent on nicotine and are less likely to quit than those without these disorders.[4][5][6] Notably, between 2004 and 2011, after controlling for risk factors such as income, education, and employment, current smoking rates dropped from 19.2% (18.7% to 19.7%) to 16.5% (16.0% to 17.0%) in US residents without mental illness but not in those with mental illness.[6] Consequently, about 50% of deaths in patients with chronic mental illness are due to tobacco related cancers, respiratory diseases, and cardiovascular conditions.[7][8]

This review critically assesses the effectiveness of smoking cessation treatments for people with schizophrenia, unipolar and bipolar depression, anxiety disorders, and post-traumatic stress disorder (PTSD). Because the development of novel treatments for smoking cessation in people with chronic mental illness may be facilitated by the identification of factors that contribute to their smoking, we also critically examine biopsychosocial mechanisms thought

to underlie these people's high smoking rates. Finally, given the current commercial and regulatory interest in electronic cigarettes (e-cigarettes) and very low nicotine content cigarettes, we describe recent studies of these products in people with chronic mental illness and discuss how such products might be used to improve smoking cessation outcomes for these people.

Sources and selection criteria

This review examines the effects and mechanisms of smoking cessation treatment in adults (≥18 years) with schizophrenia, unipolar or bipolar depression, anxiety disorders, or PTSD. References were identified through searches of publications listed in PubMed and ScienceDirect from inception to 1 December 2014. We used the following keywords: "schizophrenia", "depression", "unipolar", "bipolar", "anxiety", "panic" "PTSD", "smoking", "smoking cessation", "clinical trial", "nicotine replacement", "bupropion", "varenicline", "withdrawal", "abstinence", "cigarette", "electronic cigarette" "very low nicotine cigarette", and "denicotinized cigarette". References were also identified from relevant reviews, meta-analyses, and the authors' files. JWT and MEM independently reviewed the titles retrieved from the search and prepared an initial list of articles to be included in the review. Both authors then reviewed the abstracts and selected the most pertinent studies to include in the review. Because this is not a systematic review, we did not grade the included studies, but rather summarized outcomes. Only peer reviewed articles published in English were reviewed. We examined current guidelines for treating smoking in people with mental illness by searching the websites of international health organizations and by searching Google using the keywords "smoking cessation guidelines", "tobacco treatment guidelines", "mental illness", and "mental disorders".

Schizophrenia

Interest in the association between schizophrenia and smoking was galvanized by a report published almost 30 years ago indicating that people with chronic mental illness had substantially higher smoking rates than control samples across age, sex, marital, socioeconomic, and alcohol use subgroups. The report also found that the smoking rate was particularly high (88%) in patients with schizophrenia.[9]

A second finding that triggered intense interest in the schizophrenia-smoking comorbidity was the observation that urinary concentrations of the major nicotine metabolite, cotinine, were 1.6 times higher in smokers with schizophrenia than in control smokers without schizophrenia.[10] These findings prompted two parallel lines of research, one aimed at finding potential treatments for tobacco dependence in smokers with schizophrenia and the other aimed at identifying biopsychosocial mechanisms that might account for this comorbidity.

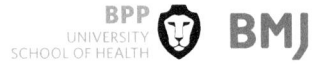

Smoking cessation studies

Nicotine replacement therapy plus psychosocial treatment
Several observational studies of open label nicotine replacement therapy (NRT) plus psychosocial treatment with motivational interviewing and cognitive behavioral therapy (CBT) components have been conducted in smokers with schizophrenia (table 1).

Three studies in 24-65 outpatients found quit rates of 9-14% at six month follow-up assessments,[11] [12] [13] and one study in 68 outpatients found a 23% continuous abstinence rate at three month follow-up.[14] In the largest smoking study in this population, 298 outpatients with a psychotic disorder (57% with schizophrenia) were randomized to routine care or to 10 weeks of treatment with motivational interviewing and CBT plus NRT.[15] At the 12 month follow-up assessment, abstinence was not significantly higher in the treatment group (10.9 v 6.6% for the control condition; odds ratio 1.72, 99% confidence interval 0.58 to 5.09), but significantly more people in the treatment group had reduced the number of cigarettes they smoked each day by half (2.09, 99% confidence interval 1.03 to 4.27). When people in this study were re-contacted four years after treatment, 18% were abstinent. Abstinence at the 12 month follow-up was significantly associated with abstinence at four years, but treatment group did not predict four year outcomes.[16] Overall, these studies indicate that average six to 12 month quit rates with treatments that include NRT are

about 13% in smokers with schizophrenia. However, it is difficult to draw definitive conclusions from these studies owing to the lack of a placebo group.

One placebo controlled study investigated the efficacy of NRT for the prevention of relapse in smokers with schizophrenia.[17] Fifty outpatients received nicotine patches that delivered 14-63 mg per day for 90 days along with weekly group motivational support. Those who quit (36%) were then randomized to continue receiving nicotine patches (same dose) or to receive placebo patches, along with biweekly group support, for another six months. At the end of this period, significantly more people receiving NRT remained abstinent compared with those receiving placebo (67% v 0%; P<0.01). These results show that prolonged NRT is feasible and reduces relapse in this population.

Bupropion
Bupropion, a weak dopamine and norepinephrine (noradrenaline) reuptake inhibitor and antagonist at $\alpha3\beta2$ and $\alpha4\beta2$ nicotinic acetylcholine receptors (nAChRs), attenuates withdrawal symptoms and nicotine reinforcement.[18] Table 2 shows the outcomes from open label and placebo controlled trials with bupropion in smokers with schizophrenia.

An early observational study (2001; n=9) with open label bupropion found that although no patients achieved abstinence, average breath carbon monoxide (CO) levels were reduced by half.[19] A placebo controlled trial (n=19) performed at the same time also reported that although

Table 1 Outcomes of cessation treatment trials of NRT in outpatients with schizophrenia*

Study	N	Intervention	Abstinence rates	Other outcomes
Ziedonis and George 1997[11]	24	10 week treatment with open label NRT (21 mg patch and gum) plus weekly behavioral, psychoeducational, and motivational enhancement therapy (no control group)	50% completed the program and 13% were abstinent for 6 months	40% of patients decreased CPD by half; there were no changes in psychiatric symptoms
Addington et al 1998[12]	65	10 week treatment with open label NRT (21 mg patch), plus 7 weekly group sessions based on the ALA "Freedom from Smoking" program, tailored for people with schizophrenia (no control group)	77% completed treatment; 42% of completers (32% of enrolled) were abstinent at end of treatment, 16% (12% of enrolled) at 3 month follow-up, and 12% (9% of enrolled) at 6 month follow-up	Group session attendance was associated with abstinence at follow-ups; there were no changes in psychiatric or extrapyramidal symptoms
George et al 2000[13]	45	10 week treatment with open label NRT (21 mg patch) plus randomization to the ALA "Freedom from Smoking" program or a tailored program with motivational, behavioural, and psychoeducational components	32.1% attained 4 week continuous abstinence at end of treatment in the tailored program v 23.5% in the ALA program (P<0.06); 17.6% abstinent at 6 months in the ALA program v 10.7% in the tailored program (P<0.03)	Use of atypical antipsychotics was associated with longer treatment retention and higher abstinence rates; there were no effects of treatment or abstinence on psychiatric symptoms dyskinesia or extrapyramidal symptoms
Chou et al 2004[14]	68	8 week treatment with open label NRT (14 mg patch) or assessment only control	26.9% point prevalence abstinence and 23.1% continuous abstinence in the NRT group at 3 months v 0% in the control group (significance level not reported)	Daily smoking rates were reduced by over half at 3 months in the experimental group; no change in the control group
Baker et al 2006[15]	298	Randomization to 10 week treatment including open label NRT (21 mg patch), 8 sessions of individual motivational interviewing, and CBT, or to routine care consisting of booklets and access to community treatments	Abstinence rates were nominally but not significantly higher for the intervention group at each assessment (point prevalence abstinence at 6 months 9.5% v 4%, odds ratio 2.54, 99% CI 0.70 to 9.28; at 12 months 10.9% v 6.6%, 1.72, 0.58 to 5.09); those in the active arm who attended all sessions had significantly higher abstinence rates than controls at each follow-up point (point prevalent abstinence at 6 months: 18.6%, 5.51, 1.45 to 20.91)	More patients in the treatment group achieved 50% reductions in smoking rate than those in the control group; atypical medication status did not moderate abstinence or attendance; in both groups, NRT use was associated with smoking reduction; functioning and symptoms improved across time in both groups
Horst et al 2005[17]	50	12 week treatment with open label NRT (up to 63 mg/day patch) plus weekly group psychoeducation; those who quit entered single blind randomization to NRT or placebo for up to 6 additional months, with biweekly psychoeducation	36% abstinence at the end of the 90 day open label phase; at end of the relapse prevention phase, 67% of the NRT group remained abstinent v 0% of the placebo group (P<0.01)	Conventional v atypical antipsychotic drug type did not affect outcome; no participants on NRT discontinued due to adverse events
Williams et al 2010[33]	100	26 week treatment with a 24 session program combining motivational, cognitive behavioural, and psychoeducational elements or a 9 session medication management program; both groups received NRT (21 mg patch) for 16 weeks; treatment was provided by mental health clinicians	16% of those in the higher intensity treatment and 26% of those in the lower intensity treatment arm had continuous abstinence at 12 weeks after the target quit day (NS); continuous abstinence rates were 17% at 6 month follow-up and 14% at 12 month follow-up, with no difference between groups	No effects of treatment or abstinence on psychiatric symptoms; higher session attendance was associated with higher cessation rate at 3 month follow-up, regardless of treatment condition

Abbreviations: ALA=American Lung Association; CBT=cognitive behavioral therapy; CI=confidence interval; CPD=cigarettes per day; NRT=nicotine replacement therapy; NS=not significant.

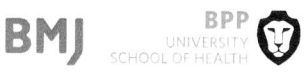

bupropion did not significantly increase abstinence, it significantly reduced breath CO levels (P<0.001) at follow-up.[20] Furthermore, a follow-up assessment two years later found that those who had reduced smoking initially were more likely to achieve abstinence P<0.005).[21]

Two placebo controlled trials in 32 and 57 smokers with schizophrenia found that bupropion significantly increased continuous abstinence during treatment (P<0.05), although these effects were not maintained at the three to six month follow-ups.[22] [23] Similarly, two trials that compared bupropion plus NRT with placebo plus NRT in smokers with schizophrenia found that bupropion plus NRT significantly increased the odds of continuous abstinence during treatment (table 2) but not at the three to 12 month follow-ups.[24] [25] Somewhat surprisingly, the effects of bupropion plus NRT were not superior to those of bupropion alone seen in an earlier study.[22]

Finally, a placebo controlled trial of bupropion in 52 patients, in which nicotine gum was also available but no patient chose to use it, found that continuous abstinence rates during the last four weeks of treatment were not significantly different.[26]

Overall, the results from most placebo controlled studies of bupropion, with or without NRT, in smokers with schizophrenia indicate that bupropion increases initial abstinence but that relapse rates are high after treatment is discontinued. This suggests that smokers with schizophrenia require prolonged treatment.

In an observational study that examined the efficacy of extended open label bupropion plus NRT, 41 smokers with schizophrenia received bupropion plus NRT (patch plus gum or lozenge) and CBT for three months. At the end of this period, those who were abstinent (42%) entered a 12 month relapse prevention phase with bupropion plus NRT and CBT.[27] At the 12 month assessment, 59% had achieved four weeks of continuous abstinence. Although this study lacked a placebo group the results, along with those from an earlier study of NRT for relapse prevention,[17] support the approach of using prolonged pharmacological treatment to reduce relapse in smokers with schizophrenia.

Varenicline

Varenicline, a partial agonist at $\alpha 4\beta 2$ nAChRs and full agonist at $\alpha 7$ nAChRs,[28] substitutes for and blocks the reinforcing effects of nicotine, and is more effective than bupropion or single forms of NRT in the general population.[29] Table 3 shows the outcomes from trials of varenicline in smokers with schizophrenia.

Table 2 Outcomes of smoking cessation trials of treatment with bupropion alone or combined with NRT in outpatients with schizophrenia*

Study	N	Intervention	Abstinence rates	Other outcomes
Weiner et al 2001[19]	9	14 week treatment with open label bupropion (150 mg BID) and 9 weekly group psychoeducational therapy sessions; no control	89% completed treatment; no patient quit smoking	Average breath CO levels decreased by half during treatment; schizophrenia symptom scores and neurocognitive measures were unchanged
Evins et al 2001[20]	19	12 week randomized double blind placebo controlled trial with bupropion (150 mg/day) and 9 weekly CBT sessions	All of those who received at least one dose of drug completed treatment; continuous abstinence rates at 6 months were 11% for bupropion v 0% for placebo (NS)	33% of bupropion group and 11% of placebo group had biochemically confirmed 50% reduction in CPD at 6 months (P<0.001); psychiatric symptoms decreased in the bupropion group and increased in the placebo group during treatment; there were no serious adverse events; 2 patients/group increased antipsychotic drug dose during the trial
George et al 2002[22]	32	10 week randomized double blind placebo controlled treatment with bupropion (150 mg BID) and weekly CBT	78% completed treatment; abstinence rates were significantly higher for bupropion at end of treatment (point prevalent abstinence 50% v 12.5%, P<0.05; continuous abstinence 37.5% v 6.3%, P<0.05) but not at 6 months (18.8% v 6.3%, P=0.29)	End of trial point prevalence abstinence rates were 67% for bupropion v 20% for placebo (P<0.01) in those taking atypical antipsychotics and 0% for both groups in those taking conventional antipsychotics; bupropion was associated with reduced negative symptoms and no effects on positive or other symptoms
Evins et al 2005[23]	57	12 week randomized double blind placebo controlled treatment with bupropion (150 mg BID) and weekly CBT	81% of those who received at least one week of drug completed treatment; point prevalence and 4 week continuous abstinence rates at end of treatment were higher in the bupropion group than in the placebo group (16% v 0% for both measures; P<0.05); at follow-up 3 months after end of the intervention, abstinence rates were 4% for bupropion and placebo (NS)	Breath CO levels were lower in the bupropion group than the placebo group during treatment, particularly in those taking atypical antipsychotics; the bupropion group tended to have greater reductions in psychiatric symptoms than the placebo group
Evins et al 2007[24]	51	12 week randomized double blind placebo controlled treatment with bupropion (150 mg BID) + NRT (21 mg patch + gum) or placebo + NRT; all received weekly CBT	71% of those who received at least one week of drug completed treatment; no significant differences between groups in abstinence rates at week 12 (36% v 19%), week 24 (20% v 8%), or week 52 (12% v 8%)	More patients in the bupropion + NRT arm had 50% reduction in CPD at 6 month follow-up (32% v 8%, P<0.05); there were no effects of bupropion or abstinence on psychiatric symptoms
George et al 2008[25]	59	10 week randomized double blind placebo controlled treatment with bupropion (150 mg BID) + NRT (21 mg) or placebo + NRT; all received weekly CBT	72% of those who received at least one drug dose completed treatment; continuous abstinence rates were higher for bupropion + NRT at end of treatment (27.6% v 3.4%, odds ratio 10.67, 95% CI 1.24 to 91.98) but not significantly higher at 6 month follow-up (13.8% v 0%)	No effects of drug treatment or abstinence on schizophrenia or depression symptoms
Weiner et al 2012[26]	52	12 week randomized double blind placebo controlled treatment with bupropion (150 mg BID) plus psychoeducation and support sessions; nicotine gum was also available but no patient chose to use it	78% of those who received at least one drug dose completed treatment; continuous abstinence rates (18% for bupropion, 11% for placebo) point prevalence abstinence, and other measures did not differ between groups	No effects of bupropion on psychiatric symptoms or neuropsychological measures
Cather et al 2013[27]	41	12 week open label treatment with bupropion + NRT (21 mg patch with gum or lozenge) and CBT; those abstinent at 3 months received another 12 months of pharmacotherapy and CBT; no control arm	42% were abstinent at 3 months and entered the relapse prevention phase; at end of the 12 month relapse prevention phase, 65% of patients had biochemically confirmed 7 day point prevalent abstinence and 59% reported 4 week continuous abstinence	No worsening of psychiatric symptoms; one participant had an adjustment in antipsychotic drugs during week 24

*Abbreviations: BID=twice a day; CBT=cognitive behavioral therapy; CI=confidence interval; CPD=cigarettes per day; NRT=nicotine replacement therapy; NS=not significant.

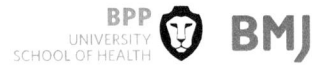

A placebo controlled trial (n=9) found that three in four smokers with schizophrenia taking varenicline achieved continuous abstinence during the last four weeks of the treatment period compared with no patients taking placebo (P=0.14). A significant reduction was seen in breath CO levels after four weeks of treatment in the varenicline group compared with the placebo group (P=0.02) and no increases were seen in psychiatric symptoms or suicidal ideation.[30]

A multi-site placebo controlled trial of varenicline with brief counseling in 128 smokers with schizophrenia found that varenicline significantly increased point prevalence abstinence at the end of treatment (19% v 4.7%; P<0.05) but not at the six month follow-up.[31] Rates of adverse events were similar across conditions (see table 3), and schizophrenia symptoms were stable or decreased in both groups.

Finally, a recent 10 site placebo controlled trial investigated whether varenicline reduces smoking relapse.[32] In total, 247 patients with schizophrenia or bipolar disorder were enrolled and 203 entered the open label treatment phase. Of these, 87 (43%) attained two weeks of continuous abstinence and entered the relapse prevention phase, in which they were randomized to varenicline or placebo with CBT. At week 52, point prevalence abstinence rates were significantly higher in people taking varenicline (60% v 19%; odds ratio 6.2, 95% confidence interval 2.2 to 19.2), and rates of continuous abstinence from week 12 to 76 were also higher (30% v 11%; 3.4, 1.02 to 13.6). Varenicline had no effect on psychiatric symptoms. Two patients in each group reported suicidal ideation during the maintenance phase but there were no suicide attempts. Thus, among smokers with schizophrenia who attained abstinence, varenicline was well tolerated and increased prolonged abstinence for as long as 76 weeks.[32]

Studies comparing psychosocial treatments

All of these studies included a psychosocial component, usually CBT, but few studies have compared the efficacy of different psychosocial treatments. One study in 45 people found that smokers with schizophrenia who received tailored treatment tended to have higher continuous abstinence at the end of treatment than those receiving the American Lung Association (ALA) "Freedom from Smoking" program, but these effects were reversed at six month follow-up.[13]

Another study in 87 people compared higher versus lower intensity behavioral treatment in smokers with schizophrenia who received NRT for 16 weeks and found no difference on abstinence.[33] Yet another study in 78 people compared the effects of a 40 minute motivational interviewing session, a 40 minute psychoeducational counseling session, and a five minute advice only session on seeking cessation treatment in smokers with schizophrenia. This study found that those who received motivational interviewing were significantly more likely to seek and attend cessation treatment than those who received the other treatments (P<0.05). This indicates that a single session of motivational interviewing increases the likelihood that these patients will seek cessation treatment.[34]

Contingency management is an approach in which monetary or other reinforcement is provided when a patient meets an objectively measured therapeutic target, such as biochemical evidence of drug abstinence. The results of proof of concept studies of this approach for smoking cessation in smokers with schizophrenia were promising.[35][36] These studies were therefore followed by a study that compared contingency management alone, contingency management plus NRT, and self help (control) in 180 smokers with schizophrenia who were treated in a behavioral healthcare setting.[37] Those receiving contingency management were significantly more likely to meet the CO criterion for abstinence than those in the control group (P<0.001) but were not more likely to meet the cotinine criterion, suggesting that they abstained only long enough to earn the monetary incentive. A study that investigated the separate and combined effects of cotinine based contingency management and bupropion over a three week period in smokers with schizophrenia found that contingency management significantly reduced cotinine levels (P<0.01). This suggests that longer trials are warranted to examine whether contingency management is an effective stand alone or adjunctive treatment for smoking cessation in this population.[38]

Table 3 Outcomes of smoking cessation trials of treatment with varenicline in outpatients with schizophrenia*

Study	N	Intervention	Abstinence rates	Other outcomes
Weiner et al 2011[30]	9	12 week randomized, double-blind, placebo controlled treatment (1 mg BID) and individualized counseling based on the ALA "Freedom from Smoking" program	89% of those randomized completed treatment; 75% of varenicline group and 0% of placebo group achieved continuous abstinence during the last 4 weeks of treatment (P=0.14)	Significant treatment by time interaction on breath CO level (P<0.05); no differences between groups on positive symptoms, anxiety, or depression; no incidence of suicidal ideation; side effects were similar to those reported in the general population
Williams et al 2012[31]	128	12 week randomized double blind placebo controlled treatment (1 mg BID) and weekly counseling	77% of those who received at least one dose of medication completed the treatment, with no difference between groups; point prevalence abstinence rates were significantly higher for varenicline at end of treatment (19% v 4.7%; P<0.05) but not at 6 month follow-up (11.9% v 2.3%; P=0.09)	Rates of adverse events were similar across conditions; 2 patients in the varenicline group had 3 serious adverse events considered to be related to treatment (1 suicide attempt) versus 0 in the placebo group; there was one unrelated death; rates of suicidal ideation during active treatment did not differ between groups; positive, negative, and extrapyramidal symptoms were stable or reduced in both groups
Evins et al 2014[32]	247	12 week randomized double blind placebo controlled relapse prevention study; those meeting abstinence criteria at the end of a 12 week phase with open label varenicline (1 mg BID) and CBT entered a relapse prevention phase, in which they received varenicline (1 mg BID) or placebo plus CBT from week 12 to week 52	Of 203 patients who engaged in treatment, 87 patients had 2 weeks' continuous abstinence at the end of the open label phase and entered the relapse prevention phase; point prevalence abstinence rates were higher for varenicline at week 52 (60% v 19%; odds ratio 6.2, 95% CI 2.2 to 19.2); continuous abstinence rates were higher for varenicline during weeks 12-52 (45% v 15%; 4.6, 1.5 to 15.7), weeks 12-64 (40% v 11%; 5.2, 1.6 to 20.4), and weeks 12-76 (30% v 11%; 3.4, 1.02 to 13.6)	No differences between groups on psychiatric symptoms, health, body mass index, or nicotine withdrawal; 11 patients were admitted to hospital during the randomized phase—2 on varenicline and 2 on placebo for medical events, and 2 on varenicline and 5 on placebo for psychiatric events; 4% reported suicidal ideation during the open label phase and 5-6% in the relapse prevention phase, but there were no suicide attempts

Abbreviations: ALA=American Lung Association; BID=twice a day; CBT=cognitive-behavioral therapy; CI=confidence interval; CO=carbon monoxide.

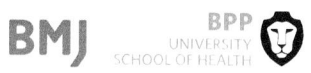

Summary of cessation outcomes in smokers with schizophrenia

No trials have directly compared the efficacy of NRT, bupropion, and varenicline in smokers with schizophrenia. However, a systematic review found that bupropion is associated with a threefold increase in cessation in smokers with schizophrenia (risk ratio 3.03, 1.69 to 5.42 at end of treatment; 2.78, 1.02 to 7.58 at six months). It also found that varenicline is associated with an almost fivefold increase in cessation (4.74, 1.34 to 16.71 at end of treatment).[39] NRT seems to have a smaller effect in smokers with schizophrenia than in the general population, although no studies have directly compared how these groups respond to NRT. Moreover, although NRT is the recommended first line treatment for smoking cessation in smokers with psychiatric comorbidities,[40] no placebo controlled trials of NRT have been carried out in this population, and such studies are long overdue.

Several other findings are also noteworthy. Firstly, several studies noted correlations between treatment attendance and abstinence.[12 15 33] Although this could be due to a direct effect of treatment or to underlying characteristics of patients who attend more versus fewer sessions, the provision of small financial incentives for treatment attendance is an effective method of increasing attendance.[20 27]

Secondly, several studies indicate that long term maintenance on smoking cessation pharmacotherapies is feasible, effective, and safe in this population.[17 27 32] Finally, several studies reported that many patients who were not able to quit completely greatly reduced their smoking. The question of whether a reduction in smoking might be an acceptable outcome for smokers with schizophrenia who were unable to quit was posed more than a decade ago,[41] and this question is still valid today. Although it is unclear whether a reduction in smoking alone improves health, a large reduction could decrease the severity of nicotine dependence and increase motivation to quit, thereby increasing the likelihood of future abstinence.[42 43] This notion is corroborated by a study that found that smokers with schizophrenia who had initially reduced their intake were more likely to have quit at a two year follow-up assessment.[21]

Mechanisms underlying the schizophrenia-smoking comorbidity

Schizophrenia is associated with social and environmental vulnerability factors for smoking, such as poverty, low education, unemployment, and lack of clinical attention to tobacco use (figure).[44] The contributions of these factors to smoking in people with schizophrenia have not been sufficiently studied, because laboratory studies have focused primarily on neurobiological factors that may contribute to smoking in this population.

Factors involved in the initiation and progression of smoking in patients with schizophrenia and the obstacles to attempts to quit and quit successThe higher nicotine metabolite levels seen in smokers with schizophrenia relative to other smokers[10] are the result of more intense cigarette puffing characteristics, particularly short inter-puff intervals.[45 46] The functional importance of these patients' higher nicotine intake is unknown, but it is often attributed to attempts to remediate psychiatric symptoms, cognitive deficits, or the sedating effects of antipsychotic drug.[47 48]

Nicotine improves sensory gating in smokers with schizophrenia through effects at α7 nAChRs,[49 50] and it may improve negative symptoms and cognitive performance through stimulation of β2 nAChRs and downstream effects on cortical dopamine.[51 52 53] In support of this idea, smokers with schizophrenia are more sensitive than smokers without psychiatric problems to the effects of nicotine abstinence and replacement with regard to some cognitive performance measures,[54 55] although this is not universally observed.[56] Smoking initiation generally precedes the onset of schizophrenia, which supports the idea that common neurobiological vulnerability factors underlie this comorbidity, but early initiation may also be a marker of the prodromal phase of schizophrenia.[57 58]

Reasons for smoking in people with schizophrenia

The neuropathology of schizophrenia might result in smokers with schizophrenia experiencing stronger reinforcing effects of nicotine.[59 60] This hypothesis is supported by a study in which smokers with schizophrenia and smokers with depression made twice as many hypothetical choices for smoking over alternative reinforcers, such as receiving candy or seeing a movie, than did controls without psychiatric disorders.[61] However, another interpretation of these findings is that smokers with schizophrenia and smokers with depression experience less pleasure from non-smoking activities (anhedonia).

Many studies have asked people with schizophrenia why they smoke in order to gain insight into the mechanisms that underlie the high smoking rates in these people. In a recent analysis of smoking motives from a large combined dataset, smokers with psychotic disorders cited coping motives (smoking to reduce craving and negative affect) as the main reason for smoking and pleasure motives as secondary. Illness motives (smoking to reduce psychiatric symptoms or side effects of antipsychotic drugs) were less commonly cited.[62] Smokers with depression ranked these motives in the same order as those with schizophrenia but endorsed them at significantly lower rates (P<0.001-0.05).[62] Studies that use ecological momentary assessment techniques to compare antecedents of smoking in patients with these disorders would help to clarify common and unique factors associated with smoking in these groups.

Reasons for relapse

During abstinence the effects of nicotine withdrawal on negative affect, cigarette craving, and cognitive functioning may contribute to early relapse in smokers with schizophrenia (figure). A study that provided high value monetary incentives for abstinence over a three day period to compare the effects of abstinence in smokers with schizophrenia and controls without a psychiatric disorder found that those with schizophrenia reported higher levels of negative affect and craving to relieve negative affect during abstinence.[63] Other than a small increase in anergia, psychiatric symptoms were not affected, consistent with a previous study.[64]

The negative effects of abstinence on cognitive functioning in smokers with schizophrenia, described above, may also contribute to early relapse, because smoking cessation requires considerable task persistence and other executive functions that are impaired in smokers with schizophrenia even before they try to quit.[65 66] In addition, patients with schizophrenia experience stronger nicotine reinforcement and a greater increase in positive mood from restarting smoking after abstinence than controls do.[63] These studies suggest that high levels of negative affect and craving,

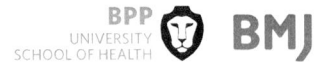

along with expectancies that smoking will improve these states; executive functioning deficits that are exacerbated during abstinence; and strong reinforcing effects of smoking after a period of abstinence may contribute to the high rates of relapse in this population.

However, conclusions from studies that examine the mechanisms underlying smoking in people with chronic mental illness are limited. Most laboratory studies do not examine the extent to which social-environmental factors contribute to differences seen between patient and control groups with regard to these biological mechanisms.

Unipolar and bipolar depression

Mood disorders such as unipolar and bipolar depression are generally associated with reduced smoking cessation rates compared with the general population,[1 5] although this difference is modest in those who enter formal cessation treatment.[67] Smokers with recurrent depression have higher levels of nicotine dependence and make fewer cessation attempts than do smokers with single episode depression,[68] and those who have difficulty tolerating distress are particularly vulnerable to early smoking lapse.[69]

Unipolar depression

A recent narrative review examined the efficacy of smoking cessation treatments in smokers with unipolar depression from 68 studies published between 1990 and 2010.[70] Although most studies found no differences in smoking cessation outcomes between people with and without depression, in those studies that did detect a difference, depression was associated with poorer outcomes, particularly in women.[70]

Regarding the relative effectiveness of particular treatment approaches, a meta-analysis of treatment trials in smokers with unipolar depression published in 2010 found that NRT was more effective than placebo, and that adding behavioral mood management to cessation counseling improved treatment outcomes.[71] In addition, bupropion and nortriptyline are effective treatments for smoking in people with unipolar depression.[72 73] It is important to note that most studies have focused on lifetime depression; very few have examined the effects of current depression on smoking cessation.[70 71] Although relapse rates are high in this population, long term treatment with bupropion reduces relapse rates in those who attain abstinence.[74]

A recent multisite placebo controlled trial examined the effects of 12 weeks of treatment with varenicline on smoking in 525 people with stable current or past major depression.[75] Attrition from the study was high (almost a third) but did not differ between groups. Varenicline significantly increased continuous abstinence during the last four weeks of treatment (35.9% v 15.6%; odds ratio 3.35, 2.16 to 5.21) and up to week 52 (2.36, 1.40 to 3.98), without exacerbating depression or anxiety.[75] Thus, although early concerns about associations with suicidality and depression[76] led to a Food and Drug Administration black box warning, this study provides evidence that varenicline is a well tolerated and effective treatment for smoking cessation in people with stable current or past depression.

Bipolar depression

Fewer studies have examined smoking cessation treatments for smokers with bipolar disorder. Two placebo controlled trials of bupropion and varenicline with only five patients per study, and an open label trial of varenicline in nine patients, showed promising results and no exacerbation of psychiatric symptoms.[77 78 79] These were followed by a placebo controlled trial of varenicline in 60 stable patients with bipolar disorder, which found that varenicline significantly increased abstinence at the end of treatment (48% v 10%; 8.13, 2.03 to 32.53), although this difference was no longer significant at six months (19% v 7%; 3.2, 0.60 to 17.6).[80] Varenicline was associated with a higher frequency of abnormal dreams (P=0.04) and a non-significant trend toward more negative mood events (P=0.08), but otherwise the groups did not differ with regard to treatment emergent or serious adverse events. Eight people in the varenicline group and five in the placebo group had suicidal ideation during the trial (not significant).[80] Maintenance treatment with varenicline has also been found to reduce relapse in smokers with bipolar disorder who attained abstinence.[32]

Mechanisms underlying the depression-smoking comorbidity

Associations between unipolar or bipolar depression and cigarette smoking may be due to biological and social-environmental factors that increase the risk of both disorders, smoking to reduce psychiatric symptoms, effects of nicotine or smoke exposure on the development of these disorders, or bidirectional causality.[81 82 83 84 85] Like smokers with schizophrenia, smokers with unipolar depression indicate that they smoke primarily to cope with craving and negative affect, and secondarily for pleasure.[62] However, they are as worried as smokers without depression about the effects of smoking on their health and equally motivated to quit.[86 87]

Effects of withdrawal

When they try to quit, smokers with unipolar depression, particularly women, report more severe withdrawal than those without depression and are more likely to attribute the reinitiation of smoking to withdrawal.[88 89 90]

The effects of smoking and abstinence on mood are regulated through the effects of nicotine on monoamines and the neuroendocrine system.[91] Chronic nicotine desensitizes or inactivates nAChRs, and this has an antidepressant effect through actions on dopamine and other monoamines.[91 92] Furthermore, abstinence increases levels of monoamine oxidase A (MAO-A), an enzyme that metabolizes dopamine and other monoamines, and this is correlated with a shift towards depressed mood.[93]

Once withdrawal symptoms fade, abstinence does not seem to be associated with exacerbation of depression for most smokers, although considerable heterogeneity exists, and those who do experience worsening of symptoms have poorer cessation outcomes.[94] Recent epidemiological studies and systematic reviews have concluded that in people with stable depression successful cessation may be associated with improvement in mood.[95 96] However, the direction of causality in this association has not been determined—cessation may improve mood, or those who do not experience mood deterioration while attempting to quit may be more likely to remain abstinent.

Reinforcing effects of smoking

In addition to experiencing stronger withdrawal symptoms during initial abstinence, smokers with depression may experience stronger relative reinforcing effects of smoking. Experimental studies indicate that smokers with a history of depression are more likely than smokers without depression to choose smoking over various alternative reinforcers,

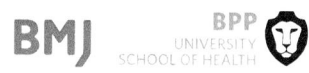

such as seeing a movie or receiving candy.[61] They are also more likely to smoke more cigarettes in laboratory sessions regardless of mood,[97] and they have higher levels of appetitive cigarette craving (craving for the positive reinforcing effects of smoking) shortly after smoking than do controls.[98]

Depression is associated with low resting levels of intrasynaptic dopamine,[99][100] and smokers with depression experience larger increases in striatal dopamine after smoking a cigarette than those without a history of depression, which may underlie these heightened reinforcing effects.[101] Regardless of diagnosis, anhedonia, defined as a deficit in positive emotion in response to pleasant stimuli, is associated with enhanced sensitivity to the effects of nicotine on positive mood, appetitive craving during abstinence, and rapid relapse.[102][103][104]

In addition, people with anhedonia have more difficulty identifying reinforcing activities to substitute for smoking during quit attempts.[105] Together, these studies suggest that high levels of withdrawal related negative affect, low tolerance of discomfort, vulnerability to smoking reinforcement, and insensitivity to alternative reinforcers contribute to cessation failure in people with depression (figure). Therefore, in addition to pharmacotherapy and mood management, smokers with depression may benefit from treatments that help them to identify and engage in alternative reinforcing activities.

Other factors that contribute to persistence of smoking
Far fewer human laboratory studies have examined mechanisms that underlie smoking in people with bipolar disorder than in those with schizophrenia or unipolar depression. Smoking is associated with greater severity of mood symptoms, comorbid psychiatric and addictive disorders, and suicidality in people with bipolar disorder.[106][107][108][109][110][111] Furthermore, in an online survey of 685 patients with bipolar disorder, almost half reported that they smoked to manage symptoms of their mental illness.[112] This study also found that although 74% of the patients surveyed wanted to quit smoking, only 33% had received medical advice to quit, suggesting that lack of clinical attention probably contributes to smoking persistence in this population.[112] Unlike some studies in smokers with schizophrenia, smokers with bipolar and unipolar depression do not differ from controls with regard to the effects of smoking status on neuropsychiatric performance. This suggests that pro-cognitive effects of nicotine may not contribute to smoking in this population.[113]

Anxiety disorders
Whereas smoking rates significantly declined from 2004 to 2011 in people without psychiatric illness, they did not decrease in those with anxiety disorders.[6] Consequently, the presence of anxiety disorders among current smokers has significantly increased, more markedly in women.[114]

A secondary analysis of data collected from a large trial of 1504 smokers that compared monotherapy and combination pharmacotherapies for smoking focused on whether psychiatric disorders moderated treatment response.[115] After controlling for treatment, age, sex, and ethnicity, smokers with lifetime anxiety disorder had significantly lower rates of abstinence than those with no psychiatric history at eight weeks (39.9% v 47.4%; odds ratio 0.72, 0.55 to 0.94) and six months (28.7 v 35.4%; 0.72, 0.54 to 0.95) after their target quit date. Lifetime history of anxiety disorder remained a predictor of poorer outcome at both follow-up points after controlling for lifetime mood or substance use disorders.

A more detailed analysis of smoking outcomes and risk factors in patients with specific anxiety diagnoses (panic attacks, social anxiety disorder, and generalized anxiety disorder) indicated that those with social anxiety or generalized anxiety disorders had more severe nicotine dependence at baseline. In addition, patients with any of the three diagnoses had higher negative affect and withdrawal symptoms before quitting than did smokers without anxiety disorders.[116]

Smokers with anxiety disorder also reported greater increases in cessation fatigue (being tired of trying to quit smoking) before and after the quit day, suggesting that these patients may not have adequate coping resources. Interestingly, although combination pharmacotherapy doubled the likelihood of abstinence compared with placebo in smokers without anxiety disorders, neither monotherapy nor combination pharmacotherapy was more effective than placebo in those with a lifetime history of anxiety disorder.[116] Similarly, in smokers with unipolar depression, the presence of comorbid anxiety disorder was associated with poorer response to combined bupropion and NRT.[117]

Mechanisms underlying the anxiety-smoking comorbidity
Studies suggest that people with anxiety disorder may smoke to reduce anxiety, that smoking or smoke exposure in early life may increase the likelihood of developing an anxiety disorder, and that shared vulnerabilities may increase the risk of both.[118][119]

Biological mechanisms that have been proposed to underpin the association between anxiety disorders and smoking include effects on several neurotransmitter systems, oxidative and nitrosative stress, and epigenetic effects.[120] In particular, given that a reduction in acetylcholine transmission improves affect, dysregulation of this system is probably one of the causes of anxiety disorders.[92]

Negative reinforcement models
Most research on smoking and anxiety focuses on negative reinforcement models, such as smoking to cope with negative affect or to feel comfortable in social situations.[121][122][123][124] For example, a longitudinal study of peer use as a moderator of the associations between anxiety and substance use in adolescence found that girls with high social anxiety were more likely to smoke when they believed that peer approval of smoking was high, and less likely when they believed it was low.[125] However, girls with generalized anxiety symptoms responded to perceptions about peer smoking in the opposite direction, highlighting the variability across anxiety diagnoses.[125] People who have high anxiety sensitivity, or fear of anxiety or related sensations, are also highly motivated to smoke to reduce negative affect and anxiety related distress.[121][122][124]

When smokers with anxiety disorder try to quit they report more severe withdrawal symptoms than those without an anxiety disorder,[88][90][126] although data on whether increased withdrawal in this population influences relapse to smoking are conflicting.[88][127]

Reasons for relapse
Laboratory and treatment studies have also found that smokers with anxiety disorder have higher levels of cigarette craving and nicotine withdrawal symptoms during abstinence than those without anxiety disorder.[116][126][128]

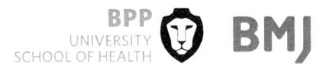

However, these differences are also seen before cessation and may reflect exaggerated tonic levels of withdrawal-like symptoms.[116] Taken together, these studies suggest that high levels of negative affect during abstinence, combined with beliefs that these symptoms are associated with harm (anxiety sensitivity[129] [130]) and the expectancy that smoking will reduce negative affect, probably contribute to rapid relapse during cessation attempts (figure).

PTSD

Only four randomized clinical trials have investigated the efficacy of smoking cessation interventions in smokers with PTSD. Two of these studies focused on integrating cessation treatment into ongoing mental healthcare, an approach that leverages pre-existing therapeutic relationships and an established visit schedule. In the first trial, 66 veterans with PTSD were randomized to integrated care modeled on clinical practice guidelines or to standard care. Abstinence was five times higher in the integrated care group nine months after randomization.[131] A larger, multi-site trial in 943 smokers with PTSD found that the integrated care group achieved significantly higher abstinence at six months (16.5% v 7.2% for standard care; P<0.001), but more than 90% were not abstinent at 12 months.[132]

The integrated care interventions offered smoking cessation pharmacotherapy to those who were interested but did not randomize patients to drugs versus placebo. The only randomized placebo controlled trial of smoking cessation pharmacotherapy in smokers with PTSD was a pilot study in 15 veterans who received 12 weeks of treatment with bupropion.[133] Bupropion was well tolerated and associated with 40% abstinence, versus 20% for placebo at six months of follow-up (level of significance not reported).

More recently, 22 smokers with PTSD were randomized to a four week contingency management intervention or a control group that received reinforcement independent of abstinence.[134] All participants also received two smoking cessation counseling sessions, along with NRT and bupropion. At three months, abstinence rates were not significantly different (55% in the contingency management group v 18% in the control group).[134] However, the size of the difference suggests that the lack of significance may be due to the small sample size and that fully powered trials should be conducted to examine whether contingency management is an efficacious cessation treatment for smokers with PTSD.

Mechanisms underlying the PTSD-smoking comorbidity

Smokers with PTSD have higher levels of depression, anxiety, and PTSD symptoms than non-smokers with PTSD.[135] [136] Both a diagnosis of PTSD and symptom severity are associated with stronger desire to smoke in order to reduce negative affect.[122] [136] [137] [138] Using baseline data from the multi-site study described above,[132] the expectancy that smoking would reduce negative affect was found to mediate the association between severity of PTSD and nicotine dependence and the negative association between severity of PTSD and abstinence self efficacy in situations involving affective distress.[139] Studies using ecological momentary assessment in the natural environment show that smokers with PTSD smoke in response to negative affect and trauma reminders.[140] [141] Taken together, these studies strongly suggest that people with PTSD smoke to cope with negative affect and anxiety. Cognitive and attentional deficits

associated with PTSD may also contribute to smoking in this population.[142] [143] Because nicotine enhances cognition and attention, smoking cessation may exacerbate cognitive deficits,[144] although one study found that smokers with PTSD did not experience stronger deleterious effects of abstinence on prepulse inhibition than did other smokers.[145] Finally, smokers with PTSD report higher craving and withdrawal during abstinence than do smokers without PTSD.[146]

Emerging treatments

Smoking cessation is clearly the most effective way to reduce the risk of tobacco related disease. However, reductions in smoking or a switch to non-combustible sources of nicotine may be acceptable proximal outcomes for those who are unable to quit, if these reduce exposure to tobacco toxicants or lead to eventual abstinence.[41] [42]

E-cigarettes

E-cigarettes may have fewer cardiovascular and respiratory effects than traditional cigarettes and may help people quit smoking,[147] [148] although we currently have little empirical evidence about their safety and efficacy. A small uncontrolled study found that 50% of smokers with schizophrenia who were provided with e-cigarettes for 52 weeks reduced their smoking by 50%, and 14% quit, with no increases in psychiatric symptoms.[149] These preliminary findings are noteworthy because none of the participants was initially seeking treatment for smoking, and they indicate that randomized controlled trials of the effects of e-cigarettes on smoking in this population are warranted.

Regulatory approaches

One potential regulatory approach to reducing tobacco dependence is to decrease the nicotine content of cigarettes to reduce their addictiveness.[150] The 2009 Family Smoking Prevention and Tobacco Control Act gave the US FDA the authority to regulate tobacco products, including the allowable levels of nicotine in cigarettes. Similarly, under Article 9 of the Framework Convention on Tobacco Control, the Conference of the Parties is charged with establishing guidelines for measuring and regulating the contents and emissions of tobacco products.[151]

A reduction in the nicotine content of cigarettes to a non-addictive level could reduce the severity of tobacco dependence, potentially making it easier for smokers to quit.[152] [153] This approach could be particularly beneficial to those who have inadequate access to and success with cessation treatments. However, one concern about this regulatory approach is that smokers with chronic mental illness may experience dysfunction as a result of nicotine withdrawal or may attempt to compensate for nicotine reduction by increasing their smoking intensity.

An initial study found that acute use of very low nicotine content cigarettes decreased withdrawal symptoms, cigarette craving, and smoking of usual brand cigarettes in smokers with schizophrenia without affecting psychiatric symptoms.[154] Trials are under way to examine the effects of extended use of these cigarettes on smoking rates, toxicant exposure, psychiatric symptoms, and cognitive functioning in smokers with schizophrenia and affective disorders.

Conclusions

Treatment for tobacco addiction must be prioritized in clinical practice to reduce the high rates of tobacco related disease and premature death in people with chronic

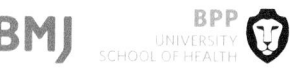

RESEARCH QUESTIONS

- What are the antecedents and consequences of smoking in people with schizophrenia, depression, and anxiety disorders during cessation attempts?
- Do reductions in smoking rates reduce biomarkers of tobacco related harm in people with chronic mental illness?
- Do reductions in smoking rates increase the likelihood of future cessation attempts or cessation success in people with chronic mental illness?

mental illness. The research reviewed here indicates that smokers with chronic mental illness can quit with standard cessation approaches, with minimal effects on psychiatric symptoms. In particular, recent randomized controlled trials have shown that bupropion and varenicline are effective in people with schizophrenia,[31 32 39] and that varenicline is effective in people with unipolar and bipolar depression.[75 80]

Treatments for people with anxiety disorders and PTSD have been less well studied and the effects of these drugs in smokers with these disorders have not been determined using adequately powered randomized controlled trials. Small scale studies suggest that contingency management approaches may be effective in smokers with schizophrenia and PTSD if feasibility challenges associated with extending the duration of these interventions can be overcome.[38 134]

Most of the studies reviewed enrolled stable patients treated in university affiliated behavioral health programs. Whether similar effects will be seen with less stable patients and in settings with less patient contact remains to be determined. An important next step for treating smoking in people with chronic mental illness will therefore be to promote the adoption, implementation, and assessment of empirically supported smoking treatments within community behavioral healthcare settings.

Researchers who study the comorbidity between psychiatric disorders and tobacco often specialize in a particular psychiatric disorder, yet clinicians treat people with a variety of illnesses and multiple comorbidities. Thus, a goal of this review was to highlight commonalities between the biopsychosocial mechanisms involved in the initiation and persistence of smoking in patients with different disorders. An appreciation of these common factors may facilitate the identification of novel prevention and tobacco treatment approaches for these patients. Finally, given that many patients reduce their smoking rates during treatment and the use of novel tobacco and nicotine products may also reduce smoking rates, it is important to determine whether reductions in smoking increase the likelihood of eventual cessation in people with chronic mental illness.

Treatment guidelines

Treatobacco.net (http://treatobacco.net/en/index.php) is an independent source of evidence based information and support for the treatment of tobacco dependence throughout the world. The site's resource library contains links to treatment guidelines from more than 30 countries, including the US Public Health Service sponsored Clinical Practice Guideline[40] and the 2014 update to the 2011 guideline from the Royal Australian College of General Practitioners.[155] Both of these guidelines include sections on treating smoking in people with mental illness and other vulnerable populations, and the Australian guideline has up to date information on the efficacy and safety of bupropion and varenicline in these populations. Other useful resources provided on the website include slide kits and summaries

of efficacy and safety information, with links to relevant research studies.

Contributors: Both authors helped in all aspects of the review, approved the version to be published, and agreed to be accountable for all aspects of the work.

Funding: The preparation of this paper was supported by grants U54DA031659 and P50DA036114 from the National Institute on Drug Abuse and the FDA Center for Tobacco Products, and grant P20GM103644 from the National Institute of General Medical Sciences. The content is solely the responsibility of the authors and does not necessarily represent the official views of the National Institutes of Health or the FDA.

Competing interests: We have read and understood BMJ policy on declaration of interests and declare the following interests: JWT has received a consulting fee from Giner (2013).MEM has no competing interests.

Patient involvement: No patients were involved in the preparation of this article.

1   Lasser K, Boyd JW, Woolhandler S, et al. Smoking and mental illness: a population-based prevalence study. JAMA2000;284:2606-10.
2   Lawrence D, Mitrou F, Zubrick SR. Smoking and mental illness: results from population surveys in Australia and the United States. BMC Public Health2009;9:285.
3   Hartz SM, Pato CN, Medeiros H, et al. Comorbidity of severe psychotic disorders with measures of substance use. JAMA Psychiatry2014;71:248-54.
4   Smith PH, Mazure CM, McKee SA. Smoking and mental illness in the US population. Tob Control2014;23:e147-53.
5   Weinberger AH, Pilver CE, Desai RA, et al. The relationship of major depressive disorder and gender to changes in smoking for current and former smokers: longitudinal evaluation in the US population. Addiction2012;107:1847-56.
6   Cook BL, Wayne GF, Kafali EN, et al. Trends in smoking among adults with mental illness and association between mental health treatment and smoking cessation. JAMA2014;311:172-82.
7   Callaghan RC, Veldhuizen S, Jeysingh T, et al. Patterns of tobacco-related mortality among individuals diagnosed with schizophrenia, bipolar disorder, or depression. J Psychiatr Res2014;48:102-10.
8   Kelly DL, McMahon RP, Wehring HJ, et al. Cigarette smoking and mortality risk in people with schizophrenia. Schizophr Bull2011;37:832-8.
9   Hughes JR, Hatsukami DK, Mitchell JE, et al. Prevalence of smoking among psychiatric patients. Am J Psychiatry1986;143:993-7.
10 Olincy A, Young DA, Freedman R. Increased levels of the nicotine metabolite cotinine in schizophrenic smokers compared to other smokers. Biol Psychiatry1997;42:1-5.
11 Ziedonis DM, George TP. Schizophrenia and nicotine use: report of a pilot smoking cessation program and review of neurobiological and clinical issues. Schizophr Bull1997;23:247-54.
12 Addington J, el-Guebaly N, Campbell W, et al. Smoking cessation treatment for patients with schizophrenia. Am J Psychiatry1998;155:974-6.
13 George TP, Ziedonis DM, Feingold A, , et al. Nicotine transdermal patch and atypical antipsychotic medications for smoking cessation in schizophrenia. Am J Psychiatry2000;157:1835-42.
14 Chou K-R, Chen R, Lee J-F, et al. The effectiveness of nicotine-patch therapy for smoking cessation in patients with schizophrenia. Int J Nurs Stud2004;41:321-30.
15 Baker A, Richmond R, Haile M, et al. A randomized controlled trial of a smoking cessation intervention among people with a psychotic disorder. Am J Psychiatry2006;163:1934-42.
16 Baker A, Richmond R, Lewin TJ, et al. Cigarette smoking and psychosis: naturalistic follow up 4 years after an intervention trial. Aust N Z J Psychiatry2010;44:342-50.
17 Horst WD, Klein MW, Williams D, et al. Extended use of nicotine replacement therapy to maintain smoking cessation in persons with schizophrenia. Neuropsychiatr Dis Treat2005;1:349-55.
18 Carroll FI, Blough BE, Mascarella SW, et al. Bupropion and bupropion analogs as treatments for CNS disorders. Adv Pharmacol2014;69:177-216.
19 Weiner E, Ball MP, Summerfelt A, et al. Effects of sustained-release bupropion and supportive group therapy on cigarette consumption in patients with schizophrenia. Am J Psychiatry2001;158:635-7.
20 Evins AE, Mays VK, Rigotti NA, et al. A pilot trial of bupropion added to cognitive behavioral therapy for smoking cessation in schizophrenia. Nicotine Tob Res2001;3:397-403.
21 Evins AE, Cather C, Rigotti NA, et al. Two-year follow-up of a smoking cessation trial in patients with schizophrenia: increased rates of smoking cessation and reduction. J Clin Psychiatry2004;65:307-11.
22 George TP, Vessicchio JC, Termine A, et al. A placebo controlled trial of bupropion for smoking cessation in schizophrenia. Biol Psychiatry2002;52:53-61.
23 Evins AE, Cather C, Deckersbach T, et al. A double-blind placebo-controlled trial of bupropion sustained-release for smoking cessation in schizophrenia. J Clin Psychopharmacol2005;25:218-25.
24 Evins AE, Cather C, Culhane MA, et al. A 12-week double-blind, placebo-controlled study of bupropion SR added to high-dose dual

143

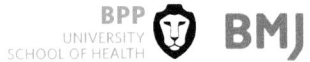

nicotine replacement therapy for smoking cessation or reduction in schizophrenia. J Clin Psychopharmacol2007;27:380-6.

25 George TP, Vessicchio JC, Sacco KA, et al. A placebo-controlled trial of bupropion combined with nicotine patch for smoking cessation in schizophrenia. Biol Psychiatry2008;63:1092-6.

26 Weiner E, Ball MP, Buchholz AS, et al. Bupropion sustained release added to group support for smoking cessation in schizophrenia: a new randomized trial and a meta-analysis. J Clin Psychiatry2012;73:95-102.

27 Cather C, Dyer MA, Burrell HA, et al. An open trial of relapse prevention therapy for smokers with schizophrenia. J Dual Diagn 2013;9:87-93.

28 Mihalak KB, Carroll FI, Luetje CW. Varenicline is a partial agonist at alpha4beta2 and a full agonist at alpha7 neuronal nicotinic receptors. Mol Pharmacol2006;70:801-5.

29 Cahill K, Stevens S, Lancaster T. Pharmacological treatments for smoking cessation. JAMA2014;311:193-4.

30 Weiner E, Buchholz A, Coffay A, et al. Varenicline for smoking cessation in people with schizophrenia: a double blind randomized pilot study. Schizophr Res2011;129:94-5.

31 Williams JM, Anthenelli RM, Morris CD, et al. A randomized, double-blind, placebo-controlled study evaluating the safety and efficacy of varenicline for smoking cessation in patients with schizophrenia or schizoaffective disorder. J Clin Psychiatry2012;73:654-60.

32 Evins AE, Cather C, Pratt SA, et al. Maintenance treatment with varenicline for smoking cessation in patients with schizophrenia and bipolar disorder: a randomized clinical trial. JAMA2014;311:145-54.

33 Williams JM, Steinberg ML, Zimmermann MH, et al. Comparison of two intensities of tobacco dependence counseling in schizophrenia and schizoaffective disorder. J Subst Abuse Treat2010;38:384-93.

34 Steinberg ML, Ziedonis DM, Krejci JA, et al. Motivational interviewing with personalized feedback: a brief intervention for motivating smokers with schizophrenia to seek treatment for tobacco dependence. J Consult Clin Psychol2004;72:723-8.

35 Roll JM, Higgins ST, Steingard S, et al. Use of monetary reinforcement to reduce the cigarette smoking of persons with schizophrenia: a feasibility study. Exp Clin Psychopharmacol1998;6:157-61.

36 Tidey JW, O'Neill SC, Higgins ST. Contingent monetary reinforcement of smoking reductions, with and without transdermal nicotine, in outpatients with schizophrenia. Exp Clin Psychopharmacol2002;10:241-7.

37 Gallagher SM, Penn PE, Schindler E, et al. A comparison of smoking cessation treatments for persons with schizophrenia and other serious mental illnesses. J Psychoactive Drugs2007;39:487-97.

38 Tidey JW, Rohsenow DJ, Kaplan GB, et al. Effects of contingency management and bupropion on cigarette smoking in smokers with schizophrenia. Psychopharmacology (Berl)2011;217:279-87.

39 Tsoi DT, Porwal M, Webster AC. Interventions for smoking cessation and reduction in individuals with schizophrenia. Cochrane Database Syst Rev2013;2:CD007253.

40 Clinical Practice Guideline Treating Tobacco Use and Dependence 2008 Update Panel, Liaisons, and Staff. A clinical practice guideline for treating tobacco use and dependence: 2008 update. Am J Prev Med2008;35:158-76.

41 McChargue DE, Gulliver SB, Hitsman B. Would smokers with schizophrenia benefit from a more flexible approach to smoking treatment? Addiction2002;97:785-93.

42 Hughes JR, Carpenter MJ. Does smoking reduction increase future cessation and decrease disease risk? A qualitative review. Nicotine Tob Res2006;8:739-49.

43 Asfar T, Ebbert JO, Klesges RC, et al. Do smoking reduction interventions promote cessation in smokers not ready to quit? Addict Behav2011;36:764-8.

44 Ziedonis D, Hitsman B, Beckham JC, et al. Tobacco use and cessation in psychiatric disorders: National Institute of Mental Health report. Nicotine Tob Res2008;10:1691-715.

45 Tidey JW, Rohsenow DJ, Kaplan GB, et al. Cigarette smoking topography in smokers with schizophrenia and matched non-psychiatric controls. Drug Alcohol Depend2005;80:259-65.

46 Williams JM, Gandhi KK, Lu SE, et al. Shorter interpuff interval is associated with higher nicotine intake in smokers with schizophrenia. Drug Alcohol Depend2011;118:313-9.

47 Dalack GW, Healey DJ, Meador-Woodruff JH. Nicotine dependence in schizophrenia: clinical phenomena and laboratory findings. Am J Psychiatry1998;155:1490-501.

48 Kumari V, Postma P. Nicotine use in schizophrenia: the self-medication hypothesis. Neurosci Biobehav Rev2005;29:1021-34.

49 Adler LE, Hoffer LD, Wiser A, et al. Normalization of auditory physiology by cigarette smoking in schizophrenic patients. Am J Psychiatry1993;150:1856-61.

50 Martin LF, Freedman R. Schizophrenia and the a7 nicotinic acetylcholine receptor. Int Rev Neurobiol2007;78:225-46.

51 Esterlis I, Ranganathan M, Bois F, et al. In vivo evidence for B2 nicotinic acetylcholine receptor subunit upregulation in smokers as compared with nonsmokers with schizophrenia. Biol Psychiatry2013;76:495-502.

52 D'Souza DC, Esterlis I, Carbuto M, et al. Lower B2*-nicotinic acetylcholine receptor availability in smokers with schizophrenia. Am J Psychiatry2012;169:326-34.

53 Wing VC, Wass CE, Soh DW, et al. A review of neurobiological vulnerability factors and treatment implications for comorbid tobacco dependence in schizophrenia. Ann N Y Acad Sci2012;1248:89-106.

54 George TP, Vessicchio JC, Termine A, et al. Effects of smoking abstinence on visuospatial working memory function in schizophrenia. Neuropsychopharmacology2002;26:75-85.

55 Barr RS, Culhane MA, Jubelt LE, et al. The effects of transdermal nicotine on cognition in nonsmokers with schizophrenia and nonpsychiatric controls. Neuropsychopharmacology2008;33:480-90.

56 Hahn B, Harvey AN, Concheiro-Guisan M, et al. A test of the cognitive self-medication hypothesis of tobacco smoking in schizophrenia. Biol Psychiatry2013;74:436-43.

57 Beratis S, Katrivanou A, Gourzis P. Factors affecting smoking in schizophrenia. Compr Psychiatry2001;42:393-402.

58 Riala K, Hakko H, Isohanni M, et al. Is initiation of smoking associated with the prodromal phase of schizophrenia? J Psychiatry Neurosci2005;30:26-32.

59 Chambers RA, Krystal JH, Self DW. A neurobiological basis for substance abuse comorbidity in schizophrenia. Biol Psychiatry2001;50:71-83.

60 Brunzell DH, McIntosh JM. Alpha7 nicotinic acetylcholine receptors modulate motivation to self-administer nicotine: implications for smoking and schizophrenia. Neuropsychopharmacology2012;37:1134-43.

61 Spring B, Pingitore R, McChargue DE. Reward value of cigarette smoking for comparably heavy smoking schizophrenic, depressed, and nonpatient smokers. Am J Psychiatry2003;160:316-22.

62 Thornton LK, Baker AL, Lewin TJ, et al. Reasons for substance use among people with mental disorders. Addict Behav2012;37:427-34.

63 Tidey JW, Colby SM, Xavier EM. Effects of smoking abstinence on cigarette craving, nicotine withdrawal, and nicotine reinforcement in smokers with and without schizophrenia. Nicotine Tob Res2014;16:326-34.

64 Dalack GW, Becks L, Hill E, et al. Nicotine withdrawal and psychiatric symptoms in cigarette smokers with schizophrenia. Neuropsychopharmacology1999;21:195-202.

65 Moss TG, Sacco KA, Allen TM, et al. Prefrontal cognitive dysfunction is associated with tobacco dependence treatment failure in smokers with schizophrenia. Drug Alcohol Depend2009;104:94-9.

66 Steinberg ML, Williams JM, Gandhi KK, et al. Task persistence predicts smoking cessation in smokers with and without schizophrenia. Psychol Addict Behav2012;26:850-8.

67 Hitsman B, Papandonatos GD, McChargue DE, et al. Past major depression and smoking cessation outcome: a systematic review and meta-analysis update. Addiction2013;108:294-306.

68 Strong DR, Cameron A, Feuer S, et al. Single versus recurrent depression history: differentiating risk factors among current US smokers. Drug Alc Depend2010;109:90-5.

69 Leventhal AM, Zvolensky MJ. Anxiety, depression, and cigarette smoking: a transdiagnostic vulnerability framework to understanding emotion-smoking comorbidity. Psychol Bull2014;141:176-212.

70 Weinberger AH, Mazure CM, Morlett A, et al. Two decades of smoking cessation treatment research on smokers with depression: 1990-2010. Nicotine Tob Res2013;15:1014-31.

71 Gierisch JM, Bastian LA, Calhoun PS, et al. Smoking cessation interventions for patients with depression: a systematic review and meta-analysis. J Gen Intern Med2011;27:351-60.

72 Brown RA, Niaura R, Lloyd-Richardson EE, et al. Bupropion and cognitive-behavioral treatment for depression in smoking cessation. Nicotine Tob Res2007;9:721-30.

73 Hall SM, Reus VI, Muñoz RF, et al. Nortriptyline and cognitive-behavioral therapy in the treatment of cigarette smoking. Arch Gen Psychiatry1998;55:683-90.

74 Cox LS, Patten CA, Niaura RS, et al. Efficacy of bupropion for relapse prevention in smokers with and without a past history of major depression. J Gen Intern Med2004;19:828-34.

75 Anthenelli RM, Morris C, Ramey TS, et al. Effects of varenicline on smoking cessation in adults with stably treated current or past major depression: a randomized trial. Ann Intern Med2013;159:390-400.

76 US Food and Drug Administration. Drug safety newsletter. www.fda.gov/downloads/Drugs/DrugSafety/DrugSafetyNewsletter/ucm107318.pdf.

77 Frye MA, Ebbert JO, Prince CA, et al. A feasibility study of varenicline for smoking cessation in bipolar patients with subsyndromal depression. J Clin Psychopharmacol2013;33:821-3.

78 Weinberger AH, Vessicchio JC, Sacco KA, et al. A preliminary study of sustained-release bupropion for smoking cessation in bipolar disorder. J Clin Psychopharmacol2008;28:584-7.

79 Wu BS, Weinberger AH, Mancuso E, et al. A preliminary feasibility study of varenicline for smoking cessation in bipolar disorder. J Dual Diagn2012;8:131-2.

80 Chengappa KN, Perkins KA, Brar JS, et al. Varenicline for smoking cessation in bipolar disorder: a randomized, double-blind, placebo-controlled study. J Clin Psychiatry2014;75:765-72.

81 Kendler KS, Neale MC, MacLean CJ, et al. Smoking and major depression. A causal analysis. Arch Gen Psychiatry1993;50:36-43.

82 Brown RA, Lewinsohn PM, Seeley JR, et al. Cigarette smoking, major depression, and other psychiatric disorders among adolescents. J Am Acad Child Adolesc Psychiatry1996;35:1602-10.

83 Breslau N, Peterson EL, Schultz LR, et al. Major depression and stages of smoking. A longitudinal investigation. Arch Gen Psychiatry1998;55:161-6.

84 Martínez-Ortega JM, Goldstein BI, Gutiérrez-Rojas L, et al. Temporal sequencing of nicotine dependence and bipolar disorder in the

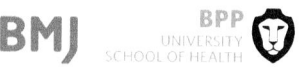

National Epidemiologic Survey on Alcohol and Related Conditions (NESARC). J Psychiatr Res2013;47:858-64.

85 Hartz SM, Lin P, Edenberg HJ, et al. Genetic association of bipolar disorder with the (3) nicotinic receptor subunit gene. Psychiatr Genet2011;21:77-84.

86 Weinberger AH, George TP, McKee SA. Differences in smoking expectancies in smokers with and without a history of major depression. Addict Behav2011;36:434-7.

87 Siru R, Hulse GK, Tait RJ. Assessing motivation to quit smoking in people with mental illness: a review. Addiction2009;104:719-33.

88 Breslau N, Kilbey MM, Andreski P. Nicotine withdrawal symptoms and psychiatric disorders: findings from an epidemiologic study of young adults. Am J Psychiatry1992;149:464-9.

89 Weinberger AH, Maciejewski PK, McKee SA, et al. Gender differences in associations between lifetime alcohol, depression, panic disorder, and posttraumatic stress disorder and tobacco withdrawal. Am J Addict2009;18:140-7.

90 Weinberger AH, Desai RA, McKee SA. Nicotine withdrawal in US smokers with current mood, anxiety, alcohol use, and substance use disorders. Drug Alcohol Depend2010;108:7-12.

91 Philip NS, Carpenter LL, Tyrka AR, et al. Nicotinic acetylcholine receptors and depression: a review of the preclinical and clinical literature. Psychopharmacology (Berl)2010;212:1-12.

92 Mineur YS, Picciotto MR. Nicotine receptors and depression: revisiting and revising the cholinergic hypothesis. Trends Pharmacol Sci2010;31:580-6.

93 Bacher I, Houle S, Xu X, et al. Monoamine oxidase A binding in the prefrontal and anterior cingulate cortices during acute withdrawal from heavy cigarette smoking. Arch Gen Psychiatry2011;68:817-26.

94 Burgess ES, Brown RA, Kahler CW, et al. Patterns of change in depressive symptoms during smoking cessation: who's at risk for relapse? J Consult Clin Psychol2002;70:356-61.

95 Cavazos-Rehg PA, Breslau N, Hatsukami D, et al. Smoking cessation is associated with lower rates of mood/anxiety and alcohol use disorders. Psychol Med2014;44:2523-35.

96 Taylor G, McNeill A, Girling A, et al. Change in mental health after smoking cessation: systematic review and meta-analysis. BMJ2014;348:g1151.

97 Perkins KA, Karelitz JL, Giedgowd GE, et al. Differences in negative mood-induced smoking reinforcement due to distress tolerance, anxiety sensitivity, and depression history. Psychopharmacology 2010;210:25-34.

98 Malpass D, Higgs S. Acute psychomotor, subjective and physiological responses to smoking in depressed outpatient smokers and matched controls. Psychopharmacology (Berl) 2007;190:363-72.

99 D'haenen HA, Bossuyt A. Dopamine D2 receptors in depression measured with single photon emission computed tomography. Biol Psychiatry1994;35:128-32.

100 Shah PJ, Ogilvie AD, Goodwin GM, et al. Clinical and psychometric correlates of dopamine D2 binding in depression. Psychol Med 1997;27:1247-56.

101 Brody AL, Olmstead RE, Abrams AL, et al. Effect of a history of major depressive disorder on smoking-induced dopamine release. Biol Psychiatry2009;66:898-901.

102 Cook JW, Spring B, McChargue D. Influence of nicotine on positive affect in anhedonic smokers. Psychopharmacology (Berl)2007;192:87-95.

103 Cook J, Spring B, McChargue D, et al. Effects of anhedonia on days to relapse among smokers with a history of depression: a brief report. Nicotine Tob Res2010;12:978-82.

104 Leventhal AM, Waters AJ, Kahler CW, et al. Relations between anhedonia and smoking motivation. Nicotine Tob Res2009;11:1047-54.

105 Goelz PM, Audrain-McGovern JE, Hitsman B, et al. The association between changes in alternative reinforcers and short-term smoking cessation. Drug Alcohol Depend2014;138:67-74.

106 Berk M, Ng F, Wang WV, et al.. Going up in smoke: tobacco smoking is associated with worse treatment outcomes in mania. J Affect Disord2008;110:126-34.

107 Goldstein BI, Birmaher B, Axelson DA, et al. Significance of cigarette smoking among youths with bipolar disorder. Am J Addict2008;17:364-71.

108 Heffner JL, DelBello MP, Fleck DE, et al. Cigarette smoking in the early course of bipolar disorder: association with ages-at-onset of alcohol and marijuana use. Bipolar Disord2008;10:838-45.

109 Heffner JL, Anthenelli RM, Adler CM, et al. Prevalence and correlates of heavy smoking and nicotine dependence in adolescents with bipolar and cannabis use disorders. Psychiatry Res2013;210:857-62.

110 Ostacher MJ, Nierenberg AA, Perlis RH, et al. The relationship between smoking and suicidal behavior, comorbidity, and course of illness in bipolar disorder. J Clin Psychiatry2006;67:1907-11.

111 Waxmonsky JA, Thomas MR, Miklowitz DJ, et al. Prevalence and correlates of tobacco use in bipolar disorder: data from the first 2000 participants in the Systematic Treatment Enhancement Program. Gen Hosp Psychiatry2005;27:321-8.

112 Prochaska JJ, Reyes RS, Schroeder SA, et al. An online survey of tobacco use, intentions to quit, and cessation strategies among people living with bipolar disorder. Bipolar Disord 2011;13:466-73.

113 Morisano D, Wing VC, Sacco KA, et al. Effects of tobacco smoking on neuropsychological function in schizophrenia in comparison to other psychiatric disorders and non-psychiatric controls. Am J Addict2013;22:46-53.

114 Goodwin RD, Wall MM, Choo T, et al. Changes in the prevalence of mood and anxiety disorders among male and female current smokers in the United States: 1990-2001. Ann Epidemiol2014;24:493-7.

115 Piper ME, Smith SS, Schlam TR, et al. Psychiatric disorders in smokers seeking treatment for tobacco dependence: relations with tobacco dependence and cessation. J Consult Clin Psychol2010;78:13-23.

116 Piper ME, Cook JW, Schlam TR, et al. Anxiety diagnoses in smokers seeking cessation treatment: relations with tobacco dependence, withdrawal, outcome and response to treatment. Addiction 2011;106:418-27.

117 Evins AE, Culhane MA, Alpert JE, et al. A controlled trial of bupropion added to nicotine patch and behavioral therapy for smoking cessation in adults with unipolar depressive disorders. J Clin Psychopharmacol2008;28:660-6.

118 Jiang F, Li S, Pan L, et al. Association of anxiety disorders with the risk of smoking behaviors: a meta-analysis of prospective observational studies. Drug Alcohol Depend2014;145:69-76.

119 Moylan S, Jacka FN, Pasco JA, et al. Cigarette smoking, nicotine dependence and anxiety disorders: a systematic review of population-based, epidemiological studies. BMC Med2012;10:123.

120 Moylan S, Jacka FN, Pasco JA, et al. How cigarette smoking may increase the risk of anxiety symptoms and anxiety disorders: a critical review of biological pathways. Brain Behav2013;3:302-26.

121 Buckner JD, Zvolensky MJ, Jeffries ER, et al. Robust impact of social anxiety in relation to coping motives and expectancies, barriers to quitting, and cessation-related problems. Exp Clin Psychopharmacol2014;22:341-7.

122 Marshall EC, Zvolensky MJ, Vujanovic AA, et al. Evaluation of smoking characteristics among community-recruited daily smokers with and without posttraumatic stress disorder and panic psychopathology. J Anxiety Disord2008;22:1214-26.

123 Watson NL, VanderVeen JW, Cohen LM, et al. Examining the interrelationships between social anxiety, smoking to cope, and cigarette craving. Addict Behav2012;37:986-9.

124 Zvolensky MJ, Schmidt NB, Antony MM, et al. Evaluating the role of panic disorder in emotional sensitivity processes involved with smoking. J Anxiety Disord 2005;19:673-86.

125 Zehe JM, Colder CR, Read JP, et al. Social and generalized anxiety symptoms and alcohol and cigarette use in early adolescence: the moderating role of perceived peer norms. Addict Behav2013;38:1931-9.

126 Marshall EC, Johnson K, Bergman J, et al. Anxiety sensitivity and panic reactivity to bodily sensations: relation to quit-day (acute) nicotine withdrawal symptom severity among daily smokers making a self-guided quit attempt. Exp Clin Psychopharmacol2009;17:356-64.

127 Smith PH, Homish GG, Giovino GA, et al. Cigarette smoking and mental illness: a study of nicotine withdrawal. Am J Public Health2014;104 :e127-33.

128 Kimbrel NA, Morissette SB, Gulliver SB, et al. The effect of social anxiety on urge and craving among smokers with and without anxiety disorders. Drug Alcohol Depend2014;135:59-64.

129 Zvolensky MJ, Baker KM, Leen-Feldner E, et al. Anxiety sensitivity: association with intensity of retrospectively-rated smoking-related withdrawal symptoms and motivation to quit. Cogn Behav Ther2004;33:114-25

130 Zvolensky MJ, Vujanovic AA, Miller MO, et al. Incremental validity of anxiety sensitivity in terms of motivation to quit, reasons for quitting, and barriers to quitting among community-recruited daily smokers. Nicotine Tob Res2007;9:965-75.

131 McFall M, Saxon AJ, Thompson CE, et al. Improving the rates of quitting smoking for veterans with posttraumatic stress disorder. Am J Psychiatry2005;162:1311-9.

132 McFall M, Saxon AJ, Malte CA, et al. Integrating tobacco cessation into mental health care for posttraumatic stress disorder: a randomized controlled trial. JAMA2010;304:2485-93.

133 Hertzberg MA, Moore SD, Feldman ME, et al. A preliminary study of bupropion sustained-release for smoking cessation in patients with chronic posttraumatic stress disorder. J Clin Psychopharmacol2001;21:94-8.

134 Hertzberg JS, Carpenter VL, Kirby AC, et al. Mobile contingency management as an adjunctive smoking cessation treatment for smokers with posttraumatic stress disorder. Nicotine Tob Res2013;15:1934-8.

135 Beckham JC, Roodman AA, Shipley RH, et al. Smoking in Vietnam combat veterans with post-traumatic stress disorder. J Trauma Stress1995;8:461-72.

136 Calhoun PS, Levin HF, Dedert EA, et al. The relationship between posttraumatic stress disorder and smoking outcome expectancies among US military veterans who served since September 11, 2001. J Trauma Stress2011;24:303-8.

137 Beckham JC, Kirby AC, Feldman ME, et al. Prevalence and correlates of heavy smoking in Vietnam veterans with chronic posttraumatic stress disorder. Addict Behav1997;22:637-47.

138 Feldner MT, Babson KA, Zvolensky MJ, et al. Posttraumatic stress symptoms and smoking to reduce negative affect: an investigation of trauma-exposed daily smokers. Addict Behav2007;32:214-27.

139 Carmody TP, McFall M, Saxon AJ, et al. Smoking outcome expectancies in military veteran smokers with posttraumatic stress disorder. Nicotine Tob Res2012;14:919-26.

140 Beckham JC, Calhoun PS, Dennis MF, et al. Predictors of lapse in first week of smoking abstinence in PTSD and non-PTSD smokers. Nicotine Tob Res2013;15:1122-9.

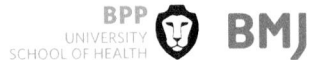

141 Dedert EA, Dennis PA, Swinkels CM, et al. Ecological momentary assessment of posttraumatic stress disorder symptoms during a smoking quit attempt. Nicotine Tob Res2014;16:430-6.

142 Shucard JL, McCabe DC, Szymanski H. An event-related potential study of attention deficits in posttraumatic stress disorder during auditory and visual Go/NoGo continuous performance tasks. Biol Psychol2008;79:223-33.

143 Vasterling JJ, Brailey K, Constans JI, et al. Attention and memory dysfunction in posttraumatic stress disorder. Neuropsychology1998;12:125-33.

144 Ashare RL, Falcone M, Lerman C. Cognitive function during nicotine withdrawal: Implications for nicotine dependence treatment. Neuropharmacology2014;76:581-91.

145 Vrana SR, Calhoun PS, McClernon FJ, et al. Effects of smoking on the acoustic startle response and prepulse inhibition in smokers with and without posttraumatic stress disorder. Psychopharmacology (Berl)2013;230:477-85.

146 Dedert EA, Calhoun PS, Harper LA, et al. Smoking withdrawal in smokers with and without posttraumatic stress disorder. Nicotine Tob Res2012;14:372-6.

147 Farsalinos KE, Polosa R. Safety evaluation and risk assessment of electronic cigarettes as tobacco cigarette substitutes: a systematic review. Ther Adv Drug Saf2014;5:67-86.

148 McRobbie H, Bullen C, Hartmann-Boyce J, et al. Electronic cigarettes for smoking cessation and reduction. Cochrane Database Syst Rev2014;12:CD010216.

149 Caponnetto P, Auditore R, Russo C, et al. Impact of an electronic cigarette on smoking reduction and cessation in schizophrenic smokers: a prospective 12-month pilot study. Int J Environ Res Public Health2013;10:446-61.

150 Benowitz NL, Henningfield JE. Reducing the nicotine content to make cigarettes less addictive. Tob Control2013;22(suppl 1):i14-7.

151 WHO. WHO framework convention on tobacco control. 2003. www.who.int/fctc/text_download/en.

152 Donny EC, Hatsukami DK, Benowitz NL, et al. Reduced nicotine product standards for combustible tobacco: building an empirical basis for effective regulation. Prev Med2014;68C:17-22.

153 Hatsukami DK, Kotlyar M, Hertsgaard LA, et al. Reduced nicotine content cigarettes: effects on toxicant exposure, dependence and cessation. Addiction2010;105:343-55.

154 Tidey JW, Rohsenow DJ, Kaplan GB, et al. Separate and combined effects of very low nicotine cigarettes and nicotine replacement in smokers with schizophrenia and controls. Nicotine Tob Res2013;15:121-9.

155 Royal Australian College of General Practitioners. Supporting smoking cessation: a guide for health professionals. 2011; updated 2014. www.racgp.org.au/your-practice/guidelines/smoking-cessation.

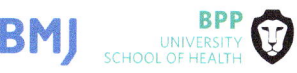

Managing and preventing depression in adolescents

Anita Thapar, professor of child and adolescent psychiatry[1], Stephan Collishaw, senior lecturer in developmental psychopathology[1], Robert Potter, consultant child and adolescent psychiatrist[2], Ajay K Thapar, general practitioner[3]

[1]Department of Psychological Medicine and Neurology, Cardiff University School of Medicine, Cardiff CF14 4XN

[2]Trehafod Child and Family Clinic (Cwm Taf NHS Trust), Cockett, Swansea SA2 0GB

[3]Taff Riverside Practice, Riverside, Cardiff CF11 9SH

Correspondence to: A Thapar
thapar@cf.ac.uk

Cite this as: BMJ 2010;340:c209

DOI: 10.1136/bmj.c209

http://www.bmj.com/content/340/bmj.c209

Depressive disorder affects 1-6% of adolescents each year worldwide,[1] [2] and early onset heralds a more severe and persistent illness in adult life.[3] Effective treatment is available, but best treatment practice is controversial because of concerns about the use of antidepressants in young people and inconsistencies in evidence. This review provides guidance for non-specialists on the assessment and management of adolescent unipolar depression and considers emerging evidence on prevention strategies.

Why is it important to identify adolescent depression?

Evidence from prospective community studies suggests that rates of underdiagnosis and undertreatment of depression are higher in adolescents than in adults.[4] Large scale, longitudinal population based and clinical cohort studies have consistently shown that rates of depression rise sharply after puberty, especially in girls, with immediate and long term risks.[5] [6] Clinical depression adversely affects schooling, educational attainment, and relationships,[7] and it has long term negative consequences on adult physical health and functioning.[8] Although most affected adolescents show initial remission, 50-70% of them will have a recurrence within five years of initial diagnosis.[5] Large prospective studies have also shown that adolescent depression is associated with a raised risk of suicide (odds ratio 11 to 27),[9] and suicide represents the third leading cause of death in this age group (aged 14-19 years).[10]

Which adolescents are most at risk of developing a depressive disorder?

Evidence from clinical and epidemiological studies shows that three groups are at increased risk of developing a depressive disorder. Firstly, adolescents who have raised levels of depressive symptoms but fall below the diagnostic threshold have a two to three times greater risk of developing future depressive episodes than those without such symptoms.[8] Secondly, the adolescent offspring of parents with a history of depression are three to four times more likely than those of parents with no psychiatric history to develop depression.[11] Thirdly, in adolescents who have previously had depression, recurrence rates are high.[8]

How is adolescent depression diagnosed?

Diagnostic criteria from either ICD-10 (international classification of diseases, 10th revision) (box) or the Diagnostic and Statistical Manual of Mental Disorders, fourth edition (DSM-IV) are currently used; these two sets of criteria are similar.

The criteria for depression in adolescents are the same as for adults (although the DSM-IV criteria allow "irritable" (easily annoyed and provoked to anger) instead of "depressed" mood in children and adolescents). Thus the clinical questioning approach with adolescents should be similar to that used in adults. In this age group, it is helpful to question both the adolescent and the parent(s) about specific symptoms and to check whether the symptoms of depression are associated with impairment—for example, an adolescent with depression may stop going out with friends or show deterioration in school work. Irritability may be a prominent symptom. In this age group, comorbidity with other psychiatric disorders—notably disruptive behaviour disorders (20-40%) and anxiety disorders—is common (occurring in 30-75% of cases), as is association with deliberate self harm and suicidality (odds ratio 51).[12] Depression may be missed if the primary reported features are behavioural problems, substance misuse, anxiety symptoms, refusal to go to school, academic failure, or unexplained physical symptoms—especially musculoskeletal pains[13]—all of which are significantly associated with adolescent depression (reported odds ratios 10 to 29).[14]

Questionnaires can be used for screening and monitoring changes in the depression symptom score. The Mood and Feelings Questionnaire (MFQ; http://devepi.duhs.duke.edu/mfq.html) is one of the most well established screening instruments for adolescent depression,[15] and it has been validated in clinical and community samples. If a parent raises the initial concerns, their reports on the adolescent can be helpful as a first screen, and the above questionnaire has both a parent version and a child version. Other questionnaires are also available.[16] It is important to ask the adolescent about suicidal thoughts and intent.

Which treatments work for adolescent depression?

Inconsistent evidence and guidelines have made best treatment practice of depression in adolescents controversial.[17] [18] Most published evaluation studies have focused on the short term effectiveness of newer generation antidepressant drugs or cognitive behavioural therapy (CBT), or both. Evidence on long term efficacy and prevention of relapse is lacking.

SUMMARY POINTS

- Depression affects 1-6% of adolescents each year worldwide
- Diagnostic criteria for depression are the same as for adults, but the primary presenting concern may be different (for example, behavioural problems, refusal to go to school)
- For mild depression, cognitive behavioural therapy seems to be effective. Because such treatment is a scarce resource, less specialised supportive treatment and guided self help can be used initially
- For moderate-severe depression, fluoxetine and routine specialist (child and adolescent mental health service) clinical care or fluoxetine plus cognitive behavioural therapy is recommended
- Suicidal risk must be carefully monitored
- Parental depression needs to be treated

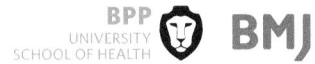

Psychological treatments

The two most commonly investigated treatments are CBT and interpersonal psychotherapy. The evidence on CBT is mixed. One meta-analysis suggests that CBT is effective for adolescent depression, although effect sizes are modest (0.3).[19] A recent systematic review and meta-analysis also shows that CBT is modestly effective for adolescent depression, but that effect sizes are smaller in more recent better designed studies and in more complicated cases.[20] In contrast, a large randomised controlled trial (TADS) from the United States found that in moderate-severe depression, CBT alone was no better than placebo,[21] and that it provided benefits only in combination with fluoxetine.

Interpersonal psychotherapy has been shown to be effective in treating adolescent depression in three randomised controlled trials.[22] However, good quality psychological treatments for adolescents are not widely available in many countries.

Taken together, the evidence on psychological treatments can be summarised as follows:

- CBT alone is probably most useful for mild depression
- Interpersonal psychotherapy, if available, is worthwhile.

Drugs

The effectiveness of selective serotonin reuptake inhibitors for children and adolescents has been systematically reviewed.[23] Two systematic reviews suggest that fluoxetine is an effective treatment for adolescent depression (41-61% response to fluoxetine v 20-35% response to placebo, relative risk 1.86; treatment effect in terms of depression symptom scores −5.63). Consistent good quality evidence on other newer generation antidepressants is currently lacking.

Treating mild depression in non-specialist settings

In most countries, including the United Kingdom, primary care plays a key part in the detection and initial management of adolescent depression, but few treatment studies are based in this setting. One randomised controlled trial in the US suggested that organisational changes in primary care through trained care managers who enhanced access to evidence based treatments (CBT and antidepressants) significantly reduced symptoms of adolescent depression in the short term.[24]

Simple, non-specific psychosocial strategies might also be helpful as an initial treatment, although good quality evidence on these is lacking. Such first line pragmatic approaches deserve proper evaluation because specialised resources such as CBT are limited. Suggested strategies include providing parental support; recognising and treating parental mental illness; educating patients about depression (this may include the use of educational leaflets); problem solving; attending to recent family or peer group conflicts; dealing with comorbidity; and liaising with schools and other agencies while monitoring mental state and using an empathic reflective approach.[25] Advice on nutrition and diet, exercise (45 minutes to one hour three times week), sleep hygiene, and anxiety management, along with guided self help and non-directive supportive counselling are also recommended.[17]

Treating moderate-severe depression

Clinical guidelines on the treatment of adolescent depression differ between Europe and the US, and some guidance is based on consensus opinion rather than evidence. Currently, evidence on the best available treatment for moderate-severe adolescent depression comes from two randomised controlled treatment versus placebo trials. One study was based on UK NHS patients (ADAPT),[25] had no sponsorship from a drug company, and found a significant treatment effect at 12 weeks. It compared fluoxetine alone (61% "much or very much improved" by 28 weeks) with CBT plus fluoxetine (53% much or very much improved); all patients received routine specialist clinical care. The other study (TADS) was from the US, and it compared 12 weeks of CBT alone (43% response), fluoxetine alone with no psychosocial care (61% response), and CBT plus fluoxetine (71% response) with placebo (35% response).[21] The evidence on treating moderate-severe depression can be summarised as follows:

- Fluoxetine is an effective treatment for adolescent depression[21 23 25]
- Evidence on the benefits of adding CBT to fluoxetine is mixed. The US study suggested that it accelerated the response to treatment and reduced suicidality,[21] whereas the UK study found no benefits.[25] This might have been because the UK study included more severe clinic derived cases and all patients received routine specialist care
- Consistent effectiveness data on newer generation antidepressants other than fluoxetine are lacking,[23] and they are currently not approved for use in patients under 18 years in the UK and Europe. Escitalopram has been approved by the US Food and Drug Administration, but consistent evidence on its effectiveness in adolescence is still limited.

Only around 60% of adolescents with depression show remission after treatment, so what about those who fail to respond to initial treatment? One large US randomised control trial of adolescents who had not responded to two months of initial treatment with a first selective serotonin reuptake inhibitor suggested that adding CBT and switching to another one of these drugs (paroxetine or citalopram) results in a higher response rate (54.8%) than switching drugs only (40.5%).[26] A switch to venlafaxine was not recommended because of adverse side effects.

Suicidal risk

One of the major concerns has been that new generation antidepressants seem to be associated with greater suicidal risk in adolescents than in adults.[27] Caution is needed in interpreting results, however, because untreated adolescent depression can itself lead to suicidality and the evidence is mixed.[23 27] A recent pooled analysis of 27 published and unpublished randomised placebo controlled trials of newer generation antidepressants in children and adolescents found that the benefits of antidepressants (number needed to treat 10) were greater than the risk of suicidal ideation and suicide attempts (number needed to harm 143).[27] Overall, the evidence supports careful monitoring for suicidal risk in adolescents with depression, regardless of treatment choice.

Can we prevent or delay onset of depression in adolescents?

Given the serious burden of depression, the poor prognosis when onset is early, and the limited treatment options available, it is increasingly being argued that preventing, or at least delaying, the onset of depression in children and adolescents is a major public health and clinical priority.

A meta-analysis of the evidence on this topic suggests that prevention strategies are likely to be effective only

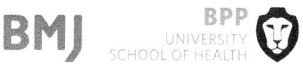

SOURCES AND SELECTION CRITERIA

We searched for papers published between 1990 and 2009 using key index terms (adolescent depression, treatment, and prevention) on PubMed (Medline and life science journals). In addition, we consulted the Institute of Medicine report "Preventing mental, emotional and behavioral disorders among young people: progress and possibilities" (published by National Academies Press 2009), NICE guidelines on adolescent depression, Cochrane systematic reviews, and BMJ *Clinical Evidence*. This was supplemented by reviews and our own knowledge.

CRITERIA FOR DEPRESSIVE EPISODE, ACCORDING TO ICD-10

Two of the first three symptoms listed below must be present. In addition, at least four symptoms (for mild episode), six symptoms (for moderate episode), or eight symptoms (for severe episode) must be present during the same two week period.

- Depressed mood for most of the day and almost every day
- Loss of interest or pleasure in activities
- Decreased energy or increased fatigability
- Loss of confidence or self esteem
- Unreasonable feelings of self reproach or excessive inappropriate guilt
- Recurrent thoughts of death or suicide, or any suicidal behaviour
- Reduced ability to think or concentrate
- Change in psychomotor activity, agitation, or retardation
- Sleep disturbance
- Change in appetite with corresponding weight change

QUESTIONS FOR FUTURE RESEARCH

- Improved understanding of the early natural history of adolescent depression including risk factors and protective factors to guide new treatments
- Randomised controlled treatment trials of adolescent depression that are not sponsored by drug companies
- Randomised controlled treatment trials of psychological therapies that can be delivered without the need for expensive and intensive training (for example, guided self help, graded activities, and guided internet packages)
- Which subgroups of patients respond better to specific treatments?
- Which treatment and prevention approaches are most effective and feasible in low resource communities and developing countries?
- Does early intervention improve longer term prognosis?
- Which interventions prevent relapse?
- Randomised controlled treatment trials of simple psychosocial strategies for prevention in non-specialist settings
- Does improving management of parental depression reduce the risk of depression in adolescents?

TIPS FOR NON-SPECIALISTS

- Consider the possibility of adolescent depression even when the adolescent does not present primarily with mood symptoms
- Remember that depression can present with behavioural problems, unexplained physical symptoms, academic failure, refusal to go to school, anxiety, and substance misuse
- Ask about suicidal thoughts
- Ask parents with depression about concerns regarding their adolescent offspring
- When depression is diagnosed, provide the adolescent and his or her parents (or carers) with information on the disorder and guided self help strategies
- If moderate-severe depression, continued mild depression, complicating psychotic features, suicidality, or other psychiatric risk factors are present, refer to child and adolescent mental health services. Monitor carefully in the interim

ADDITIONAL EDUCATIONAL RESOURCES

Resources for healthcare professionals

- Centre for Clinical Interventions (www.cci.health.wa.gov.au)—Although not specifically aimed at adolescent depression, this site has a section containing resources for general practitioners
- National Institute for Health and Clinical Excellence (www.nice.org.uk/CG28)—UK clinical guidance on depression
- American Academy of Child and Adolescent Psychiatry (www.aacap.org/cs/Depression.ResourceCenter)—US clinical guidance on adolescent depression

Resources for patients

- Youthinmind (www.youthinmind.com)—Website providing help for stressed children and teenagers and those who care for them
- Samaritans (www.samaritans.co.uk)—Confidential source of support—face to face, telephone, and email; the website also contains useful information
- Depression in Teenagers (www.depressioninteenagers.co.uk)—Aimed at teenagers; gives useful advice about depression and its treatment
- Black Dog Institute (www.blackdoginstitute.org.au/public/depression/inteenagersyoungadults.cfm)—Useful information on depression for parents and young people

A PATIENT'S PERSPECTIVE

J is a 15 year old boy who came to clinic with his mother and father. He has "always" had episodes of feeling low in mood but this has become sustained and problematic during the past 18 months and accompanied by other depressive disorder symptoms, including marked irritability. He has stopped going to school and his parents cannot get him to leave the house.

These are his own words: "I feel constantly down. I am feeling tormented. I feel sad, hate myself. This feels different from usual sadness and I can't stop crying. I don't want to go out and don't like football or computer games any more. I can't cope with activities such as rugby club. I can't concentrate on computer games. I feel exhausted all the time and can't go to school. I feel paranoid, that other people turn to look at me and I want to die. I feel I am torturing my family and I am jealous as other teenagers my age are better off. My future looks bleak."

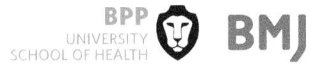

when given to high risk groups of adolescents rather than to the whole population.[28]

What sorts of prevention strategies might be useful?

The most promising prevention programme has been targeted at three high risk groups—those with raised depression symptoms, a previous episode of depression, and whose parents have a history of depression. It consists of a group based CBT approach delivered to parents and children.[29] A recent high quality randomised controlled trial in the US found that this type of intervention resulted in significantly fewer depressive episodes at one year (21.4% v 32.7% in controls).[29] However, the intervention was less effective if the parents had current depression. This could simply reflect higher inherited risk for depression in the adolescents, but it could mean that adolescent depression can arise from the direct and indirect risk effects of being exposed to current parental depression. In support of current maternal depression being an important target, the largest treatment trial of adult depression, STAR*D, found that successfully treating depression in mothers improved the mental health of children.[30] However, this finding requires confirmation. Nevertheless, these results highlight the importance of effectively monitoring and treating maternal depression and better integrating adult and child services. They also suggest future possibilities for prevention programmes.

Conclusion

Depression in adolescents is common, severe, and leads to immediate and long term morbidity and mortality. It is important for clinicians who deal with young people and families to be aware of the problem, so that high risk adolescents can be screened, assessed, and offered appropriate treatment. Prevention strategies in high risk groups are likely to become increasingly important.

Contributors: AT, AKT, and SC reviewed the literature. RP consulted guidelines and web resources. All authors helped interpret papers and write the article. AT is guarantor.

Funding: The authors' research on depression is supported by Sir Jules Thorne Medical Trust.

Competing interests: AT accepted fees from drug companies for speaking and organising educational events and received an educational grant for attention deficit hyperactivity disorder before 2006. All other authors have none to declare.

Provenance and peer review: Commissioned; externally peer reviewed.

Parental consent obtained.

1   Green H, McGinnity A, Meltzer H, Ford T, Goodman R. Mental health of children and young people in Great Britain, 2004. Palgrave Macmillan, 2005.
2   Costello EJ, Erkanli A, Angold A. Is there an epidemic of child or adolescent depression? *J Child Psychol Psychiatry* 2006;47:1263-71.
3   Lewinsohn PM, Clarke GN, Seeley JR, Rohde P. Major depression in community adolescents: age at onset, episode duration, and time to recurrence. *J Am Acad Child Adolesc Psychiatry* 1994;33:809-18.
4   Leaf PJ, Alegria M, Cohen P, Goodman SH, Horwitz SM, Hoven CW, et al. Mental health service use in the community and schools: results from the four-community MECA study. Methods for the epidemiology of child and adolescent mental disorders study. *J Am Acad Child Adolesc Psychiatry* 1996;35:889-97.
5   Lewinsohn PM, Rohde P, Seeley JR, Klein DN, Gotlib IH. Natural course of adolescent major depressive disorder in a community sample: predictors of recurrence in young adults. *Am J Psychiatry* 2000;157:1584-91.
6   Kessler RC, Avenevoli S, Ries Merikangas K. Mood disorders in children and adolescents: an epidemiologic perspective. *Biol Psychiatry* 2001;49:1002-14.
7   Birmaher B, Ryan ND, Williamson DE, Brent DA, Kaufman J, Dahl RE, et al. Childhood and adolescent depression: a review of the past 10 years. Part I. *J Am Acad Child Adolesc Psychiatry* 1996;35:1427-39.

8   Lewinsohn PM, Rohde P, Seeley JR. Major depressive disorder in older adolescents: prevalence, risk factors, and clinical implications. *Clin Psychol Rev* 1998;18:765-94.
9   Gould MS, Greenberg T, Velting DM, Shaffer D. Youth suicide risk and preventative interventions: a review of the past 10 years. *J Am Acad Child Adolesc Psychiatry* 2003;42:386-405.
10   Centers for Disease Control and Prevention. National Center for Injury Prevention and Control. Web-based injury statistics query and reporting system (WISQARS). 2009. http://webappa.cdc.gov/sasweb/ncipc/leadcaus10.html.
11   Rice F, Harold G, Thapar A. The genetic aetiology of childhood depression: a review. *J Child Psychol Psychiatry* 2002;43:65-79.
12   Foley DL, Goldston DB, Costello EJ, Angold A. Proximal psychiatric risk factors for suicidality in youth: the Great Smoky Mountains study. *Arch Gen Psychiatry* 2006;63:1017-24.
13   Egger HL, Costello EJ, Erkanli A, Angold A. Somatic complaints and psychopathology in children and adolescents: stomach aches, musculoskeletal pains, and headaches. *J Am Acad Child Adolesc Psychiatry* 1999;38:852-60.
14   Costello EJ, Mustillo S, Erkanli A, Keeler G, Angold A. Prevalence and development of psychiatric disorders in childhood and adolescence. *Arch Gen Psychiatry* 2003;60:837-44.
15   Daviss WB, Birmaher B, Melhem NA, Axelson DA, Michaels SM, Brent DA. Criterion validity of the mood and feelings questionnaire for depressive episodes in clinic and non-clinic subjects. *J Child Psychol Psychiatry* 2006;47:927-34.
16   Williams SB, O'Connor EA, Eder M, Whitlock EP. Screening for child and adolescent depression in primary care settings: a systematic evidence review for the US Preventive Services Task Force. *Pediatrics* 2009;123:e716-35.
17   National Institute for Health and Clinical Excellence. Depression in children and young people: identification and management in primary, community and secondary care. 2005. Clinical guideline CG28. guidance.nice.org.uk/CG28.
18   Birmaher B, Brent D, Bernet W, Bukstein O, Walter H, et al; AACAP Work Group on Quality Issues. Practice parameter for the assessment and treatment of children and adolescents with depressive disorders. *J Am Acad Child Adolesc Psychiatry* 2007;46:1503-26.
19   Weisz JR, McCarty CA, Valeri SM. Effects of psychotherapy for depression in children and adolescents: a meta-analysis. *Psychol Bull* 2006;132:132-49.
20   Klein JB, Jacobs RH, Reinecke MA. Cognitive-behavioral therapy for adolescent depression: a meta-analytic investigation of changes in effect-size estimates. *J Am Acad Child Adolesc Psychiatry* 2007;46:1403-13.
21   Treatment for Adolescents with Depression Study (TADS) Team. The treatment for adolescents with depression study (TADS): outcomes over 1 year of naturalistic follow-up. *Am J Psychiatry 2009* ;166:1141-9.
22   Mufson L, Dorta KP, Wickramaratne P, Nomura Y, Olfson M, Weissman MM. A randomized effectiveness trial of interpersonal psychotherapy for depressed adolescents. *Arch Gen Psychiatry* 2004;61:577-84.
23   Hetrick S, Merry S, McKenzie J, Sindahl P, Proctor M. Selective serotonin reuptake inhibitors (SSRIs) for depressive disorders in children and adolescents. *Cochrane Database Syst Rev* 2007;(3):CD004851.
24   Asarnow JR, Jaycox LH, Duan N, LaBorde AP, Rea MM, Murray P, et al. Effectiveness of a quality improvement intervention for adolescent depression in primary care clinics: a randomized controlled trial. *JAMA* 2005;293:311-9.
25   Goodyer I, Dubicka B, Wilkinson P, Kelvin R, Roberts C, Byford S, et al. Selective serotonin reuptake inhibitors (SSRIs) and routine specialist care with and without cognitive behaviour therapy in adolescents with major depression: randomised controlled trial. *BMJ* 2007;335:142.
26   Brent D, Emslie G, Clarke G, Wagner KD, Asarnow JR, Keller M, et al. Switching to another SSRI or to venlafaxine with or without cognitive behavioural therapy for adolescents with SSRI-resistant depression: the TORDIA randomized controlled trial. *JAMA* 2008:299:901-13.
27   Bridge JA, Yengar S, Salary CB, Barbe RP, Birmaher B, Pincus HA, et al. Clinical response and risk for reported suicidal ideation and suicide attempts in pediatric antidepressant treatment: a meta-analysis of randomized controlled trials. *JAMA* 2007;63:332-9.
28   Stice E, Shaw H, Bohon C, Marti CN, Rohde P. A meta-analytic review of depression prevention programs for children and adolescents: factors that predict magnitude of intervention effects. *J Consult Clin Psychol* 2009;77:486-503.
29   Garber J, Clarke GN, Weersing VR, Beardslee WR, Brent DA, Gladstone TR, et al. Prevention of depression in at-risk adolescents: a randomized controlled trial. *JAMA* 2009;301:2215-24.
30   Weissman MM, Pilowsky DJ, Wickramaratne PJ, Talati A, Wisniewski SR, Fava M, et al. Remissions in maternal depression and child psychopathology: a STAR*D-child report. *JAMA* 2006;295:1389-98.

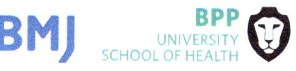

Use and misuse of drugs and alcohol in adolescence

Paul McArdle, consultant child and adolescent psychiatrist

Fleming Nuffield Unit,
Northumberland Tyne and Wear
NHS Trust, Newcastle upon Tyne
NE2 3AE

mcardlep@btinternet.com

Cite this as: *BMJ* 2008;337:a306

DOI: 10.1136/bmj.a306

http://www.bmj.com/content/337/
bmj.a306

Substance misuse is one of a group of linked behaviours that has recently become more common among young people in westernised societies.[w1] This rise has paralleled increasing rates of anxiety and depressive symptoms and of deaths related to substance misuse.[1] [w1-w3] Substance use disorders are potentially treatable and should be managed as chronic, relapsing diseases of complex origin.[2] This review examines the scale of these disorders among young people and how healthcare practitioners can intervene.

Method

We searched Medline, Google, and the websites of the UK National Treatment Agency, US National Institute on Drug Abuse, and European Monitoring Centre for Drugs and Drug Addiction for suitable evidence based material. We also consulted colleagues working with young people with substance misuse, as well as consulting young people themselves and their carers.

What constitutes substance misuse?

Substance misuse and dependence are a subset of "substance use," which includes phenomena such as experimentation and intermittent recreational use. "Substances" include alcohol as well as illicit or (if deliberately misused) prescribed drugs. See box 1 and 2 for definitions. (Substance misuse is also referred to as substance abuse—for example, by the *Diagnostic and Statistical Manual of Mental Disorders*.)

Is substance use increasing?

Drugs

Serial data from the European school survey project on alcohol and other drugs (n=103 000 in 2003) showed a broadly stable rate of 40% lifetime use of cannabis in 15 year olds in the United Kingdom up to 2003.[4] A more recent English school survey of 8200 schoolchildren aged 11-15 years showed an overall decline in drug use from 11% in 2005 to 9% in 2007[5] but also showed that 4% of 11 year olds had used illicit drugs in the past month, compared with 0% in 1998, when comparable data were first obtained.

Some southern (Cyprus, Malta, Greece) and northern (Norway, Sweden) European countries report rates for adolescents of <10% lifetime use of any illicit drug.[4] However, other regions with previously low rates such as eastern

Europe have shown considerable catch-up in lifetime use. In the United States, daily use of cannabis by 15 year olds has dropped from 6% to 5% but remains well above the 2% of the early 1990s.[w9]

Alcohol

According to survey data,[4] regular drinking is common among UK and Irish adolescents and has increased among 15 and 16 year olds from 22% in 1995 to 27% in 2003. This rise results partly from an increase from 20% to 29% in binge drinking among young females and an increase in self reported consumption of "alcopops" (fizzy, flavoured alcoholic drinks) among 15-16 year old girls. Reported rates of drinking among 11-13 year old boys and 14 year old girls have trebled since 1990.[5]

What do we know about rates of misuse and dependence?

Few large scale studies directly examine this question. However, survey data suggest that 10% of UK 15-16 year olds reported "problems" linked with substance use.[4] A diagnostic study of a representative sample of 3021 Munich adolescents and young adults found that 18% exhibited substance misuse or dependence.[6] [w10] At age 18 years, 20% of a New Zealand birth cohort of 1265 children were misusing alcohol and 6% were dependent. The corresponding figures for cannabis were 12% and 5%.[7]

Two large US cross sectional population studies of young adults showed that rates of cannabis dependence increased between 1991 and 2001.[w11] The authors attributed this rise to more potent varieties of cannabis; the rise also paralleled the increase in cannabis use during that decade.

Does substance misuse impair the developing brain?

Recent research supports the view that early adolescence is a potential "critical period" during which the long term direction of biopsychosocial development can be altered.[8] Substance use in the early teenage years may prove to have serious long term consequences.

Two studies of representative samples of over 43 000 US adults found that those who reported their first alcoholic drink before age 14 or their first drug use before age 15 were three times more likely to develop alcohol or drug dependence than those whose first use of alcohol or drugs was at age 15 or older.[9] [w12] Regular use of cannabis before age 15 seems to be linked with increased risk of subsequent psychosis.[w13]

Two small neuroimaging studies found that young adults who had misused or been dependent on alcohol in adolescence had smaller prefrontal cortices and hippocampi than healthy controls.[w14] [10] However, it is unclear whether these findings reflect alcohol neurotoxicity or pre-existing developmental vulnerabilities, or both, but animal studies support alcohol neurotoxicity.

A small longitudinal study of 113 subjects tracked from infancy showed that frequent users of cannabis in late

SUMMARY POINTS

- Substance misuse or dependence is a form of chronic, relapsing, debilitating illness
- International survey findings from a range of countries found that parental knowledge of their child's whereabouts protected against substance use, though this may be the result of a confiding parent-child relationship
- Without always consciously doing so, healthcare staff can exert substantial psychological "healing" and stabilisation, which can be valuable to troubled young people
- Healthcare organisations should actively engage young people through alliances with youth services, outreach, and continuity of care

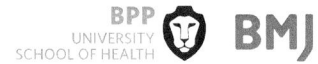

adolescence had a lower IQ than expected and poorer performance on memory tests than non-users or former users.[11] This effect on memory may be one factor in the poor educational outcomes linked with cannabis use.

How dangerous is substance misuse?

According to UK National Statistics data for 2005,[w3] 8.5% of male and 8.2% of female deaths in the 15-19 year age group were due to misuse of substances; in the male group this is similar to the proportion of deaths due to cancer (8.5%) and far ahead of deaths due to infection, for example. If deaths from self harm (often associated with substance misuse) are added, the proportions rise to 21% and 16.8% of all deaths among this age group. Deaths from accidental overdose tend to occur most often among young adults, leading to substantial "years of potential life lost."[w15] A longitudinal study of 9491 notified teenage opiate addicts indicated that their death rate was 12 times greater than the death rate in the general population of teenagers; the addicts' deaths were mainly due to accidental poisoning.[12]

Management

The capacity for healthcare workers to intervene requires first a preparedness to accept substance misuse as "their business."

Assessing the problem

Assessment searches not only for the time line, dose, type, frequency, and context of substance use, but also for predisposing, maintaining, and protective influences. In straightforward cases, this may be achievable in one interview. Ideally, the history should also enable identification of problems such as school failure, neglect, or physical or sexual abuse. Taking a careful history and explaining confidentiality (box 3) may help to establish good rapport. Consider supplementing a history with screening questionnaires (box 4) and a physical examination looking for signs of physical or sexual abuse, neglect, poor growth, pregnancy, self harm, injury, injection, and infection; also consider toxicology tests (box 5).[13]

Does watchful waiting have a role?

A large prospective study found that rates of substance dependence levelled off at age 18 years, with about 10% of illicit drug users being dependent.[7] Similar trends have been shown in relation to alcohol.[w16] Decreasing 12 month prevalence rates for misuse and dependence in one follow-up study suggested a significant rate of spontaneous recovery.[w10] After assessment, a clinician might conclude that risk is not high and that a role for watchful waiting exists.

What active interventions can healthcare staff use?

Brief intervention

In a recent randomised controlled trial a brief motivational intervention (box 6) almost halved the frequency of alcohol bingeing at 12 months' follow-up among 13-17 year olds who reported excessive drinking on presentation to an emergency department compared with those who were assessed and given literature.[16] There is recent evidence from an observational trial and a randomised controlled trial that a brief motivational interview versus information alone can substantially reduce the levels of both binge drinking and use of cocaine and ecstasy (3,4

methylenedioxymethamphetamine) among regular teenage users at one year follow-up.[w17 w18] However, reductions of substance use observed in control groups suggest that assessment and information alone may have prompted change.[w17] The following strategies may exert useful effects: a sympathetically conducted history of substance use, thoughtful, knowledgeable interpretation of the findings, and avoidance of lecturing or arguing.

What to advise parents?

A large European survey of 15 year olds found that a confiding parent-child relationship is linked with markedly lower rates of substance use.[17] International survey findings from a range of countries[4] found that parental knowledge of their child's whereabouts was a protective influence against substance use, although greater parental monitoring is likely to be a proxy for a confiding relationship in which the young person informs the parent of their whereabouts. A recent Finnish twin study found that the quality of the parent-adolescent relationship seems to moderate the effects of genetics on smoking tendency.[w19] Whatever other predisposing factors may exist, a strong parent-child relationship could be a powerful barrier to substance misuse.

A nested observation of the intervention limb of a randomised controlled trial examining the effects of multidimensional family therapy for cannabis dependence showed that a good "therapeutic alliance" with the parents as well as with the young person was the best predictor of a good outcome.[w20]

Often troublesome young people do not receive a generous response from education services or the police. Health professionals can support parents to be tenacious in obtaining a more supportive deal from education and other services.

More sustained intervention by healthcare practitioners

Research is limited on the role of healthcare providers in managing adolescent substance misuse. However, it is possible to extrapolate a general approach from relevant if tangential research. For example, a US randomised controlled trial of several interventions for young cannabis misusers reported significant reductions in use after each of these interventions. The authors concluded that the effect was the result of components that were shared between interventions.[18] Interventional studies of adolescent depression and adult alcohol dependence evaluated the effects of seeing a healthcare practitioner as part of a placebo limb compared with specialist psychotherapy for a limited number of meetings over some months. Sympathetic, informed, supportive counselling from a health practitioner approached or equalled the effectiveness of cognitive behavioural therapy for adolescent depression[19] and for adult alcoholism.[w21]

A randomised controlled trial of 90 women with personality disorder (many of the young people receiving help from substance misuse services may be developing serious personality dysfunction) showed that receiving weekly supervised support over a year led to improvement across a range of measures including self harm, depression, anxiety, and anger.[w22] The authors commented that the continuity of care or "relationship focus" buffered the extremes of instability.

Without always consciously doing so, healthcare staff can exert substantial psychological "healing" and stabilisation

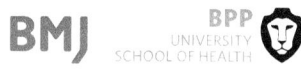

BOX 1 DEFINITIONS OF MISUSE AND DEPENDENCE*

Substance misuse

Substance misuse is a maladaptive pattern of use leading to clinically important impairment or distress, manifested by one or more of the following over 12 months:

- Failure to fulfil major obligations at work, school, or home
- Use of a substance in situations in which it is physically hazardous
- Persistent or recurrent use of the substance despite persistent or recurrent social or interpersonal problems caused or exacerbated by the effects of the substance
- Persistent or recurrent use despite legal problems related to use of the substance

Substance dependence

Substance dependence is broadly equivalent to addiction and generally suggests physiological changes related to chronic drug administration. Dependence is associated with three or more of the following over 12 months:

- Tolerance
- Withdrawal
- Taking larger amounts than intended
- Unsuccessful efforts to cut down
- Spending a great deal of time obtaining or using the substance
- Giving up important activities because of use
- Continued use despite physical or psychological problems likely to have been caused or exacerbated by the substance

*Based on the Diagnostic and Statistical Manual of Mental Disorders[w4]

BOX 2 EVIDENCE FOR A NEUROLOGICAL EXPLANATION OF DEPENDENCE

- A series of imaging studies of adults dependent on cocaine have shown abnormal responses in the prefrontal cortex and basal ganglia, including the nucleus accumbens and related structures. The studies showed that the "high" experienced by the participants coincided with rapid saturation of dopamine transporters in the basal ganglia.[3 w5-w7]
- Increased extracellular dopamine in the basal ganglia also motivates (or in animal studies prompts) the "emission of behaviours" in the pursuit of anticipated rewards such as food.[w8] Commonly misused substances seem to trigger this mechanism, which leads to the person seeking reward.
- As use progresses to dependence there is pressure to avoid uncomfortable withdrawals.[w7] This system seems to be the physiological basis for dependence or addiction, a condition in which the person's life becomes organised not by what we regard as rational considerations but by the largely subcortical drive to obtain the substance.

BOX 3 CONFIDENTIALITY

"Adolescents are more likely to provide truthful information if they believe that their information, at least detailed information, will not be shared. Before the adolescent interview, the clinician should review exactly what information the clinician is obliged to share and with whom. . . Typically, a clinician should inform the adolescent that a threat of danger to self or others will force the clinician to inform a responsible adult, usually the parents. The clinician should . . . encourage and support the adolescent's revealing the extent of substance use and other problems to parents. In other cases, the clinician should discuss what information that the adolescent will allow the clinician to reveal such as a general recommendation for treatment or impressions rather than a detailed report of specific deviant and substance use behaviors."

*Taken from Bukstein et al[13]

BOX 4 CRAFFT QUESTIONNAIRE—BRIEF SCREENING TEST FOR SUBSTANCE MISUSE IN ADOLESCENTS*[14]

C—Have you ever ridden in a Car driven by someone (including yourself) who was "high" or who had been using alcohol or drugs?

R—Do you ever use alcohol or drugs to Relax, feel better about yourself, or fit in?

A—Do you ever use alcohol or drugs while you are Alone?

F—Do you ever Forget things you did while using alcohol or drugs?

F—Do your family or Friends ever tell you that you should cut down on your drinking or drug use?

T—Have you been in Trouble while using drugs or alcohol?

*Answering "yes" to two or more questions suggests an important problem

---

BOX 5 TOXICOLOGY TESTING

"Toxicological tests of bodily fluids, usually urine but also blood, and hair samples to detect the presence of specific substances should be part of the formal evaluation and the ongoing assessment of substance use. The optimal use of urine screening requires proper collection techniques including [where possible] visualization of obtaining the sample [to ensure it is genuine], evaluation of positive results, and a specific plan of action should the specimen be positive for the presence of substance(s) . . . Because of the limited time that a drug will remain in the urine and possible adulteration, a negative result of urine testing does not [rule out drug use]."

*Taken from Bukstein et al[13]

BOX 6 MOTIVATIONAL INTERVIEWING (FRAMES)

- *Feedback*—Give structured and personalised feedback on risk and harm
- *Responsibility*—Emphasise the patient's personal responsibility for change
- *Advice*—Give clear advice to the patient to change his or her drinking habits
- *Menu*—Offer a menu of strategies for making a change in behaviour
- *Empathic*—Deliver these strategies in an empathic and non-judgmental way
- *Self efficacy*—Aim to increase the patients' confidence to change behaviour (self efficacy)[15]

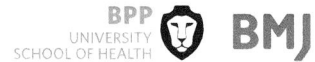

which are potentially valuable to troubled young people. The communication skills components of training could potentiate this capacity, particularly with regard to young people. Also, services working with young people need to offer continuity of care as a core feature.

An adolescent oriented service

A randomised controlled trial of 183 substance dependent adolescents showed that compared with clinic based appointments, a form of sustained flexible community outreach was linked with reduced substance use.[20] Services for adolescents could include flexible arrangements to meet, home visits, meetings in cafes, text messages, telephone calls to remind young people of appointments, and help with transport (which is crucial if some adolescents are to be engaged). This effort is required because, among those most vulnerable, lack of external routine and structure (no school, work, family, organised interests), the effects of substances, mental disorder, and perhaps learning disability may be associated with markedly poor self motivation and organisation.[21 22 w23]

Using a range of community systems

Successful intervention often requires channelling a young person away from drug using peers and lifestyle. To achieve this goal, it is often necessary to tackle obstacles such as homelessness, educational exclusion, absence of a carer, continuing mistreatment, or risk of incarceration, all of which require solutions brokered with local services.

A further key strategy is to use other networks that are designed to take the longer term strain. The components of these networks differ across jurisdictions and with age but are likely to include elements from education, social work, criminal justice, non-governmental agencies, health, and mental health. Such a multifaceted system is difficult to test in a conventional trial, but packaged multidimensional or multisystem interventions have shown sustained positive effects.[23 24]

Adjunctive interventions

Contingency management, pharmacotherapy, and motivational enhancement have been studied in healthcare settings. Voucher rewards for "clean" urine specimens and clinical attendance have been shown to be of benefit in managing addicted adults.[15] However, contingency management is expensive, and its effectiveness with younger users has not yet been adequately studied. Combining broader psychosocial and pharmacological interventions to treat adolescent addicts, as has been shown to be effective among adult alcoholics,[w21] has not yet been studied, but this might change with more medical interest in the field.

I thank the *BMJ*'s editors for their help with this article.

Contributors: PMcA is the sole contributor.

Competing interests: The author has received fees for speaking at events sponsored by the pharmaceutical industry and financial support to attend international meetings.

Provenance and peer review: Commissioned; externally peer reviewed.

1 West P, Sweeting H. Fifteen, female and stressed: changing patterns of psychological distress over time. *J Child Psychol Psychiatry Allied Disciplines* 2003;44:399-411.
2 National Insitute on Drug Abuse, National Institutes of Health, US Department of Health and Human Services. *Understanding drug abuse and addiction* . 2007. www.nida.nih.gov/Infofacts/understand.html
3 Volkow N, Wang G, Fischman M, Foltin R, Fowler J, Abumrad M, et al. Relationship between subjective effects of cocaine and dopamine transporter occupancy. *Nature* 1997;386:827-30.
4 Hibell B, Andersson B, Bjarnasson T, Ahlstrom S, Balakireva O, Kokkevi A, et al. The ESPAD Report 2003. www.sedqa.gov.mt/pdf/information/reports_intl_espad2003.pdf
5 Home Office. *Smoking, drinking and drug use among young people in England 2006: headline figures* . 2007. www.ic.nhs.uk/webfiles/publications/smokedrinkdrug06/file.pdf
6 Wittchen HU, Frohlich C, Behrendt S, Gunther A, Rehm J, Zimmermann P, et al. Cannabis use and cannabis use disorders and their relationship to mental disorders: a 10-year prospective-longitudinal community study in adolescents. *Drug Alcohol Depend* 2007;88:S60-70.
7 Fergusson D, Horwood L, Ridder E. Conduct and attentional problems in childhood and adolescence and later substance use, abuse and dependence: results of a 25 year longitudinal study. *Drug Alcohol Depend* 2007;88:S14-26.
8 Crews F, He J, Hodge C. Adolescent cortical development; a critical period of vulnerability for addiction. *Pharmacol Biochem Behav* 2007;86:189-9.
9 Hingson R, Heeren T, Winter M. Age at drinking onset and alcohol dependence. *Arch Pediatr Adolesc Med* 2006;160:739-46.

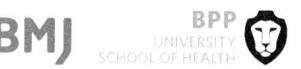

10 De Bellis M, Narasimhan A, Thatcher D, Keshavan M, Soloff P, Clark D. Prefrontal cortex, thalamus and cerebellar volumes in adolescents and young adults with adolescent-onset alcohol use disorders and comorbid mental disorders. *Alcoholism: Clinical and Experimental Research* 2005;29:1590-600.

11 Fried P, Watkinson B, Gray R. Current and former marijuana use preliminary findings of a longitudinal study of effects on IQ in young adults. *CMAJ* 2002;166:887-91.

12 Oyefeso A, Ghodse H, Clancy C, Corkery J, Goldfinch R. Drug-abuse related mortality: a study of teenage addicts over a 20 year period. *Soc Psychiatry Psych Epidemiol* 1999;34:437-41.

13 Bukstein OG, Bernet W, Arnold V, Beitchman J, Shaw J, Benson RS, et al. Practice parameter for the assessment and treatment of children and adolescents with substance use disorders. *J Am Acad Child Adolesc Psychiatry* 2005;44:609-21.

14 Knight J, Sherritt L, Schrier L, Harris S, Grace C. Validity of the CRAFFT substance abuse screening test among adolescent clinic patients. *Arch Ped Adolesc Med* 2002;156:607-14.

15 National Treatment Agency. *Drug misuse and dependence—UK guidelines on clinical management* . 2007. www.nta.nhs.uk/publications/documents/clinical_guidelines_2007.pdf

16 Spirito A, Monti P, Barnett N, Colby S, Sindelar H, Rohsenow D, et al. A randomized clinical trial of a brief motivational intervention for alcohol-positive adolescents treated in an emergency department. *J Pediatr* 2004;145:396-402.

17 McArdle P, Wiegersma A, Gilvarry E, Kolte B, McCarthy S, Fitzgerald M, et al. European adolescent substance use: the roles of family structure, function and gender. *Addiction* 2002;97:329-36.

18 Dennis M, Godley S, Diamond G, Tims F, Babor T, Donaldson J, et al. The cannabis youth treatment study: main findings from two randomised trials. *J Substance Abuse Treatment* 2004;27:197-213.

19 March J, Silva S, Petrycki S, Curry J, Wells K, Fairbank J, et al. Treatment for adolescents with depression study (TADS) randomized controlled trial. *JAMA* 2004;292:807-20.

20 Godley M, Godley S, Dennis M, Funk R, Passetti L. The effect of assertive continuing care on continuing care linkage, adherence and abstinence following residential treatment for adolescents with substance use disorders. *Addiction* 2007;102:81-3.

21 Craig TK, Hodson S. Homeless youth in London: I. Childhood antecedents and psychiatric disorder. *Psychol Med* 1998;28:1379-88.

22 Unger J, Kipke M, Simon T, Montgomery S, Johnson C. Homeless youths and young adults in Los Angeles: prevalence of mental health problems and the relationship between mental health and substance abuse disorders. *Am J Community Psychol* 1997;25:371-94.

23 Henggeler S, Halliday-Boykins C, Cunningham P, Randall J, Shapiro S, Chapman J. Juvenile drug court: enhancing outcomes by integrating evidence based treatments. *J Consult Clin Psychol* 2006;74:42-54.

24 Liddle HA, Dakof G, Parker K, Diamond G, Barrett K, Tejeda M. Multidimensional family therapy for adolescent drug abuse: results of a randomized clinical trial. *Am J Drug Alcohol Abuse* 2001;27:651-88.

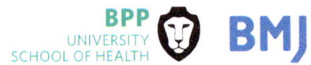

Childhood attention-deficit/hyperactivity disorder

Nienke Verkuijl, specialty trainee[1], Marian Perkins, consultant[2], Mina Fazel, NIHR postdoctoral research fellow[1], consultant[3]

[1]Department of Psychiatry, University of Oxford, Oxford OX3 7JX, UK

[2]Child and Adolescent Neuropsychiatry Service, Oxford Health NHS Foundation Trust, Oxford, UK

[3]Children's Psychological Medicine, The Children's Hospital, Oxford University Hospitals NHS Trust, Oxford, UK

Correspondence to: M Fazel mina.fazel@psych.ox.ac.uk

Cite this as: BMJ 2015;350:h2168

DOI: 10.1136/bmj.h2168

Attention-deficit/hyperactivity disorder (ADHD) is the second most common psychiatric disorder of childhood.[1] The 2010 Global Burden of Disease Study found that worldwide point prevalence rates of childhood ADHD were 2.2% in males and 0.7% in females.[2] However, the diagnosis rates of and treatment approaches to ADHD vary worldwide, which feeds some of the uncertainties that have become a hallmark of the management of ADHD.

ADHD presents with persistent and impairing symptoms of inattention, hyperactivity, and impulsivity. Children with ADHD can be negatively labelled or treated differently at school and at home, as they struggle to concentrate, sit still, and think before acting, which can make learning and functioning in a typical classroom environment challenging. Furthermore, social interactions can be difficult, leading to rejection by peers[3] and an often strained relationship with parents.[4] In combination, these factors can create secondary adversities, such as greater risk of poor school attainment and exclusion, misuse of substances, and involvement with the criminal justice system (fig 1).[5][6][7][8]

ADHD is a disorder that attracts considerable debate and controversy. Data indicate that in some areas overdiagnosis is a problem,[9] with concerns about the misuse of psychostimulants raised within the healthcare profession and elsewhere. However, the negative impact of unrecognised and untreated symptoms of severe ADHD must not be underestimated for children and their families. Both behavioural interventions and drugs improve outcomes compared with no intervention, although the functioning of affected children in the long term remains below that of their age and demographically matched peers.[7]

This review aims to provide an evidence based overview of the assessment and management of ADHD for clinicians. We also discuss some of the driving factors that may be behind the conflicting picture produced in the academic literature and popular science about ADHD, although a comprehensive assessment of these issues is beyond the scope of this review.

THE BOTTOM LINE

- ADHD is diagnosed in a child with persistent symptoms of inattention, hyperactivity, and impulsivity leading to impairment in multiple settings
- Associated problems include conduct disorder, learning difficulties, and autism spectrum disorders
- Psychosocial interventions, such as parent training and classroom interventions, can have an important role in improving self esteem, engagement with the school curriculum, and relationships with family and peers
- Drugs can improve core symptoms, school performance, and peer relationships; choice and monitoring of treatment is best conducted in specialist clinics in collaboration with primary care
- The rates of diagnosis and prescriptions of drugs for the treatment of ADHD have increased sharply in certain parts of the world and need to be better understood

What causes it?

ADHD is due to both heritable and non-heritable factors.[10] Twin studies indicate a high heritability, of around 70-80%.[11] ADHD is associated with several genes, some of which are common to other psychiatric disorders[12]; the genes are linked to dopaminergic and serotonergic pathways. Further associations with ADHD include maternal alcohol and substance misuse during pregnancy, low birth weight, prematurity, nutritional deficiencies, exposure to environmental toxins, and early psychosocial adversity.[10]

What are the current debates and controversies surrounding ADHD?

The diagnosis and treatment of ADHD have caused debate in many arenas, including within health and education professions,[13][14][15] the media, and the general public.[16] Although the core symptoms of ADHD lie at one end of the normal distribution of behaviour, a major debate has taken place as to whether ADHD is actually a disorder, and, if it is a disorder, where the diagnostic cut-off lies.[15][17] However, it is noted that a large body of family, twin, and adoption studies converge to show that ADHD is highly heritable.[17] Twin studies have consistently shown that ADHD has a heritability of around 80% for monozygotic and 40% for dizygotic twins.[10][18][19][20]

Some of the reasons for this conflicting picture include:

Variation in prevalence and treatment rates

The wide variation in reported global prevalence and treatment rates is of concern and has been described as precipitating a confidence crisis in psychiatric diagnosis.[21][22] This variation was highlighted by two studies from the United States and United Kingdom; both explored parent reported ADHD diagnosis "ever" made. The US study reported a 42% increase in ADHD diagnoses from 2003-11, with 8.8% having a current diagnosis of ADHD.[23] The UK study reported a prevalence of 1.7%, with no evidence of an increase between 1999 and 2009.[1][24] Overall, 6.1% of children in the US receive drugs for ADHD, in contrast with an estimated 0.8% in the UK.[25]

Location

Over and under diagnosis and treatment in certain geographical and population groups are additional factors. This is illustrated by the Great Smoky Mountain longitudinal study in the US. To identify those with ADHD, 4500 children were screened and those with behavioural problems were interviewed and observed as well as parent and teacher reports collected. Overall, 3.4% of the children were found to have ADHD, although 7.3% were taking psychostimulants.[9] Interestingly, children living below the poverty line were less than half as likely to receive drugs.

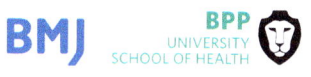

Cultural expectations of behaviour

Current diagnostic frameworks for ADHD inevitably leave a subjective element, determining the degree to which functioning is affected. There is therefore a "zone of ambiguity" affecting diagnosis.[13] [14] The judgment made by parents, teachers, and clinicians is influenced by cultural expectations of children's behaviour.[14] Recent debate has also raised the problem that psychostimulants in some countries or socioeconomic groups are being misused as cognitive enhancers for young people, for which there is some evidence in normal controls.[26] [27] [28] The clinician's role is to identify those children with a history of functional impairment as a result of attentional difficulties who might best benefit from drug treatment, balancing the benefits and potential side effects of drugs.

Classification

The two different diagnostic classification systems, the *International Classification of Diseases* (ICD) and the *Diagnostic and Statistical Manual of Mental Disorders* (DSM), may contribute to the variation in prevalence rates. This is because they each use different terms and diagnostic criteria for ADHD. When the criteria change, as in the recent move from DSM-IV to DSM-5, the changes can make comparisons between studies difficult.[14] [24] [29] The DSM is used mainly in North America and is also used internationally for research, whereas the ICD-10 is mostly used in clinical contexts outside the USA. DSM-5 utilises the term "ADHD" and has made several changes to the classification of the disorder when compared to its predecessor, whereas the ICD-10

does not use ADHD but the term "hyperkinetic disorder," which is equivalent to severe ADHD. International efforts are attempting to unify the main diagnostic categories across these two classification systems.[30]

Involvement of industry

Financial interests and constraints can contribute to the complex interplay of factors. The pharmaceutical industry is reported to have influenced the current diagnostic inflation.[21] [22] In addition, many researchers and patient support groups, as well as 37% of websites about ADHD, have received ADHD related grants from the pharmaceutical industry.[31] [32] In the USA, drugs for ADHD are heavily advertised, and pharmaceutical companies are allowed to advertise directly to potential consumers and teachers, which can also influence consumption rates.[33] Limited access to behavioural and psychological treatments may sway doctors and patients towards using drugs earlier in the ADHD management pathway. Furthermore, some health insurance policies require a diagnosis to be present for any reimbursement of treatment.[14]

Strength of the evidence base

There is a paucity of good quality experimental data on drug treatments from which to draw firm conclusions. This problem is not specific to ADHD and affects many decisions about drugs across child psychiatry, reflecting the difficulty in both securing funding and studying child populations under ideal experimental conditions.[34] Therefore areas that would benefit from a stronger evidence base include the natural progression of ADHD and numerous questions around drug treatments, including long term effects, those subgroups most likely to benefit from treatment, and longitudinal outcomes of those receiving drugs compared with other treatments.[35]

How is it assessed and diagnosed?

Making the diagnosis

Countries differ on their guidelines when stipulating who is allowed to make an ADHD diagnosis, with many countries, such as the USA and the Netherlands, having primary care physicians making the diagnosis, and other countries, such as the UK, having a paediatrician or child psychiatrist confirm a suspected diagnosis of ADHD.[36] [37]

The three core symptoms of ADHD are inattention, hyperactivity, and impulsivity. In combination these symptoms most often manifest as children struggling with schoolwork and being disorganised. Such children are often described as "constantly on the go" and have poor awareness of danger. Social interactions can be problematic because of the high level of activity, reduced awareness of others' space, impulsivity, and inability to sustain play or a conversation for longer than a few minutes. Children are susceptible to bullying or are easily encouraged to do "silly" things that get them into trouble. Parents, especially mothers, often feel blamed for their child's behaviour, which can lead either to a reluctance to approach a doctor for help or to an eagerness to seek a diagnosis.[38] [39] [40] The children may overhear negative comments, such as being described as "the most difficult" or the "worst behaved," and this can potentially impact on self esteem (fig 2).

It is important at this stage to rule out common disorders that can lead to similar presentations, such as problems with sleep, hearing, and vision.[5] Behavioural problems

Fig 1 Possible developmental impacts of attention-deficit/hyperactivity disorder

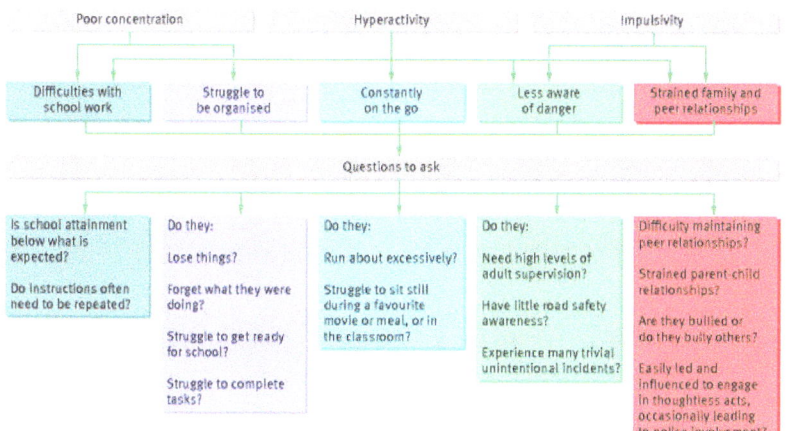

Fig 2 How to assess children for attention-deficit/hyperactivity disorder

should be of a severity to cause significant stress and disruption at home and in the classroom. If other causes are ruled out and the problems persist with moderate impairment, referral to specialist services for a diagnosis is recommended. Younger children, more commonly boys, can present with difficulties at school and, in extremis, school exclusion,[6] whereas girls have more attentional difficulties and ADHD can often remain undiagnosed until later when academic demands become greater. A referral to secondary care will be greatly aided by additional multidisciplinary reports—for example, from professionals working within the education sector, such as teachers, educational psychologists, and pastoral support staff.[36 41] Referral to a parenting course can be made for the parents of children aged less than 11 years awaiting specialist assessment. Professionals recommending a parenting course need to be mindful of implying that parents have poor parenting skills. They should instead stress that children with these difficulties often benefit from more intensive parenting.

Box 1 highlights the DSM-5 criteria for a diagnosis of ADHD. A thorough history and examination are essential to determine the correct diagnosis and assess commonly associated conditions and comorbidities (box 2).

In addition to questions on core symptoms using diagnostic criteria, the clinical interview should include:

- Presenting problems, history of difficulties, and current functioning. It should consider the children's experiences of their symptoms and include general questions around risk taking
- Pregnancy, birth history, and history of early neurodevelopment (milestones, language, attachment, sleep, feeding problems, early temperament, social-communication development)
- Medical history (tics, epilepsy, cardiac symptoms, gross and fine motor skills, vision, and hearing), drug history, and family medical history, especially cardiac, such as sudden death below 40 years or death associated with exercise
- Assessment of the level of global impairment at school, at home, and in a social context (a well validated tool for this is the Children's Global Assessment Scale)[54]

Standardised questionnaires are widely used in the assessment and management of ADHD (see table on thebmj.com). Psychometric assessments can be useful if learning or communication difficulties are present. Chromosomal analysis and functional brain imaging are not routinely recommended.

How is ADHD treated?

The management of children with ADHD has to take place within a full understanding of the severity of their current difficulties, their socio-emotional needs, family circumstances, and educational environment.[36 47] In view of the lifelong trajectory of children with severe impairments, the role and timing of drugs at different ages will need to be considered. For example, children being managed with behavioural and family strategies may be additionally supported by the use of drugs at key periods of transition or other stressors. Importantly, the management of ADHD in some families can potentially be complicated by undiagnosed and untreated ADHD in the parents.[25] Many supports available to families increasingly lie within education, social services, and the voluntary sector or the community, as well as in the healthcare setting.

Although the broad framework of assessment across the globe is relatively consistent for ADHD, countries do vary in the degree to which psychosocial interventions are prioritised compared with drug interventions, for reasons described above. The ADHD guidelines in the UK, which are broadly similar to the European and US guidelines recommend parent training programmes and behavioural strategies.[36] For severe ADHD, it is recommended that drugs should be offered alongside psychosocial interventions in children who are 6 years and older.[36 47] The recommended investigations when starting drugs are:

- Physical examination—a cardiac examination to exclude any obvious abnormalities. Baseline pulse, blood pressure, height, and weight should be recorded
- Tests—electrocardiography only if there is a medical or family history of serious cardiac disease, a history of sudden death in young family members, or abnormal findings on cardiac examination. Blood tests are not routinely recommended

Psychosocial interventions for ADHD

The evidence base for many psychosocial interventions such as parent training, social skills training, cognitive training, or specific classroom interventions is limited.[55 56 57 58 59]

Findings from a systematic review and meta-analysis in 2013 of randomised controlled trials of non-drug treatments for ADHD found no evidence for the efficacy of behavioural interventions involving children, parents, or teachers on core ADHD symptoms when using blinded assessors. There was evidence for a small but significant effect of behavioural interventions when studies used non-blinded assessors such as parents.[55]

BOX 1 DSM-5 DIAGNOSTIC CRITERIA FOR ADHD[87]

Six or more symptoms from each category are required for a diagnosis

Inattention

- Makes careless mistakes
- Has difficulty sustaining attention in tasks or play activities
- Does not seem to listen when spoken to directly
- Does not follow through on instructions and fails to finish homework
- Has trouble organising tasks and activities
- Avoids tasks that require sustained mental effort
- Loses things necessary for tasks or activities
- Easily distracted
- Forgetful

Hyperactivity and impulsivity

- Fidgets with hands or feet or squirms in seat
- Leaves seat in situations where remaining seated is expected
- Runs about or climbs excessively in situations where these are inappropriate
- Has difficulty playing or engaging in leisure activities quietly
- Talks excessively
- "On the go" or often acts as if "driven by a motor"
- Has difficulty waiting turns
- Blurts out answers before a question has been completed
- Interrupts or intrudes on others

Symptoms are

- Present for at least six months
- Presenting before age 12 years (if .17 years, only five symptoms in each category are required for a diagnosis)
- Present in at least two settings (for example, at school, at home, with friends, or in other activities) and symptoms interfere with quality of social or school functioning
- Maladaptive and inconsistent with developmental level
- Cannot be better explained by another mental disorder

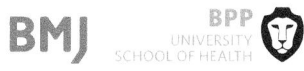

In considering the long term role of behavioural interventions compared with drugs, the Multimodal Treatment study of children with ADHD (MTA) is the largest randomised clinical trial, with eight years' follow-up.[7] The behavioural treatment studied was extensive and included parent, child, and school based elements. The drug arm consisted of tightly titrated treatment regimens. After 14 months of treatment, core ADHD symptoms were better in the drug arm than both behavioural treatment and routine community care. The combined treatment of behavioural intervention and drugs did not yield significantly greater benefits, but provided some advantages for non-ADHD symptoms such as social interactions and internalising symptoms. After 14 months the study became a naturalistic observation. At 24 months (10 months after trial completion) those children who had received a combination of drugs and behavioural management needed significantly lower drug doses.[60] At the eight year follow-up, however, the treatment groups did not differ on measures, including school attainment, criminal arrests, admissions to hospital for psychiatric disorders, or other relevant outcomes.[7] The strongest positive predictor of long term outcome was behavioural and sociodemographic advantage and having a good response to any treatment.

Psychosocial interventions have, however, been shown to play an important role in the longer term management and treatment of comorbidities associated with ADHD, which can lead to improved overall functioning of children by improving their self esteem and peer and family relationships and making it easier for them to access the school curriculum.[59]

Parent training for ADHD

Many parents report benefits from parent training, although a meta-analysis and Cochrane review have highlighted how its evidence base remains poor.[55] [57] In the UK, however, NICE guidelines recommend it as a first line treatment for children aged 3 to 11 years.[36] Parent training, as for example in the New Forest Parenting programme[61] (ADHD focused) and the Incredible Years programme (broad behavioural focus), includes psycho-education and techniques for managing challenging behaviours.[57] [62] The training is usually group based and emphasises three areas[63]:

Focus on making wanted behaviours explicit—This can be through praise and reward rather than through criticising unwanted behaviour, such as telling children to sit down instead of shouting at them to stop being naughty, and by ignoring screaming and tantrums. A more positive relationship can be promoted through activities such as play.

Making a clear set of rules for the family—The rules should be explicit, succinct, and consistently enforced by parents. Disobedience and aggression need to be firmly and calmly dealt with—for example, by temporarily removing children from a situation.

Anticipating potentially difficult times of the day—In the context of busy family life, this entails proactively placing structure, distraction, or different activities at these times—for example, during key transitions, such as when returning home from school.

Social skills training

Social skills training includes learning appropriate verbal and non-verbal communication in social situations, understanding how to share and take turns, listening, and recognising other people's emotions. A recent Cochrane review on social skills training for children aged 5-18 years with ADHD found no evidence for or against this type of training.[56] This may be because the deficit in children with ADHD is not in their social knowledge but in acting on a thought or idea before thinking about the consequences of this behaviour.[64]

Cognitive training and cognitive behavioural therapy

Cognitive training involves the training of attention and working memory, which are often considered part of "executive function." A systematic review and meta-analysis of randomised controlled trials of cognitive training for ADHD symptoms found no evidence of efficacy when using "probably" blinded assessors.[55] Cognitive training was found to be effective when non-blinded assessors were used. For cognitive behavioural therapy (CBT), a review of the literature in 2010 found no studies indicating that CBT was helpful for ADHD symptoms in children.[58] However, evidence from a subsequent non-randomised controlled trial indicates that CBT may be helpful for adolescents

---

BOX 2 COMORBIDITIES AND ASSOCIATED CONDITIONS IN ADHD

Oppositional defiant disorder and conduct disorder
The defiant and aggressive behaviour that defines oppositional defiant disorder and the more severe conduct disorder, is highly comorbid with ADHD,[42] and distinguishing between the two disorders can be difficult as the impulsivity that comes with ADHD often makes children act aggressively. Careful teasing out of the core symptoms of ADHD will enable differentiation

Autism spectrum disorder
Estimations vary substantially but prevalence rates of 20-50% have been reported for children with ADHD also meeting criteria for autism spectrum disorder.[43] It is therefore essential to include screening questions such as how able is the child to appreciate another person's perspective

Tic disorders
Compared with controls, children with ADHD are at an increased risk of developing tic disorders[42]

Poor motor coordination
ADHD is often accompanied by delays in motor milestones, difficulties with writing, clumsiness, and poor performance in sports[44]

Specific learning difficulties
Dyslexia is commonly associated with ADHD. Reading comprehension is reduced in children with ADHD; linked to deficits in working memory[45]

Sleep disorders
Sleep disorders are commonly associated with ADHD and often overlooked.[46] It is important to determine whether there is a primary sleep disorder leading to problems with attention and concentration or whether the child has trouble settling to sleep because of ADHD. In the history it is also important to rule out obstructive sleep apnoea

Emotional disorders
Anxiety and depression are often concomitant with ADHD.[42] These symptoms may be related to ADHD or problems in interpersonal relationships

Early adversity
Prolonged disruption of relationships in early childhood can lead to attachment disorders. These may present as indiscriminate behaviours towards adults and peers and inattentive behaviours that resemble ADHD.[47] However, having an attachment disorder does not rule out ADHD. Children who have experienced extreme institutional deprivation, as in the case of the Romanian orphans, have both significantly increased levels of inattention and overactivity and disinhibited attachment.[48] It is unclear whether less extreme forms of deprivation are associated with ADHD[49]

Bipolar disorder
Controversial studies indicate a large overlap between bipolar disorder in children and ADHD,[50] [51] with no consensus on treatment implications

Substance use disorder
ADHD is present in almost a quarter of adults with substance use disorder,[52] with patterns of misuse often starting in adolescence

Fetal alcohol syndrome
ADHD symptoms are seen in children with fetal alcohol syndrome and the hyperactivity symptoms often respond to ADHD drugs[53]

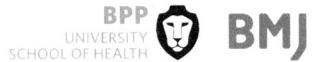

BOX 3 MANAGING THE ADVERSE EFFECTS OF DRUG TREATMENT

Neurological

Headaches, irritability, and dizziness

- Disappear spontaneously or on dose reduction[36]

Insomnia

- Evidence is inconsistent and clinical experience suggests that there is considerable individual variability in how children's sleep is affected: some experience no effect while others can settle more easily a few hours after taking psychostimulants and some are unable to sleep because of the stimulating effects of the drugs and so will need to either change the drug or ensure shorter acting preparations are taken[77 80]

Tics

- Not a contraindication to drug treatment, tics can sometimes be worsened by psychostimulant drugs and can be improved by atomoxetine.[77] Observe over three months, as the natural, fluctuating course of tics can lead them to be more and less prominent over time, independent of drugs

Epilepsy

- ADHD drugs lower the seizure threshold but can be used in children with established epilepsy with specialist monitoring[77]

Cardiovascular

Blood pressure

- All ADHD drugs have the potential to increase blood pressure and pulse and so both must be routinely monitored. In most cases the changes are small (average increases of 1-4 mm Hg for systolic and 1-2 mm Hg for diastolic pressure and 1-2 beats/min for pulse), however in a subset of children (5-15%) the increases in blood pressure and pulse may be above the 95th centile (measured three times within one visit with an age adjusted cuff) and children should be referred to specialist care[81]

Severe cardiovascular events

- Children with a congenital heart defect, a history of cardiac symptoms (for example, syncope on exercise), or a positive family history of sudden death below the age of 40 years, are at risk of sudden death.[77] For these children extra caution needs to be taken with ADHD drugs and the involvement of a paediatric cardiologist is needed

Gastrointestinal

Nausea

- Can disappear spontaneously or on dose reduction

Weight loss and reduced appetite

- Psychostimulants reduce appetite with weight loss usually most pronounced in the first six months of treatment.[82] Drugs are therefore best taken with or after food (advise additional snacks early in the morning or late in the evening)

Liver damage

- May be a rare, idiosyncratic, and mostly reversible effect of atomoxetine.[83] Routine blood screening and monitoring are not recommended but advise seeking urgent medical opinion if abdominal pain, nausea, dark urine, or jaundice emerge[36]

Growth

Reduced height

- Variable effect of psychostimulants on growth, with a delay of approximately 1 cm/year in the first three years. The effect may be dose dependent and reversible when treatment is stopped. It is unclear whether stimulants have an effect on final adult height. Atomoxetine has similar effects on growth to stimulants.[84] If height measurements drop on the centile charts then a dose reduction is recommended, as can be switching to an alternative formulation or including some drug holidays in the treatment regimen. If height is significantly affected then referral to an endocrinologist is warranted[77]

Psychological symptoms

Psychotic symptoms

- Very rarely delusions, hallucinations, and mania can emerge during treatment[77]

Suicidal thoughts

- There is a reported slight increase in suicidal thoughts when starting atomoxetine; therefore mood must be monitored on initiation of treatment. Suicidal thoughts are not a contraindication to treatment, but dose reduction might be warranted[77]

Other

Drug misuse

- There is no evidence that treatment with psychostimulants increases the risk for later drug misuse.[85] A subsample of children with ADHD may be prone to misuse of psychostimulants. Dexamphetamine has the highest potential for misuse, and, in high risk cases, modified release methylphenidate, lisdexamfetamine, or atomoxetine should be considered[77]

Sexual dysfunction

- Erectile and ejaculatory dysfunction and dysmenorrhoea are potential side effects of atomoxetine

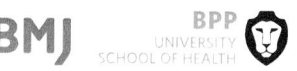

Table 1 Evidence for non-drug treatment for attention-deficit/hyperactivity disorder (ADHD)

Treatment	Level of evidence	Evidence
Parent training	1*	Insufficient evidence[55]
Cognitive training	1	More evidence needed[55]
Cognitive behavioural therapy	3†	Shown to be effective in adolescents receiving ADHD drug treatments[65]
Social skills training	1	Insufficient evidence[56]
Free fatty acid supplementation	1	Small but significant effects; clinical significance to be determined[55]
Artificial food colour exclusion	1	Statistically significant, modest effects on ADHD symptoms[55]
Restricted elimination diets	1	Insufficient evidence[55]

Levels of evidence from Oxford Centre for Evidence Based Medicine, 2011.
*Evidence from meta-analysis of randomised controlled trial.
†Evidence from non-randomised controlled cohort studies.

with ADHD who are receiving drugs and have residual difficulties.[65] The effects were better for adolescents with comorbid anxiety and depression compared with those with comorbid conduct disorder or oppositional defiant disorder.

Classroom interventions

In traditional educational settings, children with ADHD can struggle to control their behaviour, achieve academically, and manage peer relationships.[64] There is some evidence for the positive effects of school based intervention, although contextual factors and the perceptions of students and staff play an important role.[66] Advice for teachers has been shown to be useful in managing children with ADHD, delivered, for example, in leaflets, with significant positive effects on attitudes and behaviour but not on attainment.[67] Examples of effective classroom strategies include giving pupils a choice of two or more concurrently presented classroom activities,[67] sitting pupils near teachers so that they can be prompted if attention wanders, breaking down tasks and instructions,[64] and using immediate rewards (stickers or points) for wanted behaviour and mild penalties when "off task."[68] Teachers find using daily report cards, which enhance teacher-parent collaboration, a useful intervention.[66] A further study has shown how certain types of movement, for example sitting on an activity ball, can actually assist in focusing a child's attention, contrary to concerns that such activity might exacerbate inattention.[69] There have been some positive academic effects with a class peer tutoring system.[70] There is no evidence that classroom social skills training helps peer interactions for those with ADHD,[56] but peer mediated resolution of conflicts has been associated with school-wide reductions in playground violence and negative interactions.[71] Class-wide interventions—for example, to reduce distraction—are probably the least stigmatising to implement.[66]

Dietary advice

The importance of a healthy, balanced diet and regular exercise needs to be emphasised for all children, including those with ADHD. If there is a history suggesting the negative influence of certain foods then a food diary can help to determine these links. In the UK, NICE recommends that when certain foods are linked with difficult behaviour then specific elimination diets should be jointly managed by a dietician and the treating specialist.[36] A randomised controlled trial using non-blinded assessors (parents) suggests that a "restricted elimination diet," whereby the diet was reduced to a few basic foods and then gradually broadened to assess other foods, found a dramatic reduction in ADHD symptoms in children not receiving drugs.[72] However, a subsequent systematic review and

meta-analysis of randomised controlled trials using blinded assessors found insufficient evidence for the efficacy of restricted elimination diets,[55] although the exclusion of artificial food colourants had a moderate positive effect on ADHD symptoms. The authors commented that children in both the restricted elimination diet and the artificial food colour exclusion trials were often preselected on the basis of sensitivity to certain food types, so the positive results may be applicable only to children with suspected food sensitivities.[55] The use of free fatty acid supplementation can benefit some children with ADHD, as supported by the same meta-analysis of randomised controlled trials, with an effect size around 0.3, which is significant but small compared with drugs, which can have effect sizes of 0.7-1.0.[55] We have summarised the evidence for non-drug treatment for ADHD in table 1.

Drugs

Drugs can improve the three core symptoms of inattention, overactivity, and impulsivity,[36] and there is evidence from randomised controlled trials to support the use of drugs for symptomatic and functional improvement in the short term. As described above, children without ADHD treated with drugs also show improvements in attention and focus,[27][28] leading to drugs being considered performance enhancing rather than as specific treatment for the psychopathology of ADHD.[34]

There are two main groups of clinically effective drugs for ADHD: psychostimulants, which increase available central dopamine and noradrenaline (for example, methylphenidate and dexamfetamine), and others, which include noradrenergic reuptake inhibitors (for example, atomoxetine). The choice of drug depends on the needs of the young person, formulation of the drug, ratio of immediate to extended release components, side effect profile, and cost (table 2).

A systematic review of randomised controlled trials provides evidence that psychostimulants and atomoxetine improve the core symptoms of ADHD and improve quality of life, although limitations of the studies for dexamphetamine and methylphenidate were noted.[73] Short and long acting formulations of methylphenidate have been found to be equally effective.[74] The overall effect size for methylphenidate is estimated at 1.0[75] and for atomoxetine at 0.7,[76] with other studies reporting a number needed to treat of 3 for methylphenidate (extended release) and 5 for atomoxetine.[74] A few studies have explored the experiences of children with ADHD receiving drugs—for example, one small study reported generally positive experiences of treatment.[36] The children described putting up with the "annoying" aspects of drugs in return for improved relationships with peers as a result of less disruptive behaviour. The more common adverse effects of drugs for ADHD are nausea, headaches, sleep problems, slight increases in heart rate and blood pressure, and decreased appetite with associated weight loss and reduction in height; more details are provided in box 3.[77]

Although there is evidence that current and active psychostimulant treatment (of any duration) is associated with symptomatic and functional improvement, longer term follow-up studies were not able to show beneficial effects of stimulant use on ADHD symptoms and overall functioning in the longer term.[78] None of the studies accounted for the variable course of the disorder over childhood, drug adherence, and selection bias in treatment.[35]

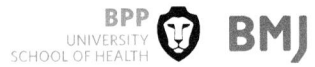

Table 2 Drugs and dosage for treating attention-deficit/hyperactivity disorder (ADHD)[86]

	Dexamphetamine	Lisdexamfetamine Elvanse (Shire, UK)	Methylphenidate Ritalin (Novartis, Switzerland) or methylphenidate hydrochloride	Medikinet XL (Medice, Germany)	Equasym XL (UCB Pharma, Belgium)	Concerta XL Janssen-Cilag, USA)	Atomoxetine (Strattera; Eli Lilly, USA)
Formulation	Tablet	Capsule, dissolvable	Tablet*	Capsule†	Capsule‡	Tablet	Capsule
Immediate release: extended release ratio of methylphenidate			100% immediate release	50% immediate release, 50% extended release	30% immediate release, 70% extended release	22% immediate release, 78% extended release	
Approximate duration of action (hours)	4	13	4	8	8	12	24
Titration, starting dose	2.5 mg 2-3 times a day	30 mg	5 mg 1-2 times a day	5-10 mg	10 mg/day	18 mg/day	<70 kg 0.5 mg/kg/day for 7 days
Titration, weekly increase	5 mg a day	20 mg	5-10 mg	10 mg	10 mg	9-18 mg	As much as 1.2 mg/kg/day
Equivalent daily dose of 30mg methylphenidate hydrochloride	15 mg		30 mg	30 mg	30 mg	36 mg	NA, must follow atomoxetine protocol
Frequency of dose/day	2-3	1	2-3	1	1	1	1 or 2 divided doses
Maximum licensed dose/day	20 mg	70 mg	60 mg	60 mg	60 mg	54 mg	<70 kg, 1.8 mg/kg/day
Controlled drug	Yes	Yes	Yes	Yes	Yes	Yes	No
Approximate cost for 30 tablets (UK 2015 rates)	£26 (5 mg)	£62 (30 mg)	£5.50 (10 mg)	£25 (10 mg)	£25 (10 mg)	£31 (18 mg)	£67 (10 mg)
Other		Licensed in Europe for those with inadequate response to methylphenidate				Continuation license for adult use	

*Can be crushed, put in water, and drunk straight away.

†Can be sprinkled over tablespoon of apple sauce or yogurt (then swallowed without chewing).

‡Can be sprinkled over tablespoon of apple sauce (then swallowed without chewing).

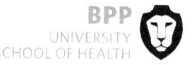

Table 3 How to manage different drugs for attention-deficit/hyperactivity disorder (ADHD)

Drug	General comments	How to start	How to change and stop
Short acting methylphenidate	Allows greatest flexibility to adjust the drug to the needs of children over the course of a day. Administering the drug away from home can be difficult. Parents can top-up with additional doses at their discretion; for example, when children attend clubs after school	Younger children could start on a single morning dose of 5 mg, with gradual dose increases until a response is observed. The same process can then be started for the afternoon dose, as different doses are often needed throughout the day	Can do a straight swap to closest equivalent dose of long acting (usually to lower of two doses if a choice exists). Relatively simple to stop as can reduce doses quickly, with higher doses needing to be tailed off.
Long acting methylphenidate	Preparations can cover the school day and are simpler as they do not need to be taken at school and might improve compliance in older children. Can cover just the school day or longer, depending on which preparation chosen	Often first line treatment with older children to avoid the complexities of adjusting doses (which can negatively impact on compliance). Treatment should start at the lowest possible dose and be reassessed weekly to fortnightly	Straight swap possible to closest equivalent dose from short to long acting (lower dose if choice exists). Relatively simple to stop as can lower doses quickly, with higher doses needing to be tailed off
Atomoxetine	Can be considered if preferred by parents or child or if psychostimulants are contraindicated. It can take longer to exert a beneficial effect and can adversely affect mood	If changing from methylphenidate, ideal to reassess baseline ADHD symptoms and side effects that might have been attributed to methylphenidate by stopping drug for at least two weeks. Can gather useful information on classroom functioning if change made during school term. Can dovetail with methylphenidate if symptoms cannot be tolerated without any drugs	Can slowly reduce by taking drug on alternate days or reducing the dose over 2-4 weeks depending on the length of time it has been taken and the dose

---

A YOUNG PERSON'S STORY

I wasn't diagnosed until I was 11 when my family moved and I had to repeat a school year. I had performed well in a well-structured parochial school but started to slide when put in a more loosely structured school. I was prescribed medication for ADHD and given counselling on how to best organise and manage my time.

I never liked to be medicated (methylphenidate); the drugs gave me a dull and disconnected sense where I felt a physical distance between others and myself. My resistance to taking medication caused an ongoing fight between my mother and me. She wanted the best for me and bought me a fancy watch with five separate alarms to help me remember to take my meds.

In secondary school I learned to manage my ADHD: I used natural stimulants like coffee, began to meditate, and participated in attention intensive sports like rowing. These practices, along with the strategies I had learned to organise my time, helped me cope. At university I abandoned medication altogether when I was tempted to use it as a diet aid. Now, 17 years since diagnosis, I don't take medicine at all, though I think it would have been helpful at times during graduate school. I've found that things that fall inside my organisational structures get done quite well, and I'm surprised when employers laud my organisational skills, which are strong enough to organise whole teams and offices.

My family has not adapted to my increased capacities, and I find that interesting and sometimes very challenging. That said, if it's not on the list, it's likely not going to get done any time soon. And if I'm in between the notebooks I keep my list in, little's going to be accomplished.

A PARENT'S STORY

In our son's last few years of school we realised that normal school challenges had become major challenges for him. Although he had managed an extremely busy school schedule, as school pressures increased we noticed that he had to work into the night to keep up with his studies. His normal fidgetiness and procrastination had become completely unmanageable. He would start new tasks before finishing others. His thoughts were scattered. He could not maintain focus for more than 10 minutes without getting up to snack or take a break. After six hours on an assignment he would have completed only 2-3 sentences.

For the first time our son lost his self esteem. He started to remark that he wasn't as smart as his classmates. I remember him telling me that sometimes he had to just stare at a blank white wall for 15 minutes to clear his mind.

Following medical review he was prescribed Concerta. Overnight his thoughts became more focused, he started to work methodically through his assignments, and normal sleep patterns came back. Most importantly, our son regained his sense of self esteem.

At university our son never lost the feeling that he should try and conquer ADHD without the benefit of medication. He began to realise that his ADHD symptoms were much more pronounced when he was forced to fulfill an academic requirement not in his core competencies. A physician counselled him to use Concerta selectively, to get through the more arduous tasks. She also helped him re-frame his perception of the condition not as a disability but as a special trait, which bestowed significant benefits on the aesthetic career path he had chosen.

QUESTIONS FOR FUTURE RESEARCH

- What is the optimal duration for drug treatments and what are their long term effects?
- What are the best classroom strategies for managing ADHD, and how can they be implemented to support children and staff?
- Is parent training best delivered individually or in groups and is it more effective for certain clusters of symptoms?
- Can treatments be tailored for specific subgroups with ADHD?
- Does screening for ADHD and associated comorbidities play a role for school children at risk of exclusion or poor academic attainment?
- Is there a role for games, apps, and digital media in the management of ADHD?
- What are the long term outcomes of ADHD when children become adults, and which are the best treatment options for adults?

SOURCES AND SELECTION CRITERIA

We searched PubMed for meta-analyses, systematic reviews, and randomised controlled trials on epidemiology and drug and non-drug treatments of ADHD published from January 2004 to December 2013 (and updated December 2014). We also read the national and international guidelines for ADHD by the National Institute for Health and Care Excellence, the European Guidelines for Hyperkinetic Disorders, the American Academy of Pediatrics, and the American Academy of Child and Adolescent Psychiatry. Further landmark studies were added, and we also sought additional expert opinion.

HOW PATIENTS WERE INVOLVED IN THE CREATION OF THIS ARTICLE

We sought accounts from children, adolescents, and young adults with ADHD and their parents on their experience of healthcare and include some of these accounts as part of this review to provide essential information on the perceptions of drugs and care. This review was changed as a result of child and parent feedback, with greater emphasis then placed on different treatments and more information given on different drugs, as these were common areas of uncertainty.

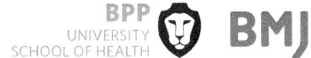

ADDITIONAL EDUCATIONAL RESOURCES

Resources for healthcare professionals

- National Institute for Health and Care Excellence guideline. Attention deficit hyperactivity disorder: diagnosis and management of ADHD in children, young people and adults (www.nice.org.uk/CG72)—evidence based guidelines on ADHD management in the UK
- Cortese S, Holtmann M, Banaschewski T, et al. Current best practice in management of adverse events during treatment with ADHD medication in children and adolescents. *J Child Psychol Psychiatry* 2013;54:227-46. http://onlinelibrary.wiley.com/doi/10.1111/jcpp.12036/epdf—guidelines on management of adverse effects of medication produced on behalf of the European ADHD Guidelines Group
- The NIMH-funded Multimodal Treatment of Attention Deficit Hyperactivity Disorder (MTA) study (www.nimh.nih.gov/funding/clinical-trials-for-researchers/practical/mta/multimodal-treatment-of-attention-deficit-hyperactivity-disorder-mta-study.shtml)—a multisite study designed to evaluate the main interventions for ADHD, including behavior therapy, drugs, and the combination of the two. First study published in 1999 and follow-up continues

Resources for young people and their families

- The National Attention Deficit Disorder Information and Support Service UK. ADDISS (www.addiss.co.uk/)—a patient and parent support organization
- Young minds (www.youngminds.org.uk/for_children_young_people/whats_worrying_you/adhd)—information on ADHD tailored for young people
- American Academy of Child and Adolescent Psychiatry and American Psychiatric Association (www.parentsmedguide.org/pmg_adhd.html)—ADHD drug information for parents
- NHS choices. Attention Deficit Hyperactivity Disorder (ADHD) (www.nhs.uk/conditions/Attention-deficit-hyperactivity-disorder/Pages/Introduction.aspx)—includes a video clip of an interview between a psychiatrist and a child with ADHD and his parents
- Green C, Chee K. Understanding ADHD. A parent's guide to attention deficit hyperactivity disorder in children. Vermilion, 1997–a book with useful information and helpful strategies for parents and teachers
- Hoopman K. All dogs have ADHD. Jessica Kingsley, 2008–a useful, light hearted book illustrating some aspects of ADHD
- www.healthline.com/health-slideshow/top-adhd-android-iphone-apps—a review of some of the ADHD apps available in 2015. Healthline (www.healthline.com/health/adhd)—has information and links to a range of blogs on ADHD and selected videos on YouTube and Tedx for young people and their families
- ADHDVoices. YouTube. What's it like to have ADHD? (www.youtube.com/watch?v=Hl7Ro1PUJmE)—short animated video of what it is like to have ADHD from a young person's perspective

In light of the evidence on the effectiveness of drugs for ADHD, the choice to start treatment should primarily be considered in severe cases where impairment is demonstrable in multiple areas of the child's life. An honest discussion with parents and older children about the benefits and uncertainties of treatment and possible adverse effects is recommended.

Initiation, titration, and monitoring of drug treatment

When drug treatment for ADHD is initiated and monitored in secondary care by child psychiatrists or paediatricians, primary care professionals have an important role in alerting overseeing specialists to problems in the overall treatment plan, such as non-compliance, or in expediting a review of the current treatment plan if difficulties arise. NICE recommends (based on effectiveness, side effect profile, and cost) methylphenidate as first line treatment for severe ADHD, followed by atomoxetine and then dexamphetamine.[36]

Initiation—Treatment regimens usually start with immediate release methylphenidate.[36] Once-daily doses, although more costly, may be more practical and less stigmatising, and as psychostimulants are controlled drugs some schools do not want to administer them. Different preparations of immediate release and extended release are available (table 2) enabling flexibility if, for example, only the school day needs to be targeted or additional evening doses are required.

Titration—Response to treatment is initially monitored and titrated closely to determine the optimal dose, which should ideally be reached within a few weeks.[36]

Monitoring—Careful and systematic follow-up of children taking psychotropic drugs is of utmost importance. There should be clinical follow-up to monitor the psychological and behavioural effects of drugs after each change in dose, then at three months and routinely every six months, when height, weight, heart rate, and blood pressure should also be recorded (see box 3). These reviews should also include information from teachers to establish how well the symptoms are being controlled at school. Rating scales can be used to monitor clinical and behavioural change (see table on thebmj.com for examples of ADHD rating scales).[79]

Duration of treatment and managing comorbidities

After an adequate treatment response, drug treatment should be continued for as long as it remains effective, with at least biannual review. Drug holidays are not routinely recommended. The decision as and when to stop drugs is one that must be informed by what the children and parents want along with clinically perceived efficacy of treatment. If children no longer want to take drugs or the parents think they would like their child to try a period without drugs, then it is important to support this request. Drugs should ideally not be stopped at times of transition or increased stress (for example, when moving schools or sitting examinations), and summer holidays can be an opportune time for dose reduction. Table 3 provides more information on how to manage different drugs.

Often specialist advice is needed in the drug treatment of psychiatric comorbidities. Selective serotonin reuptake inhibitors for depression and some anxiety disorders are tolerated with methylphenidate. For sleep disorders, sleep hygiene should be considered a first line treatment, and specialist drug intervention, such as melatonin, may be useful, but only under specialist care.

We thank David Coghill, Tamsin Ford, Brian Green, Sandra Hallett, Ilja Holland-Kaye, Alison Maycock, Neysan Pucks, and Ruth Reed for helpful comments on earlier drafts of the review; the reviewers for their thoughtful and comprehensive comments; the BMJ editors who provided considerable input to the review, and all who in combination contributed to a much improved publication. We are grateful for permission from Professor Asherson and UKAAN for allowing us to revise a slide on ADHD impact. We thank the young adult and parent who kindly shared their experience with us.

Contributors: NV analysed the data. MF and NV wrote the first draft of the review. NV, MF, and MP revised drafts of the paper. MF is the guarantor.

Competing interests: We have read and understood the BMJ policy on declaration of interests and declare the following: none.

Provenance and peer review: Not commissioned; externally peer reviewed.

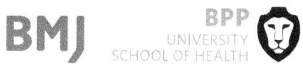

1   Ford T, Goodman R, Meltzer H. The British Child and Adolescent Mental Health Survey 1999: the prevalence of DSM-IV disorders. J Am Acad Child Adolesc Psychiatry2003;42:1203-11.

2   Erskine HE, Ferrari AJ, Nelson P, et al. Epidemiological modelling of attention-deficit/hyperactivity disorder and conduct disorder for the Global Burden of Disease Study 2010. J Child Psychol Psychiatry2013;54:1263-74.

3   Gardner DM, Gerdes AC. A review of peer relationships and friendships in youth with ADHD. J Atten Disord2013; published online 23 Sep.

4   Pimentel MJ, Vieira-Santos S, Santos V, et al. Mothers of children with attention deficit/hyperactivity disorder: relationship among parenting stress, parental practices and child behaviour. Atten Defic Hyperact Disord2011;3:61-8.

5   Babinski LM, Hartsough CS, Lambert NM. Childhood conduct problems, hyperactivity-impulsivity, and inattention as predictors of adult criminal activity. J Child Psychol Psychiatry1999;40:347-55.

6   Parker C, Whear R, Ukoumunne OC, et al. School exclusion in children with psychiatric disorder or impairing psychopathology: a systematic review. Emot Behav Difficult2014; published online 20 Aug. doi:10.1080/13632752.2014.945741.

7   Molina BS, Hinshaw SP, Swanson JM, et al. The MTA at 8 years: prospective follow-up of children treated for combined-type ADHD in a multisite study. J Am Acad Child Adolesc Psychiatry2009;48:484-500.

8   Sayal E, Washbrook E, Propper C. Childhood behavior problems and academic outcomes in adolescence: longitudinal population-based study. J Am Acad Child Adolesc Psychiatry2015;54:360-8.

9   Angold A, Erkanli A, Egger HL, et al. Stimulant treatment for children: a community perspective. J Am Acad Child Adolesc Psychiatry2000;39:975-84.

10 Thapar A, Cooper M, Eyre O, et al. Practitioner review: what have we learnt about the causes of ADHD? J Child Psychol Psychiatry2013;54:3-16.

11 Faraone SV, Perlis RH, Doyle AE, et al. Molecular genetics of attention-deficit/ hyperactivity disorder. Biol Psychiatry2005;57:1313-23.

12 Cross-Disorder Group of the Psychiatric Genomics Consortium. Identification of risk loci with shared effects on five major psychiatric disorders: a genome-wide analysis. Lancet2013;381:1371-9.

13 Shah PJ, Morton MJ. Adults with attention-deficit hyperactivity disorder—diagnosis or normality? Br J Psychiatry2013;203:317-9.

14 Parens E, Johnston J. Facts, values, and attention-deficit hyperactivity disorder (ADHD): an update on the controversies. Child Adolesc Psychiatry Ment Health2009;3:1.

15 Batstra L, Nieweg EH, Hadders-Algra M. Exploring five common assumptions on attention deficit hyperactivity disorder. Acta Paediatr2014;103:696-700.

16 Schwarz A, Cohen S. A.D.H.D. seen in 11% of U.S. children as diagnoses rise. New York Times2013 Mar 31.

17 Asherson P, Trzaskowski M. Attention-deficit/hyperactivity disorder is the extreme and impairing tail of a continuum. J Am Acad Child Adolesc Psychiatry2015;54:249-50.

18 Levy F, Hay DA, McStephen M, et al. Attention-deficit hyperactivity disorder: a category or a continuum? Genetic analysis of a large-scale twin study. J Am Acad Child Adolesc Psychiatry1997;36:737-44.

19 Stergiakouli E, Martin J, Hamshere ML, et al. Shared genetic influences between Attention-Deficit/ Hyperactivity Disorder (ADHD) traits in children and clinical ADHD. J Am Acad Child Adolesc Psychiatry2015;54:322-7.

20 Larsson H, Anckarsater H, Råstam M, et al. Childhood attention-deficit hyperactivity disorder as an extreme of a continuous trait: a quantitative genetic study of 8,500 twin pairs. J Child Psychol Psychiatry2012;53:73-80.

21 Frances A. The past, present and future of psychiatric diagnosis. World Psychiatry 2013;12:111-2.

22 Monynihan R. A new deal on disease definition. BMJ2011;342:1136.

23 Visser SN, Danielson ML, Bitsko RH, et al. Trends in the parent-report of health care provider-diagnosed and medicated attention-deficit/ hyperactivity disorder: United States, 2003-2011. J Am Acad Child Adolesc Psychiatry2014;53:34-46.

24 Russell G, Rodgers LR, Ukoumunne OC, et al. Prevalence of parent-reported ASD and ADHD in the UK: findings from the Millennium Cohort Study. J Autism Dev Disord2014;44:31-40.

25 McCarthy S, Wilton L, Murray ML, et al. The epidemiology of pharmacologically treated attention deficit hyperactivity disorder (ADHD) in children, adolescents and adults in UK primary care. BMC Pediatr2012;12:78.

26 Singh I, Filipe AM, Bard I, et al. Globalization and cognitive enhancement: emerging social and ethical challenges for ADHD clinicians. Curr Psychiatry Rep2013;15:385.

27 Rapoport JL, Buchsbaum MS, Weingartner H, et al. Dextroamphetamine. Its cognitive and behavioral effects in normal and hyperactive boys and normal men. Arch Gen Psychiatry1980;37:933-43.

28 Del Campo N, Fryer TD, Hong YTA, et al. Positron emission tomography study of nigro-striatal dopaminergic mechanisms underlying attention: implications for ADHD and its treatment. Br ain2013;136:3252-70.

29 Swanson JM, Sergeant JA, Taylor E, et al. Attention-deficit hyperactivity disorder and hyperkinetic disorder. Lancet1998;351:429-33.

30 First MB. Harmonisation of ICD-11 and DSM-V: opportunities and challenges. Br J Psychiatry2009;195:382-90.

31 Moncrieff J, Timimi S. The social and cultural construction of psychiatric knowledge: an analysis of NICE guidelines on depression and ADHD. Anthropol Med2013;20:59-71.

32 Mitchell J, Read J. Attention-deficit hyperactivity disorder, drug companies and the internet. Clin Child Psychol Psychiatry2012;17:121-39.

33 INCB. Report of the International Narcotics Control Board 2013. New York: United Nations, 2014.

34 Singh I. Beyond polemics: science and ethics of ADHD. Nat Rev Neurosci2008;9:957-64.

35 Hazell P. The challenges to demonstrating long-term effects of psychostimulant treatment for attention-deficit/hyperactivity disorder. Curr Opin Psychiatry2011;24:286-90.

36 National Institute for Health and Care Excellence. Attention deficit hyperactivity disorder: diagnosis and management of ADHD in children, young people and adults. (Clinical guideline C72.) 2008, modified 2013. www.nice.org.uk/guidance/CG72.

37 American Academy of Pediatrics. ADHD: clinical practice guideline for the diagnosis, evaluation, and treatment of attention-deficit/hyperactivity disorder in children and adolescents. Pediatrics2011;128:1007-22.

38 Klasen H, Goodman R. Parents and GPs at cross-purposes over hyperactivity: a qualitative study of possible barriers to treatment. Br J Gen Pract2000;50:199-202.

39 Singh I. Doing their jobs: mothering with Ritalin in a culture of mother-blame. Soc Sci Med2004;59:1193-205.

40 Sayal K, Taylor E, Beecham J, et al. Pathways to care in children at risk of attention-deficit hyperactivity disorder. Br J Psychiatry 2002;181:43-8.

41 Sayal K, Goodman R, Ford T. Barriers to the identification of children with attention deficit/hyperactivity disorder. J Child Psychol Psychiatry 2006;47:744-50.

42 Yoshimasu K, Barbaresi WJ, Colligan RC, et al. Childhood ADHD is strongly associated with a broad range of psychiatric disorders during adolescence: a population-based birth cohort study. J Child Psychol Psychiatry2012;53:1036-43.

43 Rommelse NN, Franke B, Geurts HM, et al. Shared heritability of attention-deficit/hyperactivity disorder and autism spectrum disorder. Eur Child Adolesc Psychiatry2010;19:281-95.

44 Fliers E, Vermeulen S, Rijsdijk F, et al. ADHD and poor motor performance from a family genetic perspective. J Am Acad Child Adolesc Psychiatry2009;48:25-34.

45 Miller AC, Keenan JM, Betjemann RS, et al. Reading comprehension in children with ADHD: cognitive underpinnings of the centrality deficit. J Abnorm Child Psychol2013;41:473-83.

46 Sung V, Hiscock H, Sciberras E, et al. Sleep problems in children with attention-deficit/hyperactivity disorder: prevalence and the effect on the child and family. Arch Pediatr Adolesc Med2008;162:336-42.

47 Taylor E, Dopfner M, Sergeant J, et al. European clinical guidelines for hyperkinetic disorder—first upgrade. Eur Child Adolesc Psychiatry2004;13(Suppl 1):I7-30.

48 Rutter M, Beckett C, Castle J, et al. Effects of profound early institutional deprivation: an overview of findings from a UK longitudinal study of Romanian adoptees. Eur J Dev Psychol2007;4:332-50.

49 Kreppner JM, Rutter M, Beckett C, et al. Normality and impairment following profound early institutional deprivation: a longitudinal follow-up into early adolescence. Dev Psychol2007;43:931-46.

50 Biederman J, Faraone S, Mick E, et al. Attention-deficit hyperactivity disorder and juvenile mania: an overlooked comorbidity? J Am Acad Child Adolesc Psychiatry1996;35:997-1008.

51 Hassan A, Agha SS, Langley K, et al. Prevalence of bipolar disorder in children and adolescents with attention-deficit hyperactivity disorder. Br J Psychiatry2011;198:195-8.

52 Van Emmerik-van Oortmerssen K, van de Glind G, van den Brink W, et al. Prevalence of attention-deficit hyperactivity disorder in substance use disorder patients: a meta-analysis and meta-regression analysis. Drug Alcohol Depend2012;122:11-9.

53 Peadon E, Rhys-Jones B, Bower C, et al. Systematic review of interventions for children with fetal alcohol spectrum disorders. BMC Pediatr2009;9:35.

54 Shaffer D, Gould MS, Brasic J, et al. A Children's Global Assessment Scale (CGAS). Arch Gen Psychiatry1983;40:1228-31.

55 Sonuga-Barke EJ, Brandeis D, Cortese S, et al. Nonpharmacological interventions for ADHD: systematic review and meta-analyses of randomized controlled trials of dietary and psychological treatments. Am J Psychiatry2013;170:275-89.

56 Storebo OJ, Skoog M, Damm D, et al. Social skills training for Attention Deficit Hyperactivity Disorder (ADHD) in children aged 5 to 18 years. Cochrane Database Syst Rev2011;12:CD008223.

57 Zwi M, Jones H, Thorgaard C, et al. Parent training interventions for Attention Deficit Hyperactivity Disorder (ADHD) in children aged 5 to 18 years. Cochrane Database Syst Rev2011;12:CD003018.

58 Young S, Amarasinghe M. Practitioner review: non-pharmacological treatments for ADHD: a lifespan approach. J Child Psychol Psychiatry2010;51:116-33.

59 MTA Cooperative Group. A 14-month randomized clinical trial of treatment strategies for attention-deficit/hyperactivity disorder. Arch Gen Psychiatry1999;56:1073-86.

60 MTA Cooperative Group. National Institute of Mental Health Multimodal Treatment Study of ADHD follow-up: 24-month outcomes

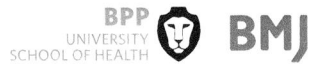

of treatment strategies for attention-deficit/hyperactivity disorder. Pediatrics2004;113:754-61.

61 Sonuga-Barke EJ, Daley D, Laver-Bradbury C, et al. Parent-based therapies for preschool Attention-Deficit/Hyperactivity Disorder: a randomized, controlled trial with a community sample. J Am Acad Child Adolesc Psychiatry2001;40:402-8.

62 Webster-Stratton C, Hancock L. Parent training for young children with conduct problems: content, methods and therapeutic process. In: Briesmeister JM, Schaefer CE, eds. Handbook of parent training: parents as co-therapists for children's behaviour problems. 2nd ed. Wiley, 1998.

63 National Institute of Health and Care Excellence. Antisocial behaviour and conduct disorders in children and young people: recognition, intervention and management. (Clinical guideline CG158.) 2013. www. nice.org.uk/guidance/cg158.

64 DuPaul GJ, Weyandt LL. School-based intervention for children with attention deficit hyperactivity disorder: effects on academic, social, and behavioural functioning. Int J Dis Dev Educ2006;53:161-76.

65 Antshel KM, Faraone SV, Gordon M. Cognitive behavioural treatment outcomes in adolescent ADHD. J Atten Disord2012;18:483-95.

66 Moore D, Richardson M, Gwernan-Jones R, et al. Non-pharmacological interventions for ADHD in school settings: an overarching synthesis of systematic reviews. J Attention Dis2015; published online 9 Mar.

67 Dunlap G, dePerczel M, Clarke S, et al. Choice making to promote adaptive behavior for students with emotional and behavioral challenges. J Applied Behav Anal1994;27:505-18.

68 DuPaul GJ, Guevremont DC, Barkley RA. Behavioral treatment of attention-deficit hyperactivity disorder in the classroom. The use of the attention training system. Behav Modif1992;16:204-25.

69 Sarver DE, Rapport M, Kofler MJ, et al. Hyperactivity in Attention-Deficit/Hyperactivity Disorder (ADHD): impairing deficit or compensatory behavior? J Abnorm Child Psychol2015; published online 12 Apr.

70 DuPaul GJ, Ervin RA, Hook CL, et al. Peer tutoring for children with attention deficit hyperactivity disorder: effects on classroom behaviour and academic performance. J Appl Behav Anal1998;31:579-92.

71 Cunningham CE, Cunningham LJ, Martorelli V, et al. The effects of primary division, student-mediated conflict resolution programs on playground aggression. J Child Psychol Psychiatry1998;39:653-62.

72 Pelsser LM, Frankena K, Toorman J, et al. Effects of a restricted elimination diet on the behaviour of children with attention-deficit hyperactivity disorder (INCA study): a randomised controlled trial. Lancet2011;377:494-503.

73 King S, Griffin S, Hodges Z, et al. A systematic review and economic model of the effectiveness and cost-effectiveness of methylphenidate, dexamfetamine and atomoxetine for the treatment of attention deficit hyperactivity disorder in children and adolescents. Health Technol Assess2006;10:iii-iv, xiii-146.

74 Banaschewski T, Coghill D, Santosh P, et al. Long-acting medications for the hyperkinetic disorders. A systematic review and European treatment guideline. Eur Child Adolesc Psychiatry2006;15:476-95.

75 Pliszka S, AACAP Work Group on Quality Issues. Practice parameter for the assessment and treatment of children and adolescents with attention-deficit/hyperactivity disorder. J Am Acad Child Adolesc Psychiatry2007;46:894-921.

76 Michelson D, Allen AJ, Busner J, et al. Once-daily atomoxetine treatment for children and adolescents with attention deficit hyperactivity disorder: a randomized, placebo-controlled study. Am J Psychiatry2002;159:1896-901.

77 Cortese S, Holtmann M, Banaschewski T, et al. Practitioner review: current best practice in the management of adverse events during treatment with ADHD medications in children and adolescents. J Child Psychol Psychiatry2013;54:227-46.

78 Riddle MA, Yershova K, Lazzaretto D, et al. The Preschool Attention-Deficit/Hyperactivity Disorder Treatment Study (PATS) 6-year follow-up. J Am Acad Child Adolesc Psychiatry2013;52:264-78.e2.

79 Collett BR, Ohan JL, Myers KM. Ten-year review of rating scales. V: scales assessing attention-deficit/hyperactivity disorder. J Am Acad Child Adolesc Psychiatry2003;42:1015-37.

80 Cortese S, Faraone SV, Konofal E, et al. Sleep in children with attention-deficit/hyperactivity disorder: meta-analysis of subjective and objective studies. J Am Acad Child Adolesc Psychiatry2009;48:894-908.

81 Hammerness PG, Perrin JM, Shelley-Abrahamson R, et al. Cardiovascular risk of stimulant treatment in pediatric attention-deficit/hyperactivity disorder: update and clinical recommendations. J Am Acad Child Adolesc Psychiatry2011;50:978-90.

82 Poulton A, Briody J, McCorquodale T, et al. Weight loss on stimulant medication: how does it affect body composition and bone metabolism? A prospective longitudinal study. Int J Pediatr Endocrinol2012;2012:30.

83 Bangs ME, Jin L, Zhang S, et al. Hepatic events associated with atomoxetine treatment for attention-deficit hyperactivity disorder. Drug Saf2008;31:345-54.

84 Kratochvil CJ, Wilens TE, Greenhill LL, et al. Effects of long-term atomoxetine treatment for young children with attention-deficit/hyperactivity disorder. J Am Acad Child Adolesc Psychiatry2006;45:919-27.

85 Chang Z, Lichtenstein P, Halldner L, et al. Stimulant ADHD medication and risk for substance abuse. J Child Psychol Psychiatry2014;55:878-85.

86 Yemula C, Besag F, Coghill D. How is standard ADHD medication used in clinical practise and how is this supported by research? Cut Edge Psychiatry Pract2013;2:35-45.

87 American Psychiatric Association. Diagnostic and statistical manual of mental disorders. 5th ed. APA, 2013.

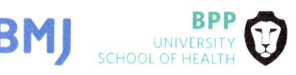

New recreational drugs and the primary care approach to patients who use them

Adam R Winstock, consultant addiction psychiatrist and honorary senior lecturer[1],
Luke Mitcheson, consultant clinical psychologist[2]

[1]South London and Maudsley NHS Trust, Institute of Psychiatry King's College London, Blackfriars Road Community Drug and Alcohol Team, London SE1 8EL, UK

[2]South London and Maudsley NHS Trust, London

Correspondence to: A R Winstock adam.winstock@slam.nhs.uk

Cite this as: BMJ 2012;344:e288

DOI: 10.1136/bmj.e288

http://www.bmj.com/content/344/bmj.e288

In recent years, hundreds of new drugs have appeared on the recreational drugs market in Europe.[1] Some of these substances, such as ketamine and γ-hydroxybutyrate (GHB), have legitimate medical purposes. These compounds have been joined by many novel psychoactive substances that, combined with their online marketing, pose a challenge for policy makers and health providers.[2]

The origins of these new drugs vary from synthetic compounds (such as 4-methylmethcathinone, or mephedrone) to traditional herbal products (such as salvia divinorum and kratom). The synthetic compounds are often designed and promoted to avoid contravening drug, medicine, and consumer protection laws. Although mephedrone, other cathinones, and various other synthetic compounds (including several cannabinoids) were classified in the United Kingdom as class B drugs in April 2010, many other new substances with psychoactive potential remain legally available. Rapid changes in legislation, combined with diverse branding and poor quality control, have led to a marked variation in the composition of these products, making it difficult for users and clinicians to identify exactly what is being consumed.

We review some common examples of these new drugs, and provide a framework for conducting an interview in the primary care setting with people who may have problems with their use. Since evidence relating to these substances is inevitably limited, we have based this article on case series, observational studies, consensus guidelines, our own clinical experiences, and those of our colleagues.

What are the characteristics of some of the new drugs?

To summarise the modes of action, routes of use, sought after effects, and possible clinical effects of these new drugs, we focused on three groups: γ-hydroxybutyrate (GHB) and its prodrugs, γ-butyl-lactone (GBL) and 1,4-butanediol; ketamine; and newer synthetic stimulants such as mephedrone, flephedrone (4-fluoromethcathinone), and methylenedioxypyrovalerone (MDPV) (tables 1-3). Most of these drugs are consumed with other substances, especially alcohol. Such combined use, along with underlying mental health problems, can greatly increase the risk of harms.

Cathinone stimulants

Mephedrone is a synthetic stimulant that is chemically related to cathinone, the psychoactive compound present in the khat plant.[3] Other synthetic cathinone stimulants include methylone. A recent crime survey in England and Wales reported mephedrone misuse in 4.4% of people aged 16-24 years in 2010-11 (the same proportion as cocaine misuse).[4] Perceived effects of cathinone stimulants are dose related and include euphoria, increased energy, feelings of empathy, increased libido, sweating, tachycardia, headache, and teeth grinding.[5] For mephedrone, the limited research so far suggests that its patterns of use and potential for misuse are similar to those of cocaine,[6] and that excessive consumption can result in emergency presentations characterised by extreme agitation, chest pain, and sweating.[7] Reported deaths, including suicide by hanging, have usually involved the use of other substances or underlying health problems.[8]

GHB, GBL, and 1,4-butanediol

GHB (G, GBH, liquid ecstasy) was originally developed as an anaesthetic and has been used to treat substance withdrawal and insomnia. GBL is found in solvent cleaning products. GHB and its precursors GBL and 1,4-butanediol share broadly similar effect profiles. Dose dependent, subjective effects (including euphoria, disinhibition, and increased sexual arousal) begin within 15 minutes of oral consumption and peak after 30-60 minutes.[9] GHB has a short half life of 27 minutes—and frequent redosing is common. Users might seem drunk, although agitation and self injurious behaviours have been reported. A steep dose-response curve exists with a narrow margin between euphoria and overdose, which is characterised by a rapid onset of respiratory depression and profound unconsciousness. High risk sexual behaviour might also occur. A retrospective review of emergency department cases found that the probability of overdose increased substantially with concomitant alcohol use[10] and that overdoses were typically self limiting, although fatal overdoses are seen. GHB was declared a class C drug in the UK in 2003, followed by GBL and 1,4-butanediol in December 2009.

Although dependence is rare, users of these compounds can develop tolerance, loss of control, and craving, and those who become dependent could dose continually every two hours.[11] Tolerance does not protect users against overdose. From a small case series, dependent users have reported personal and emotional isolation, a considerable loss of relationships, severe insomnia, and deterioration in physical health.[11] Withdrawal symptoms have been described as severe, unpredictable, and potentially life threatening, sharing features with alcohol withdrawal syndrome and starting 2-8 hours after last use of the drug. Evidence for the management of withdrawal symptoms comes from several small case series by specialist centres and consensus guidelines.[10][11][12] Many patients had persistent insomnia,

SUMMARY POINTS

- New drugs of misuse, including ketamine, γ-hydroxybutyrate (GHB), and a range of synthetic stimulants, have become part of global recreational drug culture
- Use in combination with other substances (especially alcohol) is common and increases the associated health risks
- These drugs are associated with non-specific risks of intoxication and substance specific toxicological harms
- Assessment and feedback using a motivational approach and provision of information about harm reduction are useful interventions that can be delivered in primary care
- Referral to specialist services might be needed to manage complex withdrawal or specific harms

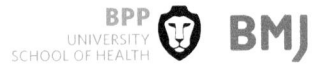

Table 1 Mode of action, routes of use, and sought after effects of new recreational drugs

	Neurobiological basis for action	Typical route and single dose amounts	Common routes of use	Sought after effects	Duration of effect
GHB, GBL, or 1,4-butanediol	Dopamine release and action at γ-amino-butyric acid (GABA) A and B receptor; primary effect as agonist at GABA B receptor	Colourless, odourless liquid of variable potency (GHB 2.5-5 mL, GBL 1-2 mL)	Oral*	Euphoria and stimulation*, prosocial effects, talkativeness disinhibition, increased libido, sedation	1-4 h
Ketamine	Antagonist at N-methyl-D-aspartate receptors, μ and σ agonist at opioid receptors, and enhances monoaminergic transmission(resulting in pronounced sympathomimetic effects)	White crystalline powder (1/20-1/4 g)	Intranasal*, by injection, oral	Euphoria and stimulation*; synaesthesia; dissociation; floating sensations; tactile and visual distortion; hallucinations; intense psychedelic experiences; spiritual, out of body, and near death experiences (the "K hole")	1-2 h
New synthetic stimulants	Elevation in monoamine neurotransmitters through enhanced vesicular release, reuptake blockade, and reduced synaptic degradation	Powder, pills, and capsules of widely variable potency (1/20-1/4 g)	Intranasal*, oral*, by injection, transbuccal, by smoking, rectal	Euphoria and stimulation*, increased alertness, increased sexual desire, prosocial effects	1-12 h

*Primary route of use or primary sought after effect.

Table 2 Signs of intoxication and harms from drug use

	Signs and symptoms of intoxication and overdose	Acute harms and other associated presentations	Chronic harms
GHB, GBL, or 1,4-butanediol	Initial arousal gives way to predominantly depressant effects: rambling incoherent speech, weakness, excessive sedation, ataxia, nausea, vomiting, agitation, involuntary jerking movements, nystagmus, urinary incontinence, ataxia, profound unconsciousness, respiratory depression, aggression and disorientation (especially on waking from an overdose)	Amnesia, agitation (rhabdomyolysis), hypothermia, respiratory depression, loss of gag reflex, bradycardia, hypotension, aspiration, seizures	Loss of relationships, psychological emotional deterioration, dependence, withdrawal risks
Ketamine	Predominantly stimulant and psychedelic effects: raised pulse and blood pressure; arrhythmia; dilated pupils, blurred vision, and diplopia; ataxia; nausea and vomiting; anxiety; dizziness; excitability; insomnia; immobility; inability to speak; abdominal tenderness; frequency of micturition; white powder in nostrils	Palpitations; chest pain; anxiety; agitation; disorientation; confusion; psychotic symptoms; reduced consciousness and immobilisation can place users vulnerable to assault and theft, accidental trauma, and unawareness of injury; urinary symptoms; frequency of micturition; dysuria; haematuria; epigastric pain	Psychological wellbeing, mood related harms (anxiety, depression, chronic dissociation, and flashbacks), dependence, cognitive impairment, urinary tract symptoms with toxic cystis and renal pathology, gastritis, dilated biliary ducts
New synthetic stimulants	Predominantly stimulant effects: dilated pupils, raised pulse and blood pressure, cold peripheries, bruxism, trismus, hyperthermia, excessive sweating, tremor, hyperarousal, nausea, psychotic episodes, white powder in nostrils	Tachyarrhythmias, anxiety, agitation, chest pain, overheating, dehydration, seizures, disorientation confusion, psychotic symptoms	Dependence, withdrawal, possible long term psychiatric sequelae (for example, depression)

Table 3 Withdrawal symptoms and basic management of potential drug users

	Withdrawal symptoms	Recommended management
GHB, GBL, or 1,4-butanediol	Occurs within a few hours of last dose and resembles alcohol withdrawal; includes anxiety, tremor, nausea, vomiting, sweating, insomnia, elevated pulse and blood pressure, hallucinations, confusion, disorientation, self harming, paranoia, delirium, seizures, rhabdomyolysis, acute renal failure, death	Start benzodiazepine treatment (10-20 mg diazepam or 30 mg chlordiazepoxide) 1-2 hours before onset of withdrawal; 10-20 mg baclofen (three times daily) might also act as antispasmodic agent and reduce the need for benzodiazepines; specialist or inpatient advice might be needed to manage health risks, high doses of benzodiazepines, and close monitoring, treatment might be fatal with risk of seizures and traumatic injury; intravenous benzodiazepine doses with increased potency might also be needed. See patients daily, with gradual reduction in drug treatment titrated against symptom over 5-14 days; management in primary care not recommended
Ketamine	Poorly described and predominantly psychological symptoms, including agitation and anxiety; loss of analgesia could unmask underlying pain (for example, in the bladder) and be a motivator for continued use	Symptomatic treatment only. Use of benzodiazepines could help ease anxiety and provide adequate analgesia. If underlying urinary symptoms are identified, consider referral to specialist services for advice and inclusion of urologist services
New synthetic stimulants	Includes irritability, craving, lethargy, poor mood, increased appetite and fatigue	Avoidance of drug. Symptomatic treatment only. Education about the time limited duration and nature of withdrawal can help reduce patient anxiety and assist in accurate diagnosis of affective disorder

anxiety, and depression for several weeks after withdrawal. A key principle of withdrawal management includes starting treatment with benzodiazepines before withdrawal begins. Withdrawal from GHB and its precursors should not be managed in primary care.

Ketamine

Ketamine (K, special K, super K, ketalar, green) is a short acting dissociative compound with anaesthetic and analgesic properties,[13] which was classified as a class C drug in the UK in 2006. Ampoules of the liquid anaesthetic form are dried to produce a white or yellowy crystalline powder that is then typically snorted ("bumped"). Illicitly manufactured formulations of ketamine powder are also available, with varying purity. Ketamine's effects, which last for about 2 hours, are strongly dose related and include feelings of euphoria, dream like hallucinations, and mystical experiences.[13] [14] [15] The drug is often used in combination with other substances to modulate its effect.

Major risks related to ketamine use are accidental trauma (often unrecognised while intoxicated), immobilisation, and personal vulnerability.[14] [15] [16] Intoxication can be associated with high risk sexual behaviour, but is not typically associated with increased violence. An emergency room case series reported that the most common acute presentations were impaired consciousness, lower urinary tract symptoms, abdominal pain (also known as "K cramps"), and dizziness.[17] Transient and self limiting psychological experiences—for example, panic, paranoia, and frightening hallucinations—might also be seen.[18] Chronic consumption has been linked to severe and persistent urinary problems. In a recent cross sectional study of more than 1000 ketamine users, more than a quarter associated at least one urinary symptom with their use of the drug.[19] Symptoms seem to be dose related, but might persist on abstinence, and could progress to bladder atrophy and hydronephrosis.[19] [20] Young people who present with dysuria and do not respond to antibiotic treatment might have urinary abnormalities associated with ketamine use.[19]

Tolerance to the sought after effects of ketamine develops rapidly within a using session. As a result, escalation in both frequency and dose can develop rapidly, with

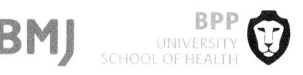

some patients reporting compulsive use and symptoms suggesting dependence (see "A patient's perspective").[19] [21] [22] Physical symptoms of withdrawal on cessation have not been consistently observed, although small case studies have reported sleep disturbance and irritability.[21] [22] Both self report studies of recreational users and lab studies of users suggest that ketamine use leads to acute impairments in mood, memory, and perception.[23] [24] A longitudinal study of 30 frequent users identified profound, dose related impairments in memory, although these effects might be reversible with abstinence.[25] [26] The same study identified pronounced depressive and prodromal symptoms among current users. More recently, evidence from small clinical trials has suggested that repeated infusions of ketamine could rapidly (albeit temporarily) improve mood in people with treatment refractory depression.[27] Ketamine, in itself, is relatively safe in overdose; users are more likely to die from having accidents while intoxicated than from overdose.[15]

Approaching the question of drug use in primary care

Consultations that address any of these behaviours present an opportunity to ask about a patient's use of these new drugs. In this scenario, we recommend a brief screening procedure, outlined in box 1.

Clinical presentations directly related to drug use could occur in one of two ways. The patient might have clear concerns about their drug use or have a problem that they think is a consequence of drug use (for example, withdrawal on cessation of GBL). Alternatively, the patient might report a problem that could be drug related, but is not recognised as such (for example, urinary symptoms related to ketamine use).

In both scenarios, as with other lifestyle behaviours that can be difficult to discuss, we recommend a guiding communication style based on motivational interviewing.[28] A good starting point is to assume that the patient might be ambivalent about change. The key to motivational interviewing is to ascertain the patient's concerns and respond accordingly; hold back from advocating change until a clearer picture is obtained. This strategy encourages the patient to actively participate in the consultation and favours a positive change in behaviour. Box 2 outlines a recommended approach if the problem of substance use is not immediately apparent but seems pertinent to exclude.

Seek the patient's permission before asking questions about substance use ("is it ok for me to ask you some questions about your GBL use?"); if permission is given, a reminder of the limits of confidentiality might still be needed. In cases where family members have raised concerns about a patient, doctors should explore the relative's concerns, the impact on them, and their coping, with signposting to relevant additional support if appropriate.

BOX 1 BRIEF SCREENING PROCEDURE FOR POSSIBLE USERS OF NEW RECREATIONAL DRUGS

- Question 1: "Have you used any drugs in the following list in the past year, such as . . . cocaine, cannabis, ecstasy?"
- If yes to any, go to question 2
- Question 2: "Have you used any other substances, such as GHB, ketamine, or newer drugs such as mephedrone in the last year?"
- If yes to any, go to question 3
- Question 3: "Which of those drugs have you used most recently?"
- Go to question 4
- Question 4: "How often would you take this [or them]?"
- Go to question 5
- Question 5: "Have you noticed any link between the problems you are having and your use of these?"

BOX 2 RECOMMENDED APPROACH TO EXPLORING PROBLEMS RELATED TO SUBSTANCE USE

- Ask what the patient wants to talk about first: "What would you like to talk about today?"
- Introduce the idea of a substance use assessment and invite the patient to accept it: "I usually ask people about their drug and alcohol use—would it be ok if we can cover that today as well?"
- Negotiate time and priorities
- For problems likely to be related to substance use, consider talking about substance use generally rather than telling the patient that you think their problem is directly attributable at this stage:
- "Often when people are feeling like you do today I like to rule out substance use as a contributing factor—would it be ok if we spend some time with me asking some questions about this?"
- "I have seen some patients in which this problem is related to drug or alcohol use—is it ok to explore this with you now?"

Table 4 Key considerations for assessing drug use and identifying associated risks

Key parameters of assessment	Descriptor	Function
Amount and change over time	Determine amount consumed per dose and total amount consumed per day	Increasing amounts per dose or per day suggest tolerance
Frequency	Determine dosing interval (number of days per week or per month) and average daily use	Increasing frequency is consistent with tolerance and could indicate physical dependence
Duration of use	Time since first ever use of drug and duration of current episode of use	Extended duration of use is associated with increased risk of harms and dependence
Route of use	Oral, intranasal, or by injection	Identify associated risks
Consumption in combination with other substances (especially alcohol and prescribed drugs)	Types of other substance taken, function, and consequence	Identify risks related to intoxication, toxicological harms, and behavioural changes
Function	Mood state sought or enhanced	Identify clues to underlying psychopathology or existence of physical dependence
Risk behaviours related to intoxication (for example, sex, driving, violence)	Determine activity and whether use of drug is in isolation or in public places	-
Major perceived health concerns (including exacerbation of underlying conditions of physical or mental health)	Describe psychological, physical, relationship, and behavioural consequences of use	Identify risks related to intoxication, as basis for advice on harm reduction, motivational interventions, referral guidance, and monitoring
Attempts to control or reduce misuse	Determine whether patient tried to stop and how many days spent recently without use	Identify loss of control, compulsive use, and withdrawal discomfort and risks on the reduction or cessation of use
Withdrawal discomfort on cessation of use	Determine psychological and physical consequences after marked reduction or cessation of use	Identify negative reinforcement of withdrawal relief and existence of high risk withdrawal symptoms (such as delirium and seizures)
Urine analysis	The new recreational drugs are not usually detected by routine drug screens, although most can be detected (if specifically requested) by specialist toxicology laboratories	

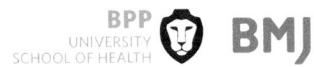

What is the approach to assessing patients who admit to problems related to drug use?

A good assessment should capture the key information outlined in table 4, and allow the patient to actively contribute. Open ended questions can achieve this aim as well as obtain relevant information ("Tell me about your drug use?", "What is your drug use over a typical week?"). Asking the patient to explain drug jargon and effects can also help to build rapport. During the assessment, use open questions to elicit and explore the patient's potential concerns ("What concerns do you have?", "You said that you experience discomfort on urination—how might that be related to your drug use?").

Simply providing feedback with specific reference to concerns the patient has identified can help the patient think about their drug use and its consequences in a new way. At this stage, substance use might still be ruled out as a problem, or the patient might deny any problems related to their drug use. If this scenario occurs, end the discussion by seeking permission to review the situation at a later date.

Any further questioning could begin with a simple open question: "Where would you like to go with this next?" If the patient does not know, invite them to consider that your medical expertise may help them; for example, ask: "Is there anything I can specifically help with?" This step could involve further information about the presenting problem or drug use, harm reduction advice, guidance about changing or reducing substance use, managing physical or psychiatric problems, or referring the patient to a specialist service.

If the patient clearly attributes an identified problem to drug use, they will probably begin to ask questions or be receptive to expert information (tables 1-3 and 5 provide substance specific information). A set of principles applies to the exchange of information at this stage, which follows the circular process of eliciting the patient's interest ("Would you like to know a bit more about how mephedrone can affect your mood?"), providing information ("When people use stimulants over a weekend and don't get any sleep, it can lead to a reduction in the chemicals in your brain that help keep our mood stable and feeling happy"), and eliciting the patient's response to that information ("How does that fit with your experience?").[29]

These principles of information exchange also apply to the provision of harm reduction information and exploration of risk behaviours related to drug use, such as sex (table 5).[30] This stage of the consultation could lead to a discussion about a possible change in substance use. Do not assume that the patient wants to change or even needs expert help to change. To introduce the idea of change, ask an open question: "We've spoken about some of the concerns you

have and how your drug use might be related to this—where do we go from here?" A direct question might be: "Would you like to do something about your drug use?"

If the patient indicates that they wish to change, ask them how they might do this and whether they think they need professional support. If the patient does not know what they should do, this stage might be an opportunity to provide harm reduction advice. Since little is known about these substances, guidance on harm reduction is usually limited to common sense advice, including limiting consumption, reviewing the progression of any health concerns with a period of cessation, and total avoidance of the drug for people in high risk groups, such as those with pre-existing mental health issues.[3] For patients who seek information on internet forums about a drug before procuring it, remind them that although online reports can be useful, they can also be unreliable or irrelevant to a particular substance. Irrespective of whether the patient expresses an interest in change, end the consultation by asking for permission to review the issue in the future.

Are psychological interventions and specialist referral needed?

The National Institute for Health and Clinical Excellence does not have literature specifically related to these new recreational drugs, but its guidelines for psychosocial interventions for drug misuse[31] and substance misuse among vulnerable young people[32] highlight the value of motivational interviewing.[28] The benefits of a single session of motivational interviewing in addressing substance misuse by young people are supported by findings from a cluster randomised trial, with effect sizes ranging from 0.34 for alcohol to 0.75 for cannabis.[33] The same study showed that this approach can be used to target use of several different substances in a generic fashion. Substance specific interventions have shown broader positive effects, for example, on mood and on the use of other substances, as shown by a randomised controlled trial of cognitive behavioural therapy in amfetamine dependence.[34] Most users of new recreational drugs will be intermittent temporary users and will not experience any serious harms. We recommend a staged approach to management that begins in the primary care setting with the type of brief intervention outlined in this article. If a clinical problem or accompanying mental health problem is identified and the patient does not respond to a brief motivational intervention, consider referral to a specialist service for substance misuse if the patient is willing. Monitoring the association between drug use, cessation, and the progression of physical and mental health symptoms over time will help to inform the need for specialist referral.

Table 5 Harm reduction advice for drug users

	Specific advice on harm reduction	General harm reduction advice
GHB, GBL, or 1,4-butanediol	Avoid drug use with alcohol. If patient is dependent on the drug, avoid sudden cessation	Avoid the development of tolerance by using infrequent dosing and reduced amounts of drugAvoid drug consumption in combination with other substances (such as CNS depressants, alcohol, or stimulants)Plan ahead to minimise the probability of behaviours related to high risk intoxication Avoid use if patient is already on prescribed drugs, particularly for psychiatric, neurological, cardiovascular, or chronic pain conditionsUse of a drug for the first time should be avoided if the person isalone or already intoxicated with another substance; recommend thathaving a non-using trusted person present can be helpful if adversereactions occurExplain what is expected on cessation of drug use and outline when help should be sought
Ketamine	Reduced risks are associated with routes of use other than injection Remain well hydrated and seek medical assistance early if patient has urinary symptoms Users should not be left alone because of the risk of accidental harm, or be left in situations in which drug use could increase personal vulnerability; ideally, a non-drug affected person should be present	
New synthetic stimulants	If patient has never taken stimulant before, be wary of variable potencies of different compounds Reduced risks are associated with routes of use other than injectionAvoid overheating and dehydrationRemind patient that what they think is legal might not beInternet purchases do not have quality control or consumer protection; remind patients that labelling on the packet might have little relation to the composition of the enclosed substance	

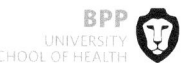

A PATIENT'S PERSPECTIVE: A USER'S ACCOUNT OF URINARY SYMPTOMS ASSOCIATED WITH USING KETAMINE

My ketamine misuse started off recreationally but escalated. The first time I visited a doctor because of problems with my bladder I was given antibiotics and sent on my way. I urinated what looked like a thick jelly, sometimes with blood in it, and had nasty involuntary bladder spasms that left me unable to walk upright. I even told the doctor about my ketamine use, but he just said I was a silly boy for taking drugs. The antibiotics did not work so I went back to the doctor and was told just to drink lots of water and cranberry juice to flush out what was left of the infection. My symptoms did not resolve so I self medicated with ketamine because it seemed to be the only thing that helped to alleviate the terrible pain, and I stopped seeing doctors for a while.

After about a year of constant ketamine misuse, I became really ill for the first time. I had intense bladder and abdominal pain and I was admitted to hospital. I managed to do about a month clean without ketamine after this, while taking the painkillers (diclofenac) that I was prescribed from the doctor at the hospital, but I started using ketamine again.

Over the next six months, I made three more attempts to stop using ketamine, all of which failed. None of the services I accessed at the time seemed to help. During this time, I passed a clot that was about the thickness of my little finger, and from this point on, I was incontinent of urine. The painkillers had stopped working. As I was a drug user, my doctor would not prescribe me anything stronger for pain. So I just continued using the one thing that helped—ketamine—knowing that every time I took it I was doing more damage. At least if I took ketamine I could walk to the shops in no pain and just about get on with things. As time went on, my bladder pain got worse. I started to get scared of eating meals because defecating was even more painful than when I was just urinating, because of contraction of the abdominal muscles, and afterwards I might urinate blood for days. Ketamine also affected my mind. I could not remember what had happened a couple of days earlier. I started to forget passwords, PIN numbers, even people's names.

I made a few attempts to kill myself and an old friend of mine, who had observed the change in me, made me register at a local general practitioner. My friend had done some investigation and found out about the specialist drug and alcohol service and the inpatient unit in the city. I asked the doctor that I was assigned to for the referrals I needed and for help.

I needed strong pain relief if I was to stop taking the ketamine completely. My doctor helped me to try different painkillers to see what worked. I tried tramadol, diclofenac, and Buscopan [hyoscine], but they did nothing. Oromorph [morphine solution] stopped the pain, but was not ideal; my doctor was not happy with my having a big bottle of morphine in the house—since my memory was not very good and because of my previous suicide attempts. I then moved on to Zomorph [morphine capsules], 10 mg twice daily with a daily collection from the chemist. I started to notice a dramatic reduction in pain lasting for roughly 6 hours after taking the first pill in the morning. This would then wear off and leave me feeling uncomfortable for the hours leading up until my next dose. From this point my ketamine intake started to decrease, as I wanted to use ketamine only when I was in pain. I explained this to my doctor, and she increased my dose of Zomorph until my admission to an inpatient addiction unit in Bristol.

After the first couple of days at the detox unit, I started to come out of my shell and participate in inpatient discussion groups. In the inpatient unit, I was put on a benzo reducing regimen to help the ketamine detox—a reducing dose of Librium [chlordiazepoxide] for a week along with my other painkillers, followed by Phenergan [promethazine hydrochloride] when needed as I came off the Librium.

I came out of the inpatient addiction unit and started to change my life. The first six months were a really slow process with regard to my bladder healing itself. It started becoming manageable six months after my last ketamine use, but it continued to be very sore and painful at times. I have to drink plenty of fluid and avoid caffeine. My bladder capacity is slowly improving but I had to wear absorbent pads at work for a long time and struggled with waking frequently in the night to go to the toilet. I am now two years clean from ketamine. My bladder and urinary functions are at about 80% of what I remember them to have been. I have not used any drugs since 10 months after my detox. I still have to drink a lot. If I do think about using ketamine, it doesn't take long to remember what it did to me.

ADDITIONAL EDUCATIONAL RESOURCES

- Talk to Frank (www.talktofrank.com)—self help website with telephone helpline providing confidential advice on drug misuse
- Erowid (www.erowid.org)—extensive database of expert and user opinions on various legal, prescribed, and illegal substances
- Substance Misuse Management in General Practice (www.smmgp.org.uk)—special interest website for general practitioners regarding drug and alcohol misuse
- European Monitoring Centre for Drugs and Drug Addiction (www.emcdda.europa.eu)—the drug monitoring agency of the European Union has many up to date and useful risk assessments and monographs
- The Party Drug Clinic (www.national.slam.nhs.uk/services/adult-services/partydrugs) at South London and Maudsley NHS Trust and the Club Drug Clinic (www.clubdrugclinic.com) at Central North West London NHS Trust—medically led specialist services providing assessment and withdrawal support for substance users
- Helpfinder at DrugScope (helpfinder.drugscope.org.uk/)—DrugScope's database of drug treatment services

SOURCES AND SELECTION CRITERIA

We searched Medline, PsycINFO, the Cochrane Library, and databases of England's National Treatment Agency and Drug Scope, the United States National Institute on Drug Abuse, and the European Monitoring Centre for Drugs and Drug Addiction, using the indexed MeSH terms "dependence", "abuse withdrawal", "harms", "death", "intervention", "assessment", "psychiatric", and "overdose" (1971-2011). We aimed to provide profiles of the use, effect, and risks of these drugs for general practitioners to identify, assess, and manage the common presentations associated with their use.

commonly used drugs, and launches in March 2012; LM is on the expert advisory group of the Global Drug Survey.

Provenance and peer review: Commissioned; externally peer reviewed.

Patient consent obtained.

We thank Fergus Law and James Bell for their advice on the sections related to ketamine and GHB, respectively; the anonymous ketamine user who provided his story; and the participants at the Substance Misuse Management in General Practice workshop for their help in the refining of this paper.

Contributors: ARW conceived the review, wrote the initial draft, prepared the final draft, and is the guarantor. LM helped with conception of the review and contributed to the sections on assessment and intervention.

Competing interests: All authors have completed the ICMJE uniform disclosure form at www.icmje.org/coi_disclosure.pdf (available on request from the corresponding author) and declare: no support from any organisation for the submitted work; no financial relationships with any organisations that might have an interest in the submitted work in the previous three years; ARW is founder and director of the Global Drug Survey, an independent data mapping and exchange hub for drug use data and provider of "drugs meter", a free online and smartphone application for self assessment on drug use that provides comparative and individually adjusted feedback on most

1 European Monitoring Centre for Drugs and Drug Addiction. The state of the drug problem in Europe. European Monitoring Centre for Drugs and Drug Addiction, 2009.

2 Winstock AR, Ramsey JD. Legal highs and the challenges for policy makers. Addiction 2010;105:1685-7.

3 Winstock AR, Marsden J, Mitcheson L. What should be done about mephedrone? BMJ 2010;340:c1605.

4 UK Home Office Statistical Bulletin. Drug misuse declared: findings from the 2010/11 British Crime Survey England and Wales. 2011. www.homeoffice.gov.uk/publications/science-research-statistics/research-statistics/crime-research/hosb1211/.

5 Winstock AR, Mitcheson L, Ramsey J, Marsden J. Mephedrone: use, subjective effects and health risks. Addiction 2011;106:1991-6.

6 Winstock AR, Mitcheson L, De Luca P, Davey Z, Schiffano F. Mephedrone, new kid for the chop? Addiction 2011;106:154-61.

7 James D, Adams RD, Spears R, Cooper G, Lupton DJ Thompson JP, et al. Clinical characteristics of mephedrone toxicity reported to the UK National Poisons Information Service. Emerg Med J 2011;28:686-9.

8 Advisory Council on the Misuse of Drugs. Novel psychoactive substances report (2011). Annex C:61-4. 2011. www.homeoffice.gov.uk/publications/agencies-public-bodies/acmd1/acmdnps2011.

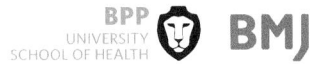

9   Rodgers J, Ashton H, Gilvarry E, Young AH. Liquid ecstasy on the dance floor. *Br J Psychiatr* 2004;184:104-6.

10   Munir VL, Hutton JE, Harney JP, Buykx P, Weiland TJ, Dent AW. Gamma-hydroxybutyrate: a 30 month emergency department review. *Emerg Med Australas* 2008;20:521-30.

11   Bell J, Collins R. Gamma-butyrolactone (GBL) dependence and withdrawal. *Addiction* 2011;106:442-7.

12   McDonough M, Kennedy N, Glasper A, Bearn J. Clinical features and management of gamma-hydroxybutyrate (GHB) withdrawal: a review. *Drug Alcohol Depend* 2004;75:3-9.

13   Lingford-Hughes A, Welch SJ, Peters L, Nutt DJ, on behalf of expert groupfor BAP. Evidence-based guidelines for the pharmacological management of substance misuse, addiction and comorbidity: recommendations from the British Association for Psychopharmacology. *J Psychopharmacol* [forthcoming].

14   Wolff K, Winstock AR. Ketamine: from medicine to misuse. *CNS Drugs* 2006;20:199-218.

15   Morgan CA, Curran HV, Independent Scientific Committee on Drugs. Ketamine use: a review. *Addiction* 2012;107:27-38.

16   Dillon P, Copeland J, Jansen K. Patterns of use and harms associated with non-medical ketamine use. *Drug Alcohol Depend* 2003;69:23-8.

17   Jansen KL. A review of the nonmedical use of ketamine: use, users and consequences. *J Psychoactive Drugs* 2000;32:419-33.

18   Ng SH, Tse ML, Ng HW, Lau FL. Emergency department presentation of ketamine abusers in Hong Kong: a review of 233 cases. *Hong Kong Med J* 2010;16:6-11.

19   Muetzelfeldt L, Kamboj SK, Rees H, Taylor J, Morgan CJ, Curran HV. Journey through the K-hole: phenomenological aspects of ketamine use. *Drug Alcohol Depend* 2008;95:219-29.

20   Winstock AR, Mitcheson L, Gillatt DA, Cottrell AM. The prevalence and natural history of urinary symptoms among recreational ketamine users. *Br J Urol Int* [forthcoming].

21   Cottrell AM, Gillatt DA. Ketamine-associated urinary tract pathology: the tip of the iceberg for urologists? *Br J Med Surgical Urol* 2008;1:136-8.

22   Jansen K, Darracot-Cankovic R. The nonmedical use of ketamine, part two: a review of problem use and dependence. *J Psychoactive Drugs* 2001;33:151-8.

23   Moore NN, Bostwick JM. Ketamine dependence in anesthesia providers. *Psychosomatics* 1999;40:356-9.

24   Copeland J, Dillon P. The health and psycho-social consequences of ketamine use. *Int J Drug Policy* 2005;16:122-31.

25   Curran HV, Morgan C. Cognitive, dissociative and psychotogenic effects of ketamine in recreational users on the night of drug use and 3 days later. *Addiction* 2000;95:575-90.

26   Morgan CJ, Muetzelfeldt L, Curran HV. Consequences of chronic ketamine self-administration upon neurocognitive function and psychological wellbeing: a 1-year longitudinal study. *Addiction* 2010;105:121-33.

27   Aan het Rot M, Collins KA, Murrough JW, Perez AM, Reich DL, Charney DS, et al. Safety and efficacy of repeated-dose intravenous ketamine for treatment resistant depression. *Biol Psychiatry* 2010;67:139-45.

28   Rollnick S, Miller WR, Butler CC. Motivational interviewing in health care: helping patients change behavior. Guilford Press, 2008.

29   Rollnick S, Butler CC, Kinnersley P, Gregory J, Mash B. Motivational interviewing. *BMJ* 2010;340:c1900.

30   Mitcheson L, McCambridge J, Bryne A, Hunt N, Winstock AR. Sexual health risk among dance drug users: cross-sectional comparisons with nationally representative data. *Int J Drug Policy* 2008;19:304-10.

31   National Institute for Health and Clinical Excellence. NICE clinical guideline 51. Drug misuse: psychosocial interventions. NICE, 2007.

32   National Institute for Health and Clinical Excellence. NICE public health intervention guidance 4. Community-based interventions to reduce substance misuse among vulnerable and disadvantaged children and young people. NICE, 2007.

33   McCambridge J, Strang J. The efficacy of single-session motivational interviewing in reducing drug consumption and perceptions of drug-related risk and harm among young people: results from a multi-site cluster randomized trial. *Addiction* 2006;101:1014-26.

34   Baker A, Lee NK, Claire M, Lewin TJ, Grant T, Pohlman S, et al. Brief cognitive behavioural interventions for regular amphetamine users: a step in the right direction. *Addiction* 2005;100:367-78.

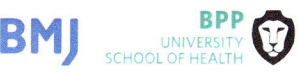

Assessment and management of alcohol use disorders

Ed Day, senior lecturer and consultant in addiction psychiatry[1], Alex Copello, professor[2], Martyn Hull, GP principal and lead GP with a special interest in substance misuse[3]

[1]Addictions Department, Institute of Psychiatry, Psychology & Neuroscience, King's College London, London SE5 8AF, UK

[2]School of Psychology, University of Birmingham, Birmingham, UK

[3]Ridgacre Medical Centres, Quinton, Birmingham, UK

Correspondence to: E Day Edward. Day@kcl.ac.uk

Cite this as: *BMJ* 2015;350:h715

DOI: 10.1136/bmj.h715

http://www.bmj.com/content/350/bmj.h715

Alcohol can impact on both the incidence and the course of many health conditions, and nearly 6% of all global deaths in 2012 were estimated to be attributable to its consumption.[1] A quarter of the UK adult population drinks alcohol in a way that is potentially or actually harmful to health.[2] Between 2002 and 2012 in England the number of episodes where an alcohol related disease, injury, or condition was the primary reason for hospital admission or a secondary diagnosis doubled.[3] Despite the large numbers of people drinking alcohol at higher risk levels, a relatively low number access treatment.[4] Possible causes for this include missed opportunities to identify problems, limited access to specialist services, and underdeveloped care pathways. International studies have shown that more than 20% of patients presenting to primary care are higher risk or dependent drinkers,[5] yet the problem of alcohol is inadequately addressed. This review focuses on practical aspects of the assessment and treatment of alcohol use disorders from the perspective of the non-specialist hospital doctor or general practitioner.

How are alcohol use disorders defined?

As the level of alcohol consumption goes up, so the risk of physical, psychological, and social problems increases. Alcohol related harm is a public health problem, and strategies that reduce average consumption across the whole population by even a small amount produce considerable health benefits. Increasing the cost of alcohol has been consistently associated with a reduction in alcohol related harm,[6] and a minimum cost for a unit of alcohol has been under consideration in the United Kingdom.[7]

Alcoholic drinks have different strengths, and so alcohol is not measured by number of drinks but by number of "units." In the United Kingdom, 1 unit comprises 8 grams of alcohol (equivalent to 10 mL of pure ethanol), but elsewhere this value is defined differently.[8] Box 1 shows how to calculate the number of units. The terminology used to define alcohol use disorders is currently evolving, with various organisations using slightly different terms.[9] [10] However, the general agreement is that there is no such thing as a "safe level" of drinking and that the risk of harm increases with either frequency of consumption or amount consumed on a

drinking occasion.[8] To plan effective intervention strategies, the categories of alcohol use disorders defined in table 1 are most commonly used. Figure 1 shows the prevalence of these categories in England.

The term "addiction" is not used in current classificatory systems, partly because it has pejorative connotations. The latest version (fifth edition) of the *Diagnostic and Statistical Manual of Mental Disorders* has removed the category of dependence, and instead describes a spectrum of alcohol use disorders of differing severity.[11] The concept of alcohol dependence is, however, important to describe people in whom the ability to control the frequency and extent of consumption has been completely eroded, while recognising that dependence may exist at different levels of severity.[12] [13]

How can alcohol use disorders be identified?

Most people with risky patterns of drinking are not dependent on alcohol (fig 1). A few minutes spent systematically identifying drinkers at increased risk of harm and delivering advice about moderating alcohol consumption has been shown to be an effective strategy in various settings,[14] [15] and the process of identification and brief advice should be offered as a first step in treatment.[4] In the United Kingdom, the National Institute for Health and Care Excellence recommends that professionals in the National Health Service should carry out alcohol screening as part of routine practice,[4] and all doctors should feel comfortable and confident in raising the topic of alcohol consumption in a consultation. However, the low level of detection and treatment suggests that generalists are not sufficiently proactive in screening groups potentially at risk, including those who have relevant physical conditions (for example, hypertension and gastrointestinal or liver disorders); mental health problems, such as anxiety or depression; been assaulted; are at risk of self harm; regularly experience unintentional injuries or minor trauma; and regularly attend genitourinary medicine clinics or repeatedly seek emergency contraception.

AUDIT, the alcohol use disorders identification test (fig 2), consists of 10 questions about drinking frequency and intensity, experience of alcohol related problems, and signs of possible dependence.[16] It is the ideal screening questionnaire for detecting drinkers at increasing or higher risk.[1] Furthermore, the AUDIT score can guide clinicians as to the best intervention, including brief advice or a referral to specialist services (box 2). Owing to the potentially more important effects of alcohol on certain populations, scores should be revised downward when screening young people aged less than 18, or adults aged more than 65 (see box 2). Biochemical measures such as liver function tests are not normally used for screening, but may be helpful in assessing the severity and progress of an established alcohol related problem, or as part of a secondary care assessment.[17]

A guiding style that aims to build motivation and avoid confrontation is recommended, and motivational interviewing has shown considerable promise in this area.

THE BOTTOM LINE

- Alcohol use disorders exist across a spectrum, and public health measures to reduce the drinking of a whole population have considerable health benefits
- All front line clinicians should be aware of the potential effects of alcohol consumption and be able to screen for alcohol use disorders using the alcohol use disorders questionnaire test
- Brief interventions are quick and easy to deliver and have a potentially large impact on reducing hazardous and harmful drinking
- Benzodiazepines are the drug of choice for medically assisted alcohol withdrawal
- Relapse to drinking is common in the first year after stopping drinking, but psychological treatments, mutual aid groups, and relapse prevention drugs increase the likelihood of remaining abstinent

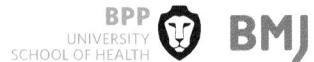

BOX 1 HOW TO CALCULATE UNITS OF ALCOHOL

- The alcohol content of a drink is usually expressed by the standard measure "alcohol by volume," or ABV. This is a measure of the amount of pure alcohol as a percentage of the total volume of liquid in a drink and can be found on the labels of cans and bottles. For example, if the label on a can of beer states "5% ABV" or "alcohol volume 5%," this means that 5% of the volume of that drink is pure alcohol.
- The number of units in any drink can be calculated by multiplying the total volume of a drink (in millilitres) by its ABV (which is measured as a percentage) and dividing the result by 1000. For example, the number of units in a pint (568 mL) of strong lager (ABV 5%) would be calculated:
- This is worth doing, as the increasing strength of many alcoholic drinks and the larger glass sizes served in bars mean that people are often drinking more alcohol than they realise.

Units calculators are available (for example, www.nhs.uk/Tools/Pages/Alcohol-unit-calculator.aspx)

BOX 2 DELIVERING ALCOHOL IDENTIFICATION AND BRIEF ADVICE IN PRACTICE

The rationale

- A large body of international research evidence indicates that 1 in 8 people drinking at increasing risk or higher risk levels who receive structured brief advice reduce their drinking to within lower risk levels.[4] Raising the problem of alcohol consumption with patients often meets with several attitudes, including indifference, confusion about what is and is not healthy, and possibly defensiveness and irritability. Clinicians should ensure that they are aware of the facts about alcohol consumption and health related harms to convey the risks of drinking to patients accurately. It is important to avoid stigmatising terms such as "alcoholic," emphasising the concept of increasing risk with increasing consumption and suggesting trying to cut down to a lower risk level rather than stopping. Clinicians should also be able to detect alcohol dependence and refer to specialist help.

Stage 1: raise the problem

- The most time and resource effective strategy in non-specialist settings is to target those at greatest risk—that is, people with relevant physical (for example, hypertension, gastrointestinal or liver problems) or mental health (anxiety or depression) conditions, at risk of self harm, or who regularly experience unintentional injuries or minor trauma.
- Ask the first three questions on the AUDIT questionnaire (see fig 2) and score the answers (known as AUDIT-C).
- *Score of .5*—suggests a high likelihood that the patient is drinking at an increasing risk level, and the full AUDIT questionnaire should be administered (this threshold may be reduced to 3 or more in young people aged less than 18 years or adults older than 65 years)[30 31]

Stage 2: administer and score the 10 item AUDIT questionnaire

- *Score ,7*—this result should be fed back in a positive manner—for example, reiterate the sensible drinking guidelines and point out that people who exceed these levels increase their chances of alcohol related health problems such as unintentional injuries, high blood pressure, liver disease, cancer, and heart disease, while congratulating them for adhering to guidance
- *Score 8-19*—this suggests that the patient's drinking pattern is in the increasing risk or higher risk band, and clinicians should move to offering brief advice as described in stage 3

Stage 3: deliver structured brief advice

- Use an open ended "transitional" statement such as "how important is it for you to change your drinking?," possibly accompanied by a simple "readiness ruler"—that is, ask patients to rate between 1 and 10 how confident they feel in making changes. This can be followed by asking what would have to happen to make the number go up.
- A structured episode of brief advice may only last 5-10 minutes and is best guided by a structured advice tool (for example, www.alcohollearningcentre.org.uk/alcoholeLearning/learning/IBA/Module4_v2/pdf/structured_advice_tool.pdf). This makes use of the FRAMES (feedback, responsibility, advice, menu, empathy, self efficacy) structure for brief interventions. The leaflet provides material to use for three of these elements:
- Feedback on patients' level of drinking when compared with others, the common effects of drinking, and the potential benefits of reduction
- A menu of options to support the attainment of their preferred drinking goal
- Advice on units and limits
- Clinicians should aim to be firm enough to ensure that patients realise that it is their responsibility to make the change (restating the need to reduce risk and encouraging patients to begin now), while also showing empathy (for example, "it can be very difficult to make these changes if everyone around you is drinking heavily") and aiming to boost their confidence and self efficacy ("You mentioned you were going to drink a non-alcoholic drink first when you get home in the evening. That sounds like an excellent start. Let's see how you get on and arrange another time to talk to discuss how you get on").
- It is a good idea to offer a follow-up appointment to assess progress. An "extended brief intervention" places greater emphasis on exploring the pros and cons of change and formulating a specific action plan. This approach is often based on the principles of motivational interviewing,[18] and again is best guided by a structured leaflet such as the one available at www.alcohollearningcentre.org.uk/alcoholeLearning/learning/IBA/Module5_v2/extended_intervention_worksheet.pdf.
- Patients should be referred for more specialist alcohol assessment and intervention if they ask for such help, already exhibit major alcohol related harm, have an AUDIT score of ›20, or exhibit features of the alcohol dependence syndrome.

A step by step teaching module and full range of materials is available at www.alcohollearningcentre.org.uk/eLearning/.

Although a review is beyond the scope of this article, useful materials can be found at www.motivationalinterviewing.org.

What treatments are available for alcohol dependence in the non-specialist setting?

Identification and brief advice is an important public health approach because of the numbers of people drinking at increasing risk or higher risk levels. However, even after gold standard brief interventions in primary care, nearly two thirds of people will still be drinking at an increasing or higher risk level.[15] At the "dependent" end of the drinking spectrum, change is even more difficult to achieve. People with a moderate to severe level of alcohol dependence may benefit from more intensive help from mutual aid groups such as Alcoholics Anonymous or specialist treatment services, or both.[4] Abstinence is the preferred goal for many such people, particularly for those whose organs have already been damaged through alcohol use, or for those who have previously attempted to cut down their drinking without success. In considering the correct level of treatment intensity it is important to consider risks, capacity to consent to treatment, the experience and outcome of previous episodes of treatment, motivation for change, and other existing problems, including harm to others.

Three interventions may assist generalists in altering the drinking trajectory: medically assisted withdrawal,

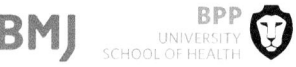

Table 1 Classification and definition of alcohol use disorders

Category of drinking	Definition	AUDIT score
Low risk	No amount of alcohol consumption can be called "safe," but risks of harm are low if consumption is below levels specified in the "increasing risk" category (below)	≤7
Increasing risk (hazardous)	Regularly drinking more than 2 or 3 units a day (women) and more than 3 or 4 units a day (men)	8-15
Higher risk (harmful)	Regularly drinking more than 6 units daily (women) or more than 8 units daily (men), or more than 35 units weekly (women) or more than 50 units weekly (men)	16-19
Dependence, as defined by ICD-10 (international classification of diseases, 10th revision)[9]	A definite diagnosis of dependence should be made only if three or more of the following have been present at the same time during the previous year: (a) a strong desire or sense of compulsion to drink alcohol; difficulties in controlling drinking behaviour in terms of its onset, termination, or levels of consumption; a physiological withdrawal state when drinking has stopped or been reduced, as evidenced by the characteristic alcohol withdrawal syndrome, or use of the same (or a closely related) substance with the intention of relieving or avoiding withdrawal symptoms—for example, benzodiazepines; (d) evidence of tolerance, such that increased quantities of alcohol are required to achieve the effects originally produced by lesser amounts; (e) progressive neglect of alternative pleasures or interests because of alcohol consumption, increased amount of time necessary to obtain or drink alcohol or to recover from its effects; (f) persisting with drinking alcohol despite clear evidence of overtly harmful consequences, such as harm to the liver, depressive mood states, or impaired cognitive functioning. It is an essential characteristic of the dependence syndrome that either alcohol consumption or a desire to drink alcohol is present; the subjective awareness of compulsion to drink alcohol is most commonly seen during attempts to stop or control substance use	≥20

AUDIT=alcohol use disorders identification test.

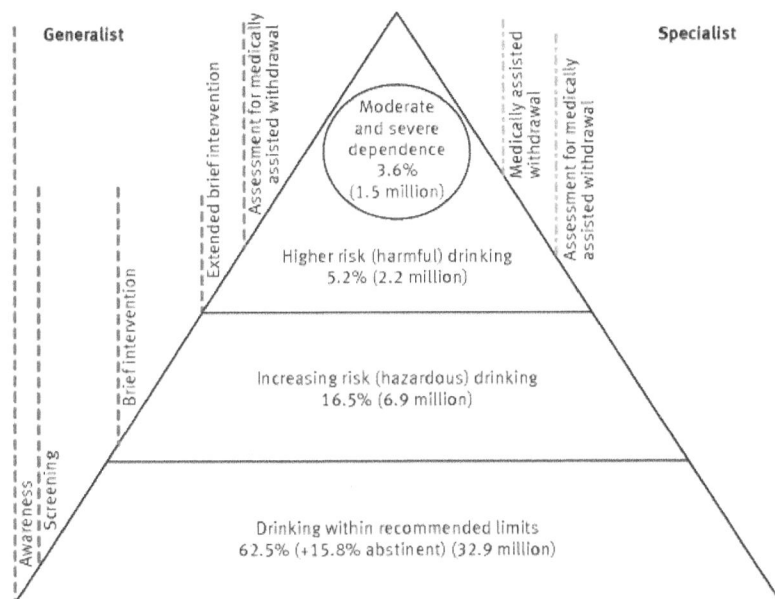

Fig 1 Prevalence of alcohol use disorders in England (taken from general household survey 2009 and psychiatric morbidity survey 2007) and recommended treatment strategies across the spectrum

facilitation through mutual aid, and use of drugs to prevent relapse.

Medically assisted withdrawal

The alcohol withdrawal syndrome develops when consumption is abruptly stopped or substantially reduced, and symptoms and signs appear within 6-8 hours. These include anxiety, tremor, sweating, nausea, tachycardia, and hypertension, usually peaking over 10-30 hours and subsiding within two or three days. Seizures may occur in the first 12-48 hours (but rarely after this), and delirium tremens is a serious condition that occurs 48-72 hours after cessation of drinking, characterised by coarse tremor, agitation, fever, tachycardia, profound confusion, delusions (characteristically frightening), auditory and visual hallucinations, and possibly hyperpyrexia, ketoacidosis, and circulatory collapse.

Minor degrees of alcohol withdrawal are common and can be managed with information, reassurance, and adequate fluid intake. However, the alcohol withdrawal syndrome is potentially life threatening; systematic reviews recommend long acting benzodiazepines (chlordiazepoxide or diazepam) as the drug of choice for managing the alcohol withdrawal syndrome and preventing serious complications such as seizures or delirium tremens.[19] [20] The aim is to titrate the initial dose to the extent of withdrawal symptoms and then slowly to reduce the dose over 7-10 days using a standard fixed dose protocol (table 2). Rating scales such as the clinical institute withdrawal assessment for alcohol (CIWA-Ar) can be used to measure the severity of the withdrawal symptoms and more accurately adjust the dose, but the use of such a regimen triggered by symptoms is only recommended if trained staff are available, such as in an inpatient setting.[21] Prescribing in the community for alcohol dependent patients without adequate assessment and support is not recommended, as successful withdrawal is unlikely and there are considerable associated clinical risks. This is a common scenario facing general practitioners, and expeditious referral to specialist services for support from a specialist alcohol nurse during medicated withdrawal is advised.

Doses of benzodiazepines should be reduced for children and young people aged less than 18 years, adults aged more than 65 years, and those with impaired liver synthetic function, such as reduced albumin or increased prothrombin time (where a benzodiazepine requiring less metabolism within the liver, such as oxazepam, may be preferred). Clinicians should be aware of complications from nutritional deficiency, such as the Wernicke-Korsakoff syndrome. This should be suspected in anyone with a history of alcohol dependence and one or more of ophthalmoplegia, ataxia, acute confusion, memory disturbance, or unexplained hypotension, hypothermia, or unconsciousness. Treatment with intramuscular or intravenous thiamine is important to prevent permanent memory loss and should continue until the symptoms and signs stop improving.[21] Most episodes of medically assisted alcohol withdrawal can take place at home, but inpatient treatment should be considered if patients drink more than 30 units of alcohol daily, have a history of epilepsy, withdrawal related seizures, or delirium tremens, or have comorbid physical or mental health conditions.[19]

Mutual aid facilitation

Treatment of alcohol withdrawal is not sufficient on its own and should be viewed as the precursor to a longer term treatment and rehabilitation process. Research consistently shows that people with alcohol dependence who have stopped drinking are vulnerable to relapse and that they may have unresolved problems that predispose them to it.[22] Mutual aid groups (for example, Alcoholics Anonymous

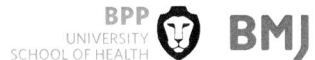

Alcohol use disorders identification test (AUDIT)

1. How often do you have a drink containing alcohol?
(0) Never
(1) Monthly or less
(2) 2-4 times a month
(3) 2-3 times a week
(4) 4 or more times a week ☐

2. How many units of alcohol do you have on a typical day when you are drinking?
(0) 1 or 2
(1) 3 or 4
(2) 5 or 6
(3) 7, 8, or 9
(4) 10 or more ☐

3. How often do you have 6 or more units if female, or 8 or more units if male, on a single occasion in the past year?
(0) Never
(1) Less than monthly
(2) Monthly
(3) Weekly
(4) Daily or almost daily ☐

4. How often during the past year have you found that you were not able to stop drinking once you had started?
(0) Never
(1) Less than monthly
(2) Monthly
(3) Weekly
(4) Daily or almost daily ☐

5. How often during the past year have you failed to do what was normally expected from you because of drinking?
(0) Never
(1) Less than monthly
(2) Monthly
(3) Weekly
(4) Daily or almost daily ☐

6. How often during the past year have you needed a first drink in the morning to get yourself going after a heavy drinking session?
(0) Never
(1) Less than monthly
(2) Monthly
(3) Weekly
(4) Daily or almost daily ☐

7. How often during the past year have you had a feeling of guilt or remorse after drinking?
(0) Never
(1) Less than monthly
(2) Monthly
(3) Weekly
(4) Daily or almost daily ☐

8. How often during the past year have you been unable to remember what happened the night before because you had been drinking?
(0) Never
(1) Less than monthly
(2) Monthly
(3) Weekly
(4) Daily or almost daily ☐

9. Have you or someone else been injured as a result of your drinking?
(0) No
(2) Yes, but not in the past year
(4) Yes, during the past year ☐

10. Has a relative or friend, doctor, or another health worker been concerned about your drinking or suggested that you cut down?
(0) No
(2) Yes, but not in the past year
(4) Yes, during the past year ☐

Total score: ☐

Fig 2 Alcohol use disorders identification test

and UK SMART Recovery) are a source of ongoing support for people seeking recovery from alcohol dependence, and for partners, friends, children, and other family members. Long term cohort studies show that people who actively participate in mutual aid are more likely to sustain their recovery,[23] and NICE recommends that treatment staff should routinely provide information about mutual aid groups and facilitate access for those who want to attend.[19]

Clinicians should be aware of the range of mutual aid groups available locally and how to access them. Level of clinician knowledge about Alcoholics Anonymous groups has been positively correlated with levels of referral,[24] and attending a meeting is an invaluable learning experience. Evidence from randomised controlled trials suggests that proactive efforts to engage patients with mutual aid groups increase attendance, particularly introducing the patient to a group member in advance of a meeting.[25] A simple three stage process to guide this is available (www.nta.nhs.uk/uploads/mutualaid-fama.pdf).

Relapse prevention drugs

Interventions based on psychological or social processes of change are the mainstay of treatment for alcohol dependence.[26] Although research suggests that such treatments lead to improved outcomes when compared with no treatment, the evidence favouring one type of psychological intervention over another is less clear. Other factors such as therapist characteristics and service variables are also important. The uptake and implementation of psychological approaches in the United Kingdom vary widely,[19] [27] and most practice involves an eclectic approach that combines strategies from various psychological approaches and typically lasts 12 weeks. In those who have decided to become abstinent from alcohol, this treatment is enhanced by both attendance at a mutual aid group and the prescribing of relapse prevention drugs. Several drugs can be prescribed in primary care, although they may all be started and monitored by a specialist.

Acamprosate and the opioid antagonist naltrexone—both these drugs are effective in increasing the time to first drink and to relapse in people with alcohol dependence who have achieved abstinence.[19] Acamprosate may also be neuroprotective and is believed to act by altering the balance between excitatory and inhibitory neurotransmission.[20] Naltrexone seems to reduce cravings by reducing the reinforcing effect of alcohol consumption. Both drugs should only be used in combination with an individual psychological intervention, started as soon as possible after withdrawal, and may be prescribed for six months or more depending on perceived benefit. Systematic reviews suggest a number needed to treat to prevent return to any drinking of between 12 and 20.[28]

Disulfiram—this drug works by interfering with the metabolism of alcohol, causing an accumulation of acetaldehyde in the body and a throbbing headache, facial flushing, palpitations, dyspnoea, tachycardia, nausea, and

Table 2 Suggested titrated fixed dose chlordiazepoxide protocol for treatment of alcohol withdrawal. From National Collaborating Centre for Mental Health[19]

Treatment day	15-25 units/day		30-49 units/day		50-60 units/day
	Moderate dependence: SADQ score 15-25		Severe dependence: SADQ score 30-40		Very severe dependence: SADQ score 40-60
Day 1 (starting dose)	15 mg four times/day	25 mg four times/day	30 mg four times/day	40 mg four times/day*	50 mg four times/day†
Day 2	10 mg four times/day	20 mg four times/day	25 mg four times/day	35 mg four times/day*	45 mg four times/day†
Day 3	10 mg three times/day	15 mg four times/day	20 mg four times/day	30 mg four times/day	40 mg four times/day*
Day 4	5 mg three times/day	10 mg four times/day	15 mg four times/day	25 mg four times/day	35 mg four times/day*
Day 5	5 mg twice/day	10 mg three times/day	10 mg four times/day	20 mg four times/day	30 mg four times/day
Day 6	5 mg at night	5 mg three times/day	10 mg three times/day	15 mg four times/day	25 mg four times/day
Day 7	—	5 mg twice/day	5 mg three times/day	10 mg four times/day	20 mg four times/day
Day 8	—	5 mg at night	5 mg twice/day	10 mg three times/day	15 mg four times/day
Day 9	—	—	5 mg at night	5 mg three times/day	10 mg four times/day
Day 10	—	—	—	5 mg twice/day	10 mg three times/day
Day 11	—	—	—	5 mg at night	5 mg three times/day
Day 12	—	—	—	—	5 mg twice/day
Day 13	—	—	—	—	5 mg at night

SADQ=severity of alcohol dependence questionnaire (www.alcohollearningcentre.org.uk/Topics/Latest/Resource/?cid=4615).

*Doses of chlordiazepoxide >30 mg four times/day should be prescribed only in severe alcohol dependence, with response to treatment monitored regularly and closely.

†Doses of chlordiazepoxide >40 mg four times/day should be prescribed only in very severe alcohol dependence. Such doses are rarely necessary in women and children and never in older people or in patients with liver impairment.

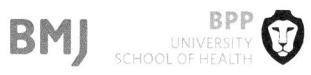

vomiting within 10 minutes of alcohol consumption. Its use as a deterrent is most suited to people who have abstinence as a goal and who have someone to supervise consumption each day. Treatment should be started at least 24 hours after the last alcoholic drink and should be used with caution in the context of pregnancy, liver disease, severe mental illness, stroke, heart disease, or hypertension. Patients need to know about the symptoms caused by the interaction between alcohol and disulfiram and the rare and unpredictable onset of hepatotoxicity, which is unrelated to dose.

Nalmefene—is an opioid antagonist that is indicated for the reduction of alcohol consumption in adults with alcohol dependence who have a high risk drinking level (>7.5 units/day in men and >5 units/day in women), but without physical withdrawal symptoms and who do not need immediate medically assisted withdrawal. The drug should be started only in patients who continue to have a high risk drinking level two weeks after initial assessment, and it should only be prescribed in conjunction with continuous psychosocial support focused on treatment adherence and reducing alcohol consumption. Such psychosocial support can be delivered in primary care, and this seems to be a cost effective approach to dealing with higher risk drinking.[29] The recommended dose is one tablet on each day the patient perceives a risk of drinking, ideally 1-2 hours before the anticipated time of drinking.

When should people with alcohol use disorders be referred?

Referral for specialist treatment should be considered if patients have failed to benefit from a brief intervention or an extended brief intervention and want to receive further help, show signs of moderate or severe alcohol dependence (see table 1), or have severe alcohol related physical impairment or a related comorbid condition (for example, liver disease or mental health problems). General practitioners should actively encourage patients to attend local mutual aid groups such as Alcoholics Anonymous, as well as access local specialist services for full assessment and management. The general practitioner's role in supporting patients and their family is crucial, as in any long term chronic disorder.

Contributors: ED was approached to write this review and produced the first draft. ED and AC were part of the guideline development group that produced the NICE clinical guideline 115, and used the searches conducted as part of the NICE process as the basis for the review. AC and MH commented on the initial draft and contributed sections on brief interventions (AC, MH), specialist treatment (AC), and drug treatment in primary care (MH). ED is the guarantor.

Competing interests: We have read and understood the BMJ policy on declaration of interests and declare: ED is a member of the Addictions Department at the Institute of Psychiatry, Psychology and Neuroscience, King's College London. The department is in receipt of or has received grants from the Medical Research Council (MRC) and the National Institute for Health Research (NIHR) to research both drug and psychosocial treatments for alcohol use disorders. He is currently a coinvestigator on NIHR Health Technology Assessment grant (13/86/03) to investigate the effectiveness of adjunctive medication management and contingency management in enhancing adherence to drugs for relapse prevention in alcohol dependence. He is a trustee of the charities Action on Addiction and Changes UK. AC is an honorary member of the School of Psychology at the University of Birmingham, and his department is in receipt or has received grants from the MRC and the NIHR to research psychosocial treatments for alcohol use disorders. He is chief investigator on a randomised controlled trial of a family and social network intervention for young people who misuse alcohol and drugs (HTA grant 11/60/01) and principal investigator on a pilot study to assess the feasibility and impact of a motivational intervention on problem drug and alcohol use in adult mental health inpatient units (NIHR—PB-PG-1010-23138). He is an expert advisor to the charity Action on Addiction. MH is a member of SMMGP (Substance Misuse Management in General Practice) and has been funded through SMMGP by Lundbeck to complete and tutor on the SMMGP advanced certificate in the community management of alcohol disorders.

Provenance and peer review: Commissioned; externally peer reviewed.

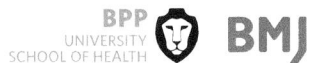

1 World Health Organization. Global status report on alcohol and health 2014. WHO, 2014.
2 Office for National Statistics. General lifestyle survey overview: a report on the 2009 general lifestyle survey. In: Dunstan S, ed. ONS, 2011.
3 Health and Social Care Information Centre. Statistics on alcohol: England, 2013. HSCIC, 2013.
4 National Institute for Health and Care Excellence. Alcohol-use disorders: preventing harmful drinking. (Public health guidance 24.) 2010. www.nice.org.uk/guidance/ph24.
5 Funk M, Wutzke S, Kaner E, Anderson P, Pas L, McCormick R, et al. A multicountry controlled trial of strategies to promote dissemination and implementation of brief alcohol intervention in primary health care: findings of a World Health Organization collaborative study. *J Stud Alcohol* 2005;66:379-88.
6 Babor T, Caetano R, Casswell S, Edwards G, Giesbrecht N, Graham K, et al. Alcohol: no ordinary commodity: research and public policy. 2nd ed. Oxford University Press, 2010.
7 Rice P, Drummond C. The price of a drink: the potential of alcohol minimum unit pricing as a public health measure in the UK. *Br J Psychiatry* 2012;201:169-71.
8 House of Commons Science and Technology Committee. Alcohol guidelines: 11th report of session 2010-2012. Stationery Office, 2012.
9 World Health Organization. The ICD-10 classification of mental and behavioural disorders. Geneva: WHO, 1992.
10 American Psychiatric Association. Diagnostic and statistical manual of mental disorders, fifth edition. American Psychiatric Publishing, 2013.
11 Hasin DS, O'Brien CP, Auriacombe M, et al. DSM-5 Criteria for Substance Use Disorders: Recommendations and Rationale. *Am J Psychiatry* 2013;170:834-51.
12 Heather N. A radical but flawed proposal: comments on Rehm et al. defining substance use disorders: do we really need more than heavy use? *Alcohol Alcohol* 2013;48:646-7.
13 Rehm J, Marmet S, Anderson P, Gual A, Kraus L, Nutt DJ, et al. Defining substance use disorders: do we really need more than heavy use? *Alcohol Alcohol* 2013;48:633-40.
14 Jackson R, Johnson M, Campbell F, Messina J, Guillaume L, Meier P, et al. Screening and brief intervention for prevention and early identification of alcohol use disorder in adults and young people. School of Health and Related Research (ScHARR) Public Health Collaborating Centre, 2010.
15 Kaner E, Bland M, Cassidy P, Coulton S, Dale V, Deluca P, et al. Effectiveness of screening and brief alcohol intervention in primary care (SIPS trial): pragmatic cluster randomised controlled trial. *BMJ* 2013;346:e8501.
16 Babor TF, Higgins-Biddle JC, Saunders JB, Monteiro MG. AUDIT: the alcohol use disorder identification test. Guidelines for use in primary health care. World Health Organization, 2001. http://whqlibdoc.who.int/hq/2001/WHO_MSD_MSB_01.6a.pdf?ua=1.
17 Drummond C, Ghodse H, Chengappa S. Use of investigations in the diagnosis and management of alcohol use disorders. In: Day E, ed. Clinical topics in addiction. RCPsych Publications, 2007:113-29.
18 Rollnick S, Butler CC, Kinnersley P, Gregory J, Mash B. Motivational interviewing. *BMJ* 2010;340:1242-5.
19 National Collaborating Centre for Mental Health. Alcohol-use disorders: the NICE guideline on diagnosis, assessment and management of harmful drinking and alcohol dependence. British Psychological Society and Royal College of Psychiatrists, 2011.
20 Lingford-Hughes AR, Welch S, Peters L, Nutt DJ; British Association for Psychopharmacology, Expert Reviewers Group. BAP updated guidelines: evidence-based guidelines for the pharmacological management of substance abuse, harmful use, addiction and comorbidity: recommendations from BAP. *J Psychopharmacol* 2012;26:899-952.
21 National Institute for Health and Care Excellence. Alcohol-use disorders: diagnosis and clinical management of alcohol-related physical complications. (Clinical guideline 100.) 2010. http://guidance.nice.org.uk/CG100.
22 Marlatt GA, Gordon JR. Relapse prevention: maintenance strategies in the treatment of addictive behaviors. Guilford Press, 1985.
23 Moos RH, Moos BS. Participation in treatment and Alcoholics Anonymous: a 16-year follow-up of initially untreated individuals. *J Clin Psychol* 2006;62:735-50.
24 Wall R, Sondhi A, Day E. What influences referral to 12-step mutual self-help groups by treatment professionals. *Eur Addict Res* 2014;20:241-7.
25 Timko C, DeBenedetti A. A randomized controlled trial of intensive referral to 12-step self-help groups: one-year outcomes. *Drug Alcohol Depend* 2007;90:270-9.
26 Raistrick D, Heather N, Godfrey C. Review of the effectiveness of treatment for alcohol problems. National Treatment Agency for Substance Misuse, 2006. www.nta.nhs.uk/uploads/nta_review_of_the_effectiveness_of_treatment_for_alcohol_problems_fullreport_2006_alcohol2.pdf.
27 Drummond C, Oyefeso A, Phillips T, Cheeta S, Deluca P, Perryman K, et al. Alcohol needs assessment research project (ANARP). The 2004 national alcohol needs assessment for England. Department of Health, 2004:1-31.
28 Jonas DE, Amick HR, Feltner C, Bobashev G, Thomas K, Wines R, et al. Pharmacotherapy for adults with alcohol use disorders in outpatient settings: a systematic review and meta-analysis. *JAMA* 2014;311:1889-900.
29 National Institute for Health and Care Excellence. Nalmefene for reducing alcohol consumption in people with alcohol dependence. (Technology appraisal guidance TA325). 2014. www.nice.org.uk/guidance/ta325.
30 Public Health England. Young people's hospital alcohol pathways: support pack for A&E departments. PHE, 2014.
31 Center for Substance Abuse Treatment. Alcohol use among older adults: pocket screening for health and social care providers. Substance Abuse and Mental Health Services Administration, 2001.

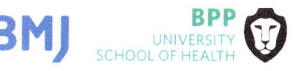

Assessing mental capacity: the Mental Capacity Act

Timothy R J Nicholson, specialist registrar in psychiatry[1], William Cutter, consultant psychiatrist[2], Matthew Hotopf, professor of general hospital psychiatry[1]

[1]Department of Psychological Medicine, Institute of Psychiatry, Western Education Centre, London SE5 9RJ

[2]Directorate of Older Persons' Mental Health Services, Hampshire Partnership NHS Trust, Southampton, Hampshire SO40 2RZ

Correspondence to: M Hotopf
m.hotopf@iop.kcl.ac.uk

Cite this as: BMJ 2008;336:322

DOI: 10.1136/bmj.39457.485347.80

http://www.bmj.com/
content/336/7639/322

ABSTRACT

Assessing mental capacity is an important part of a clinician's role, and the recent Mental Capacity Act can help doctors when making such decisions

Clinicians are often confronted with decisions about mental capacity. Healthcare workers in England and Wales should therefore be aware of the recent changes to how capacity is assessed and the way that adults lacking capacity are dealt with since the implementation in 2007 of the Mental Capacity Act 2005.[1]

What does the Mental Capacity Act do?

The act protects people who lack the mental capacity to make decisions. Until the Mental Capacity Act 2005 was implemented no statutory law covered this area. Courts previously dealt with capacity under "common law," which consists of the accumulated judgments of individual cases. The Mental Capacity Act is underpinned by five key principles (box 1), which are illustrated in a hypothetical scenario (box 2).

Why do I need to know about the Mental Capacity Act?

An assessment that a person lacks capacity has major implications; it gives clinicians influence over that person, and this influence could, potentially, be abused. The Mental Capacity Act provides important safeguards to patients' rights, and it also provides help for clinicians in dealing with capacity problems. In general hospitals, more than 30% of patients on acute medical wards may lack capacity.[2] A slightly higher proportion (44%) of psychiatric inpatients lack capacity to make the primary decision for which they were admitted.[3][4] Two million people in the UK are estimated to lack capacity through mental illness, learning difficulties, dementia, or physical illnesses that affect brain function (such as delirium or head injury).[5]

Until now, capacity has mostly been assessed in patients who refuse the management suggested by the clinical team; such patients are often referred to psychiatrists for capacity assessments.[6] Clinicians are also often unaware that their patients may have difficulty in making decisions.[2] Surveys indicate that clinicians have limited understanding of the law pertaining to capacity.[7][8]

What has the Mental Capacity Act changed?

Much of the Mental Capacity Act simply codifies previous common law, but it also changes the law in significant ways. The act introduces several new concepts and services: a code of practice; a criminal offence for wilful neglect or ill treatment of people without capacity; an independent mental capacity advocate service; and advance decisions. It has also expanded the role of several existing services, such as the court of protection and frameworks such as lasting power of attorney and court deputies.

What is the code of practice?

The code accompanies the Mental Capacity Act, and it is designed to guide those responsible for interpreting the act.[9] Clinicians are legally required to "have regard to" (have read and understood) its guidance and, if later asked, prove they did. Consequently, any departures from this will be hard to justify. The code of practice can be viewed and downloaded online.[9]

What is the independent mental capacity advocates service?

The service comprises the independent organisations that assign someone to support and represent "unbefriended" people who lack capacity. Their recommendations do not need to be adhered to by clinicians, although they should be taken into account as part of the decision making process. Each local authority (borough) has appointed its own independent mental capacity advocates service.

The code specifies when to instruct an independent mental capacity advocate. They can be instructed for care reviews or adult protection cases, but they must be instructed and then consulted when serious medical treatment is being proposed (such as ventilation, major surgery, chemotherapy, and discontinuation of artificial nutrition or hydration). They must also be involved when accommodation for more than 28 days in hospital or eight weeks in a care home is being arranged or changed.

What is a lasting power of attorney?

This replaces the enduring power of attorney system, where a person could appoint a named person (the "donee") with the authority to make decisions on their behalf if they lost capacity. Previously this only applied to property and affairs. The Mental Capacity Act widens this authority to decisions about personal welfare, including health care and social affairs. It includes all decisions except those about the withdrawal of life saving treatment, unless explicitly authorised in the agreement. Existing enduring power of attorney agreements will continue as before, but new appointments will be to the lasting power of attorney system.

SUMMARY POINTS

- The Mental Capacity Act has resulted in increased formalisation of capacity law and assessment
- The act has increased the expectation that healthcare workers should be competent at assessing capacity
- The act has also increased the need for training and education, especially awareness and understanding of the code of practice, independent mental capacity advocates, and advance decisions

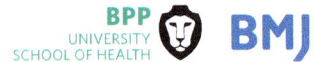

BOX 1 FIVE KEY PRINCIPLES OF THE MENTAL CAPACITY ACT

- Principle 1: Capacity should always be assumed. A patient's diagnosis, behaviour, or appearance should not lead you to presume capacity is absent
- Principle 2: A person's ability to make decisions must be optimised before concluding that capacity is absent. All practicable steps must be taken, such as giving sufficient time for assessments; repeating assessments if capacity is fluctuating; and, if relevant, using interpreters, sign language, or pictures
- Principle 3: Patients are entitled to make unwise decisions. It is not the decision but the process by which it is reached that determines if capacity is absent
- Principle 4: Decisions (and actions) made for people lacking capacity must be in their best interests
- Principle 5: Such decisions must also be the least restrictiveoption(s) for their basic rights and freedoms

BOX 2 HYPOTHETICAL SCENARIO

A 64 year old Asian man who speaks poor English presents to hospital with chest pain. Investigations reveal an ST elevation myocardial infarction and the clinical team decides to admit him. However, he is not willing to stay as he is flying to India the next day for his son's wedding. He is clearly distressed and very anxious.

In managing this case it is important to remember the principles of the Mental Capacity Act (box 1).

- Do not presume lack of capacity (principle 1) because of his anxiety or because he disagrees with the team's decision
- His capacity to make this decision should be assessed by the clinical team. To do this, his decision making ability should be optimised (principle 2) by explaining the benefits and risks of admission compared with other management options. An interpreter should be used if necessary
- If a lack of capacity cannot be proved, his decision to refuse admission must be respected, even if it is "unwise" (principle 3) or risky, because it is the decision process that is important, not the decision itself. The patient should be told how best to re-access treatment if he changes his mind or the clinical situation changes. Given the high risks associated with this decision, if the initial assessment of capacity is not clear, an expert (for example, psychiatry) opinion should be sought. The combination of angina, the realisation that he may have a serious illness, or the stress of his son's impending wedding may cause severe anxiety, although it would be rare for this to impair capacity
- If he is found to lack capacity, it must be established what is in his best interests (principle 4); this may not be what the clinical team initially thought. It may be clear, after researching his known beliefs and values, that he would have refused admission even if he still had capacity. The clinical team would be legally protected under the Mental Capacity Act if they thought it was in his best interests not to admit him
- Many options are available when acting in his best interests. These range from surgery to angioplasty to optimal drug therapy as an inpatient or outpatient. The least restrictive option must be used (principle 5) after weighing the risks, benefits, degrees of restriction, and practical consequences of each, given his clinical situation

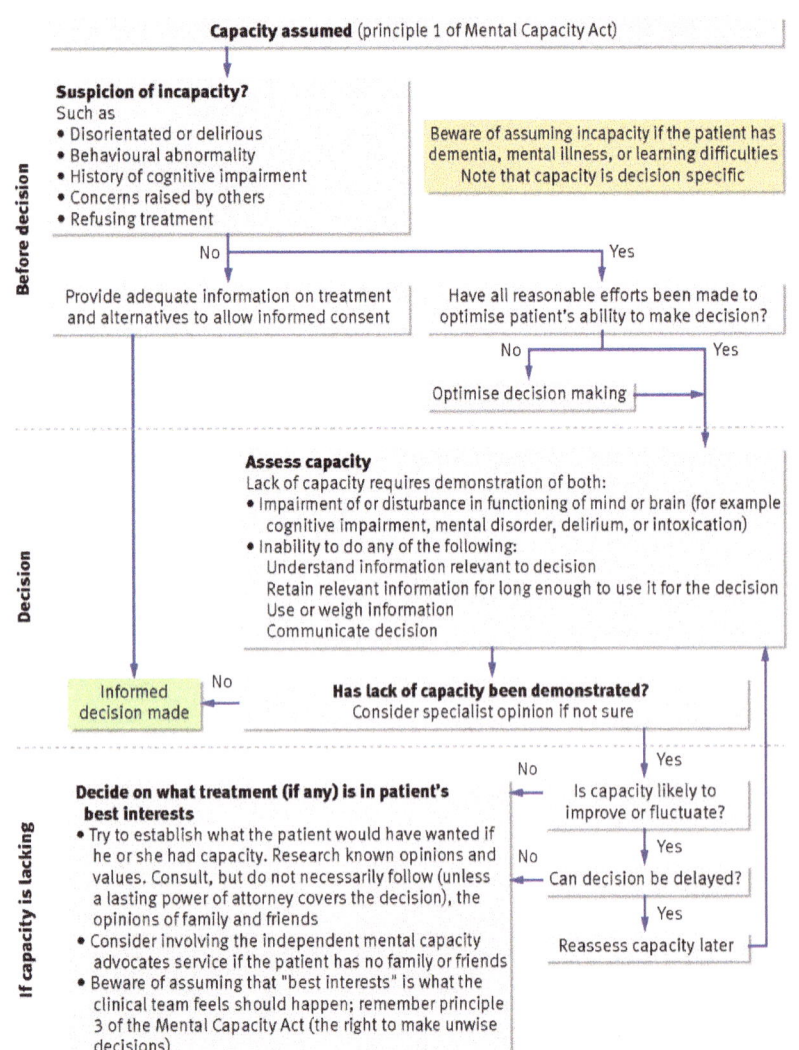

Flow chart of how to decide whether or not a person aged 16 or over has capacity

Property and affairs lasting power of attorney agreements can start before a person has lost capacity, but personal welfare ones cannot. Clinicians treating people without capacity must follow the decision of a donee, unless they are thought not to be acting in the person's best interests or to be abusing the person lacking capacity, in which case you should follow the guidance of the code of practice. In serious cases you may need to seek a decision from the court of protection.

When making a lasting power of attorney agreement, the limits of the powers granted are specified—this is known as the "nature and effect." Decisions about life sustaining treatment must be specified in the lasting power of attorney, and a signed statement from the attorney and a certificate completed by an independent third party are required.

A parallel system exists where the court of protection can appoint a deputy for someone who already lacks capacity. The deputy is likely to be a family member or director of social services. The deputy can consent on the person's behalf but can never consent to decisions that will shorten the person's life.

What are advance decisions?

Advance decisions can be drawn up by anybody to specify treatments they would not want if they lost capacity. They cannot demand treatments. Provided advance decisions are made when the person had capacity, and they are sufficiently specific to cover the patient's current predicament, clinicians must respect them. They can be made verbally and can be reversed by the individual if they regain capacity. Advance decisions that refuse life sustaining treatments (such as ventilation) have to be written, signed, and witnessed to be valid. It is incumbent on clinicians to find out if an advance decision exists and assess whether it is valid.

What is the court of protection?

This specialist court has been greatly changed by the Mental Capacity Act. It previously only adjudicated on the financial matters of people without capacity, but its role has widened

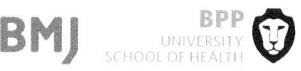

to include health and welfare decisions. It will be more accessible and available to arbitrate on disputes and is now able to "establish precedent" with the same powers as the High Court.

What legal protection do I have under the Mental Capacity Act?

Section 5 of the act protects from legal liability those providing health care (and personal care) for people without capacity, provided they had "reasonable belief" that the person lacked capacity and their actions were in the person's best interests. Documentation is key in such situations. However, the act does not protect from liability those professionals who have been negligent, or who have gone against the wishes of an attorney (or deputy) acting within the scope of their power.

How is capacity assessed?

Assessing capacity is a two stage process. For a person to lack capacity, he or she must have an impairment of or disturbance in the functioning of the brain or mind, and this defect must result in the inability to understand, retain, use, or weigh information relevant to a decision or to communicate a choice (figure). Note that there is both a diagnostic threshold and a component that is specific to a decision. Capacity can be assessed only in relation to a specific decision. This has been described as a "functional" approach rather than a "status" approach, where a person—having reached a diagnostic threshold—would be described as lacking capacity for all decisions. Capacity needs to be reassessed for each decision, particularly if the impairments fluctuate over time, as in delirium.

Under principle 3 of the Mental Capacity Act, a patient cannot be deemed to lack capacity just because the treating clinicians disagree with his or her decision. People are entitled to make unwise decisions (principle 2)—what matters is not the decision itself, but the way it was reached.

How do I decide what is in someone's best interests?

When deciding on best interests, you should consider not just the intervention likely to lead to the best clinical outcome, but you should place yourself in the patient's shoes and ask what they would have wanted if they still had capacity. The views of relatives and others who know the person well may be crucial to making this decision. Clinical problems have a variety of management options, ranging from doing nothing to radical treatments, and the least restrictive option should be used (principle 5 of the Mental Capacity Act).

Restraint can be used to achieve this, but its use is limited by the act (box 3) and it cannot amount to "deprivation of liberty" (see interaction with Mental Health Act).

How do the Mental Capacity Act and Mental Health Act interact?

This is a complex area. The Mental Health Act is relevant only when treating a mental disorder; in most circumstances it is not relevant when treating physical illnesses.

Patients detained under the Mental Health Act who refuse physical health treatments need to have their capacity assessed. Incapacity should not be assumed in such patients (principle 1 of Mental Capacity Act).

Except when a court of protection order—a consequence of which is the deprivation of liberty—is in place, the Mental Capacity Act cannot be used to give care involving

---

> **BOX 3 USE OF RESTRAINT UNDER THE MENTAL CAPACITY ACT**
> - Restraint is the use (or threat) of force to make someone do something that they are resisting
> - Restraint is also the restriction of a person's freedom of movement, whether they are resisting or not
> - Restraint must reasonably be believed to be necessary to prevent harm to the person lacking capacity
> - Restraint must be proportional to the likelihood and seriousness of harm

---

> **ADDITIONAL EDUCATIONAL RESOURCES**
>
> **General resources**
> - BMJ online learning(www.bmj.com/learningmodules/capacity)—Includes multiple choice questions for self testing
> - Department of Constitutional Affairs(www.dca.gov.uk/menincap/legis.htm#lpa)—Download the Mental Capacity Act and its code of practice
> - Public Guardianship Office(www.guardianship.gov.uk)—Administrative arm of the Court of Protection, which provides financial protection for those without capacity and information on lasting power of attorneys
> - Mental Health Act 2007 (www.opsi.gov.uk/acts/acts2007/ukpga_20070012_en.pdf)—download the new act. Its code of practice will also be available to download soon
> - Making Decisions Alliance (www.makingdecisions.org.uk)—Resource for patients and relatives who want to learn more about capacity
> - Royal College of Psychiatrists (www.rcpsych.ac.uk/pdf/Bournewoodfinalinterim.pdf)—Provides guidance on "Bournewood" patients until the new Mental Health Act is implemented
>
> **In your trust or area**
> - Senior colleagues
> - Psychiatry on call services (ideally "liaison" psychiatry if available)
> - Hospital lawyers
> - Clinical ethics committees
> - Social services
> - Court of protection
> - Your personal medical defence society

---

deprivation of liberty (see code of practice for details). Treatments that are prohibited in advance decisions or treatments that are not consented to by an attorney can still be given under the Mental Health Act if they are to treat a mental disorder.

The current Mental Health Act (1983) is due to be replaced by a new one (2007) in 2008. Among other changes, it will modify the Mental Capacity Act by clarifying how to deal with patients who lack capacity to decide whether or not to stay in hospital (or a care home), but who do not object to staying. Such patients are referred to as "Bournewood" patients, and the lack of statutory provisions for them is called the Bournewood gap.

Contributors: The authors planned the article together after discussions about patients seen in clinical practice. TRJN and WC wrote the first draft, which was revised by all three authors. MH edited the final manuscript and is guarantor.

Competing interests: None declared.

Provenance and peer review: Not commissioned; externally peer reviewed.

1   Department of Health. *Mental Capacity Act* . London: Stationery Office, 2005.
2   Raymont V, Bingley W, Buchanan A, David AS, Hayward P, Wessely S, et al. Prevalence of mental incapacity in medical in-patients and associated risk factors: cross sectional study. *Lancet* 2004;364:1421-7.

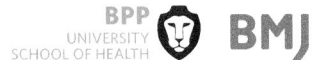

3   Cairns R, Maddock C, Buchanan A, David AS, Hayward P, Richardson G, et al. Prevalence and predictors of mental incapacity in psychiatric in-patients. *Br J Psychiatry* 2005;187:379-85.

4   Okai D, Owen G, McGuire H, Singh S, Churchill R, Hotopf M. Mental capacity in psychiatric patients: systematic review. *Br J Psychiatry* 2007;191:291-7.

5   Department of Constitutional Affairs. Mental Capacity Act 2005 factsheet. 2004. www.dca.gov.uk/menincap/mcbfactsheet.htm.

6   Ranjith G, Hotopf M. "Refusing treatment—please see:" an analysis of capacity assessments carried out by a liaison psychiatry service. *J R Soc Med* 2004;97:480-2.

7   Jackson E, Warner J. How much do doctors know about consent and capacity? *J R Soc Med* 2002;95:601-3.

8   Evans K, Jackson E, Warner J. How much do emergency healthcare workers know about capacity and consent? *Emerg Med J* 2007;24:391-3.

9   Mental Capacity Act 2005. *Code of practice* . Norwich: Stationery Office, 2007.

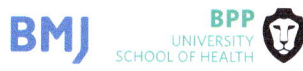

An introduction to patient decision aids

Drug and Therapeutics Bulletin

Drug and Therapeutics Bulletin
Editorial Office, London WC1H 9JR, UK

Correspondence to: dtb@bmjgroup.com

Cite this as: *BMJ* 2013;346:f4147

DOI: 10.1136/bmj.f4147

http://www.bmj.com/content/347/bmj.f4147

Patient decision aids are a means of helping people make informed choices about healthcare that take into account their personal values and preferences. Decision aids are a part of a shared decision making process, encouraging active participation by patients in healthcare decisions.[1] [2] Decision aids are relevant in many common healthcare decisions. They have been developed to make it easier for patients and healthcare professionals to discuss treatment options. Here, we give an overview of the rationale for the use of patient decision aids, what they contain, the evidence of their efficacy, and examples of their current and potential uses.

Decision aids in the context of shared decision making

Shared decision making is a process in which clinicians and patients work together to decide about interventions based on clinical evidence and the patient's informed preferences.[2] It involves the provision of evidence based information about options, benefits, risks, and uncertainties, together with decision support counselling and a system for recording and implementing patients' informed preferences. There is evidence that patients want to take part in decision making. A recent systematic review of peer reviewed journal articles found that, in 63% of articles most patients expressed a wish to actively participate in decisions around their treatment.[3] Also, the wish to participate appears to have increased over time. In studies published before 2000, only around 50% of articles found that most patients wished to be active partners in their treatment decisions, whereas from 2000, the percentage rose to 71%.[3] This was especially clear for cancer patients, where most patients in 85% of the 27 studies published since 2000 wished to be involved in treatment decisions. However, patients' preferences for involvement in decision making are variable and are affected by factors such as age, sex, and education.[4]

Shared decision making is appropriate for many types of healthcare decisions, including whether to undergo screening or a diagnostic test, whether to undergo a medical or surgical procedure, whether to participate in a self management programme, whether to take medication, or whether to attempt a lifestyle change.[2]

For patients to be able to play a part in the decision making process, they need clear, easy to understand information about the condition and the treatment or support options. A decision aid can be used to inform patients and help them think about the different options and to reach an informed preference.[2]

What is a patient decision aid?

Decision aids are available in a variety of media (online, print, video). However, they share common aims[5]:

- To inform people about the available options, from an evidence based perspective
- To encourage active engagement with the decision making process
- To help people think through what is important to them, so that they can make choices that reflect their own values and preferences.

An example for helping to decide between mastectomy or lumpectomy for early breast cancer can be found on the NHS Direct website (www.nhsdirect.nhs.uk/DecisionAids/PDAs/PDA_BreastCancer.aspx).

Most decision aids are being made available online, although some are only available as printed material. Ideally, patients need to work through the decision aids in their own time (although some are brief enough to use during the consultation). Patients may then wish to discuss use of the decision aid with the clinician, before finalising their decision.

What is in a decision aid?

At a minimum, a decision aid describes the decision to be taken, the options available, and the outcomes of these options (including benefits, harms, and uncertainties) based on a careful review of the evidence. Defining the decision involves framing it in a way that makes clear that this is a decision for the patient to make. Patients may not be aware that they have a choice but expect the clinician to tell them what treatment they "need."

Presentation of options can be done in a variety of formats. Tables that present all the options together, along with headline outcomes, have emerged as a popular format (see fig 1, more examples can be viewed at www.optiongrid.co.uk).

Explanation of risk is a key part of a decision aid, and work is ongoing as to how this can best be achieved, so as to present the information clearly and without bias. Use of visual aids such as "smiley faces" or "Cates plot" (see fig 2) is recommended (see www.nntonline.net).[6]

Decision aids go beyond simple provision of information, seeking also to help people think about their own values.[5] For example, in a decision aid for osteoarthritis of the hip, patients might be asked to consider the importance to them of returning to a high level of mobility, or of reducing pain to a minimum, compared with the importance they place on avoiding the risks of surgical complications, or a lengthy recovery from treatment. Patients are asked to explicitly address the "trade-offs" they need to make, accepting that treatments have risks as well as benefits. They can then make decisions based on an exploration of their own attitudes to risk, and to the importance they personally place on potential outcomes.

Evidence

Evidence supporting the use of decision aids is accumulating. A Cochrane systematic review of decision aids for screening or medical interventions concluded that when patients use decision aids they

- Improve their knowledge of the options
- Are helped to have more accurate expectations of possible benefits and harms
- Reach choices that are more consistent with their informed values
- Participate more in decision making.[7]

The reviewers found 86 randomised controlled trials (involving a total of over 20 000 participants) covering 35 condition-specific decisions and comparing use of a decision aid to a variety of control interventions. Improved knowledge of the options and their likely outcomes led to more accurate risk perceptions, especially when the decision aid expressed probabilities in numbers.[7]

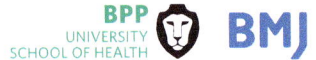

Use this grid to help you and your clinician decide whether to have mastectomy or lumpectomy with radiotherapy

Frequently asked questions	Lumpectomy with radiotherapy	Mastectomy
Which surgery is best for long term survival?	There is no difference between surgery options	There is no difference between surgery options
What are the chances of cancer coming back in the breast?	Breast cancer will come back in the breast in about 10 in 100 women in the 10 years after a lumpectomy	Breast cancer will come back in the area of the scar in about 5 in 100 women in the 10 years after a mastectomy
What is removed?	The cancer lump is removed with a margin of tissue	The whole breast is removed
Will I need more than one operation on the breast?	Possibly, if cancer cells remain in the breast after the lumpectomy. This can occur in up to 5 in 100 women	No, unless you choose breast reconstruction
How long will it take to recover?	Most women are home 24 hours after surgery	Most women are home 2-3 days after surgery
Will I need radiotherapy?	Yes, for up to 6 weeks after surgery	Unlikely, radiotherapy is not routine after mastecomy
Will I need to have my lymph glands removed?	Some or all of the lymph glands in the armpit are usually removed	Some or all of the lymph glands in the armpit are usually removed
Will I need chemotherapy?	Yes, you may be offered chemotherapy as well, usually given after surgery and before radiotherapy	Yes, you may be offered chemotherapy as well, usually given after surgery and before radiotherapy
Will I lose my hair?	Hair loss is common after chemotherapy	Hair loss is common after chemotherapy

Fig 1 An example of an Option Grid (reproduced with permission)

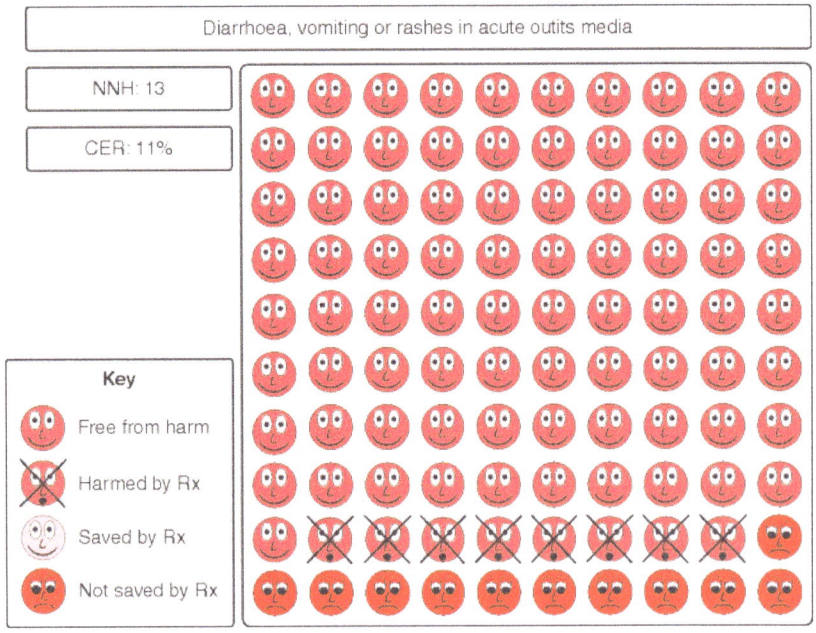

Fig 2 An example of a Cates plot illustrating the effect of antibiotic therapy for acute otitis media: out of 100 children with acute otitis media, 11 will suffer diarrhoea, vomiting, or a rash. If 100 children are given an antibiotic for the condition, an additional 8 children will suffer diarrhoea, vomiting, or a rash. The number needed to harm (NNH)=13 (CER=control event rate) (reproduced with permission)

Decision aids also reduced decisional conflict, reducing the numbers of people who felt they were unable to make a decision, either through feeling insufficiently informed or being unclear about their personal values. In line with this, people were less likely to be passive in decision making after using a decision aid.[7]

The evidence appears to show that people are more likely to choose more conservative treatment options. In studies focused on choices regarding more major elective surgery, people were 20% less likely to choose major invasive elective surgery, compared with usual care, after

using a decision aid; likewise, in studies on prostate specific antigen (PSA) testing people were 15% less likely to choose the screening test.[7] However, the results for these secondary outcomes should be treated with caution. This is because the research looked at an initial decision, and does not represent a long term assessment of decisions and cost. It is not unreasonable to assume that patients might choose a conservative route first, then opt for surgery at a later stage if the conservative option does not meet their needs. Until the results of long term research are available, we cannot assume that total healthcare resource use would be significantly different.

Development

A great many decision aid resources already exist. Pioneering work was done in this area by the Informed Medical Decisions Foundation (a US non-profit organisation, http://informedmedicaldecisions.org/), initially in the US but also in the UK. Subsequently, the International Patient Decision Aids Standards (IPDAS, http://ipdas.ohri.ca/) organisation was established to propose standards for the development of these materials.

IPDAS produced a quality criteria framework in 2006.[8] Agreed standards include the following requirements:

- A systematic development process
- The provision of information about options and probabilities
- Clarification of values
- Disclosure of conflicts of interest
- A balanced presentation of options
- Use of plain language
- Information based on current evidence.

A list of decision aids appraised against the IPDAS criteria is available on the IPDAS website (http://decisionaid.ohri.ca/AZinvent.php).

The NHS has commissioned the development of a suite of patient decision aids. Decision aids on the following topics are already available on the NHS Direct website (www.nhsdirect.nhs.uk/en/DecisionAids):

- Advanced kidney disease—planning for end of life care
- Benign prostatic hyperplasia
- Cataracts
- Localised prostate cancer
- PSA testing
- Chorionic villus sampling and amniocentesis
- Breast cancer
- Knee arthritis
- Osteoarthritis of the hip.

More decision aids, commissioned by NHS RightCare, are under development (www.rightcare.nhs.uk/index.php/shared-decision-making/).

A selection of decision aids relating to the use of medicines has been produced by the National Prescribing Centre (now known as the Medicines and Prescribing Centre, which is part of the National Institute for Health and Clinical Excellence).

Use and integration

Patients might have difficulty using decisions aids if they have difficulty reading or have no access to, or ability to use, a computer, or if they do not understand English. Alternative formats and presentations need to be developed for these people.

An important issue for clinicians is the effect of using a decision aid on the length of the consultation. A Cochrane

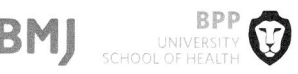

- This article was originally published in *Drug and Therapeutics Bulletin* (*DTB* 2012;50:90-2; doi:10.1136/dtb.2012.08.0121).
- *DTB* is a highly regarded source of unbiased, evidence based information and practical advice for healthcare professionals. It is independent of the pharmaceutical industry, government, and regulatory authorities, and is free of advertising.
- *DTB* is available online at http://dtb.bmj.com.

review showed a variable effect, ranging from reducing the consultation by 8 minutes to increasing it by 23 minutes compared with a standard consultation (median +2.5 minutes).[7] However, the review did not distinguish between primary or secondary care consultations. There was also considerable heterogeneity depending on the clinical condition. Of course, the effect on consultation length will depend on when decision aids are used, where in the patient journey they are introduced, and whether they are used in the consultation or outside it. This will vary depending on the decision under consideration. For example, a decision about preferred treatment options for osteoarthritis of the hip is probably best undertaken before an appointment is made with an orthopaedic surgeon. In this situation, the decision aid could be offered after probable diagnosis, but before a secondary care referral is made. The referral, if required, would follow on from the patient's expressed preferences.

Reported "facilitators" to implementing shared decision making are the motivation of health professionals and their perception that putting shared decision making into practice will lead to improved patient outcomes and improved healthcare processes.[9] The use of decision aids as part of a shared decision making process will have implications for training of healthcare professionals.[10]

Embedding decision aids into clinical systems is likely to make them more accessible to clinicians.[9] There are several initiatives to promote shared decision making in the NHS. They include

- The NHS RightCare Shared Decision Making project (www.rightcare.nhs.uk/index.php/shared-decision-making/)
- The Health Foundation's MAGIC (www.health.org.uk/areas-of-work/programmes/shared-decision-making/) and Co-Creating Health programmes (www.health.org.uk/areas-of-work/programmes/co-creating-health/).

Conclusion

People increasingly want to be involved in making decisions about treatment choices. Patient decision aids help inform patients about the options available to them and involve them in the decision making process. They also help improve communication between clinicians and patients. A number of decision aids have been produced, and a quality criteria framework and set of standards have been developed for those involved in designing them. The NHS is developing a collection of patient decision aids as a resource for clinicians. However, it is probably not enough to make decision aids easily available. If they are to become part of routine clinical practice, they need to be embraced by the clinical community as well as by patients, established as part of the clinical workflow, and included in education, training, and development programmes for healthcare professionals.

1. Barry MJ, Edgman-Levitan S. Shared decision making—the pinnacle of patient-centred care. *N Engl J Med* 2012;366:780-1.
2. Coulter A, Collins A. *Making shared decision-making a reality: no decision about me, without me* . 2011. www.kingsfund.org.uk/publications/nhs_decisionmaking.html.
3. Chewning B, Bylund CL, Shah B, Arora NK, Gueguen JA, Makoul G. Patient preferences for shared decisions: a systematic review. *Patient Educ Couns* 2012;86:9-18.
4. Say R, Murtagh M, Thomson R. Patients' preferences for involvement in medical decision making: a narrative review. *Patient Educ Couns* 2006;60:102-14.
5. International Patient Decision Aids Standards Collaboration. *Criteria for judging the quality of patient decision aids* . 2005. www.ipdas.ohri.ca/IPDAS_checklist.pdf.
6. Spiegelhalter D, Pearson M, Short I. Visualizing uncertainty about the future. *Science* 2011;333:1393-400.
7. Stacey D, Bennett CL, Barry MJ, Col NF, Eden KB, Holmes-Rovner M, et al. Decision aids for people facing health treatment or screening decisions. *Cochrane Database Syst Rev* 2011;10:CD001431.
8. Elwyn G, O'Connor A, Stacey D, Volk R, Edwards A, Coulter A, et al. Developing a quality criteria framework for patient decision aids: online international Delphi consensus process. *BMJ* 2006;333:417.
9. Légaré F, Ratté S, Gravel K, Graham ID. Barriers and facilitators to implementing shared decision-making in clinical practice: update of a systematic review of health professionals' perceptions. *Patient Educ Couns* 2008;73:526-35.
10. Elwyn G, Frosch D, Thomson R, Joseph-Williams N, Lloyd A, Kinnersley P, et al. Shared decision making: a model for clinical practice. *Gen Intern Med* 2012; doi:10.1007/s11606-012-2077-6.

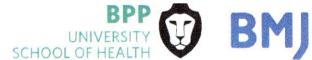

Safeguarding adults at risk of harm

Billy Boland, consultant psychiatrist and lead doctor for safeguarding adults[1],
Jemima Burnage, head of social work and safeguarding[1],
Hasan Chowhan, general practitioner[2]

[1]Hertfordshire Partnership NHS Foundation Trust, St Albans AL3 5TL, UK

[2]Creffield Medical Centre, Colchester CO2 7GH, UK

Correspondence to: B Boland billy.boland@hertspartsft.nhs.uk

Cite this as: BMJ 2013;346:f2716

DOI: 10.1136/bmj.f2716

http://www.bmj.com/content/346/bmj.f2716

What is safeguarding adults?

Safeguarding adults is about protecting those at risk of harm. It involves identifying abuse and acting where harm is occurring. The UK Department of Health's *No Secrets* guidance defines a vulnerable adult as a person aged 18 years or over "who is or may be in need of community care services by reason of mental or other disability, age or illness; and who is or may be unable to take care of him or herself, or unable to protect him or herself against significant harm or exploitation."[1]

In the United Kingdom awareness of safeguarding adults has been raised in recent years through some high profile events. In May 2011, the BBC *Panorama* programme "Undercover care, the abuse exposed" (www.bbc.co.uk/programmes/b011pwt6) revealed the abuse of people with learning disabilities at Winterbourne View Hospital.[2] More recently, the Francis inquiry into the care provided at Mid Staffordshire NHS Foundation Trust highlighted substandard care that resulted in harm to patients.[3]

Abuse is not just about an act against someone, such as physical abuse, but can also be about acts of omission and neglect, such as not listening or acting on the concerns of patients and carers, neglecting those in need, and allowing institutional harm to occur (box 1 summarises different types of abuse). This article reviews what constitutes abuse, who is at risk, and how to identify and manage suspected abuse in adults.

Who is considered an adult at risk of harm?

Many patients who use health services may be vulnerable (or "at risk of harm"[4]) in one way or another, but defining the core concept of vulnerability is a challenge. A frail elderly person and a blind adult may both be at risk, but the nature and impact of their vulnerabilities are likely to be different. Frailty or blindness, however, is not synonymous with being at risk. In both circumstances individuals may well be at liberty to make informed choices about their lives and be able to protect themselves. Rather, these factors may present additional challenges to keeping safe in particular situations, such as being in receipt of care that is substandard.

In clinical practice, be that primary or secondary care or partner agencies, adults at risk of harm can present in a variety of ways. Examples include:

- An elderly person who is frail, physically unwell, disabled, or has cognitive impairment
- A person with a severe mental illness who is in a nursing home or residential care
- A person with a learning disability
- People who lack capacity to make decisions about the care that they receive
- Somebody with drug or alcohol problems
- Someone with a physical disability, blindness, or deafness.

When should a health professional suspect abuse?

Given its nature, potential or actual abuse is not always obvious. For example, a general practitioner may visit a care home and notice that a patient seems withdrawn, unkempt, has lost weight, and has poor skin care. This should raise concerns for the general practitioner and stimulate further inquiries. Such a presentation could be due to disease that has led to deterioration, and treatment is needed. It could, however, mean that the patient is not being provided with the level of care that he or she requires and is being neglected. Points that the general practitioner might consider are whether the patient can reach a drink, can feed him or herself, and is able to ask for help and whether fluid and food intake are being monitored.

Good clinical skills can uncover abuse, but the clinician needs to be alert to this in order to recognise it. Doctors should consider not only the patient, but also the wider context, including environment, family, social networks, and culture. It is the space between the individual and the world around them where abuse can occur.

Doctors should be aware of the various "red flags" that initiate suspicions of abuse. Unexplained injuries may be discovered on examination or reported by a third party. These should be followed up and the cause of injury clarified to understand whether abuse may have occurred. Behavioural change, such as becoming withdrawn, aggressive, irritable, or emotionally labile, may be a direct result of distress caused by harm. A patient mentioning a change in personal circumstances may lead the doctor to consider the possibility of exploitation by another. For example, a person with a learning disability who was previously financially independent may talk about his or her family "stopping" the money and not allowing the person to make choices. In all such cases, doctors must assess the risk to the individuals and whether there is a need for immediate intervention. Circumstances that would require immediate action would include when someone's life is in immediate danger or there is significant risk of serious harm. Doctors assessing risk should also think about any risk posed to adults at risk other than the patient, to members of the public, or to children.

SUMMARY POINTS

- Doctors have a key role in safeguarding adults at risk from harm. Identifying and reporting safeguarding events is the duty of all clinicians, and doctors need to familiarise themselves with how to do this
- Preventing abuse is a key component of any effective safeguarding system. Listening to concerns, promoting self determination, and offering choice supports people in protecting themselves
- Be sensitive to the challenges of inquiring about abuse. Does the patient want the support of a trusted person? Have you made sure the abuser is not present at the assessment?
- Information sharing and reporting are necessary to protect adults at risk. Be aware of when the need to share information outweighs the right to confidentiality
- Working in partnership with other agencies and organisations is recognised as good practice and fundamental to ensuring that services provided are safe and of a high quality. Adults at risk may receive care from several different providers, and so a coordinated approach is most effective in safeguarding adults

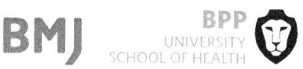

BOX 1 SUMMARY OF TYPES OF ABUSE OF VULNERABLE ADULTS*

- *Physical abuse*—including hitting; slapping; pushing; kicking; misuse of medication, restraint, or sanctions
- *Sexual abuse*—including rape and sexual assault or sexual acts to which the adult at risk has not consented, could not consent, or was pressured into consenting
- *Psychological abuse*—including emotional abuse, threats of harm or abandonment, deprivation of contact, humiliation, blaming, controlling, intimidation, coercion, harassment, verbal abuse, isolation or withdrawal from services or supportive networks
- *Financial or material abuse*—including theft; fraud; exploitation; pressure in connection with wills, property, inheritance, or financial transactions; misuse or misappropriation of property, possessions, or benefits
- *Neglect and acts of omission*—including ignoring medical or physical care needs; failure to provide access to appropriate health, social care, or educational services; the withholding of the necessities of life such as medication, adequate nutrition, and heating
- *Discriminatory abuse*—including racist, sexist, that based on a person's disability, and other forms of harassment, slurs, or similar treatment

*Adapted from Department of Health. No Secrets: Guidance on developing and implementing multi-agency policies and procedures to protect vulnerable adults from abuse.[1]

BOX 2 FACTORS TO CONSIDER WHEN INQUIRING ABOUT ABUSE*

- The vulnerability of the individual
- The nature and extent of the abuse
- The length of time it has been occurring
- The impact on the individual
- The risk of repeated or increasingly serious acts involving this or other vulnerable adults

*Adapted from Department of Health. No Secrets: Guidance on developing and implementing multi-agency policies and procedures to protect vulnerable adults from abuse.[1]

BOX 3 MANAGING THE CONVERSATION WITH AN INDIVIDUAL WHEN ABUSE IS SUSPECTED

- Make sure the abuser is not present
- Allow the victim to be accompanied by a trusted person if they wish
- Vulnerable people can have particular difficulties with communication. Ensure they have appropriate support to express themselves clearly (such as a foreign language interpreter or British Sign Language interpreter)
- Be clear what will happen with the information that the victim discloses
- Establish the facts of the allegation of abuse and acknowledge the impact of the abuse on the victim

The primary aim of safeguarding is to keep an individual safe and prevent further abuse from occurring. When assessing abuse, doctors should seek to establish the circumstances surrounding the concerns in an unbiased, objective way. It is important to be mindful of the difficulties the abused person may have in reporting abuse. The person may be frightened that the abuse will become worse if it is revealed and worried that it may leave them vulnerable to other types of harm. Making sure the potential abuser is not present when asking about concerns should help the abused person talk frankly about his or her experiences. Being accompanied by a trusted person may help a vulnerable adult feel supported and more confident in sharing information. For a summary of points to consider during assessment see boxes 2 and 3.

How common is abuse of adults?

Concerns about allegations of abuse are known to be under-reported—with issues about identification, stigma, and institutional systems[5] [6]—and so prevalence is difficult to identify. The Health and Social Care Information Centre reports that there were over 95 000 referrals for adult safeguarding in 2010-11 in England.[7] Of these, 62% were for women and 61% for adults aged 65 years or older. People with a significant health need constituted a large proportion of the total referrals, including people with a physical disability (49%), with mental health difficulties (23%), with learning disabilities (20%), and with substance misuse problems (7%). International comparisons are difficult to draw given national variations in definitions of abuse and safeguarding.

One systematic review of studies of elder abuse has found that about a quarter of vulnerable elderly people are at risk of abuse, with only a small proportion of these currently detected, and it recommends that adequate standards for abuse measures are developed.[8] In Hong Kong a study of Chinese elderly people found that 2.5% reported physical abuse,[9] while in a US study women with disabilities were found to be four times more likely to experience sexual assault than other women.[10] Accounts from carers also shed light on the prevalence of abuse. In the UK a cross sectional survey of family carers for people with dementia found around a third reported important levels of abuse,[11] and a Japanese study found 30% of care givers reported potentially harmful behaviour towards an elderly disabled family member.[12] Threshold inconsistencies in determining abuse are just one of the difficulties in safeguarding research.[13]

Who is responsible for protecting vulnerable adults?

The General Medical Council has highlighted the central role of doctors in protecting patients: "Good Medical Practice says that the safety of patients must come first at all times. If you believe that patient safety is or may be seriously compromised ... you should put the matter right if that is possible. In all other cases you should raise your concern with the organisation you have a contract with or which employs you."[14]

Safeguarding is the responsibility of all clinicians, and anyone can raise a safeguarding concern. All allegations of abuse need to be taken seriously whether made by a patient, carer, healthcare professional, or other service provider. If a third party reports concerns to a general practitioner, the doctor should make inquiries about the nature and circumstances of the allegation. It is particularly important to ask about the safety of the individual at the time the allegation is raised and any support the person has sought.

In addressing abuse, the Department of Health for England and Wales has described six safeguarding principles. Their aim is to inform how safeguarding matters should be approached (see box 4).[15] These recommendations capture the essence of good safeguarding practice and would be of use to a clinician working in any country.

What factors influence the likelihood of abuse?

Certain personal characteristics of adults at risk can increase their vulnerability, and thus susceptibility to abuse (see box 5). A lack of mental capacity to make decisions about their own safety can place individuals at the mercy of others. Those who are unable to make such decisions have impaired ability to protect themselves from bad decisions and may be impaired in asking for help if they experience an abusive act.

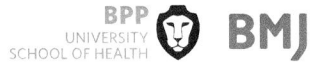

BOX 4 SIX PRINCIPLES OF GOOD SAFEGUARDING PRACTICE*

- *Empowerment*—Presumption of person-led decisions and informed consent
- *Protection*—Support and representation for those in greatest need
- *Prevention*—It is better to take action before harm occurs
- *Proportionality*—Proportionate and least intrusive response appropriate to the risk presented
- *Partnership*—Local solutions through services working with their communities. Communities have a part to play in preventing, detecting, and reporting neglect and abuse
- *Accountability*—Accountability and transparency in delivering safeguarding

*Taken from Department of Health for England and Wales. Statement of government policy on adult safeguarding.[15]

BOX 5 RISK FACTORS FOR ABUSE IN VULNERABLE ADULTS

- Lack of mental capacity
- Being physically dependent on others
- Low self esteem
- Previous history of abuse
- Negative experiences of disclosing abuse
- Social isolation
- Lack of access to health and social services or high quality information

---

Capacity may be impaired permanently, as in some cases of learning disability or brain injury. Temporary incapacity can also arise if conditions such as mental illness or physical illness involving the brain affect decision making sufficiently to disturb capacity. By contrast, people with communication difficulties may have recognised that an abusive act has taken place but are unable to communicate that it has occurred. In England and Wales, the Mental Capacity Act[16] makes it clear that a person is assumed to have capacity unless established otherwise. Where people lack capacity to make decisions to protect themselves from abuse, then any acts done or decisions made must be in their best interests. Clinicians must consider if any matters to be resolved can be deferred until capacity returns (such as when mental illness resolves), but this needs to be balanced against ongoing risk of harm. Doctors should also think about whether capacity can be supported in any way, such as through simplifying communication.

Feelings of low self worth in victims can mean that abuse goes unreported. A prior history of abuse, including abuse in childhood, can shape an individual's response to current abuse. Stigma and discrimination of vulnerable people can increase the chance of their becoming a target for abusive types of behaviour.

How should we prevent and respond to abuse?

Abuse can be prevented through services ensuring that they provide safe and effective care. Staff must be supported in raising concerns about practice and action needs to be taken in response. Organisations need to have systems in place to monitor incidents, complaints, and feedback in order to understand what is happening, and should act as early warning systems to identify systemic problems as quickly as possible.[3] Staff should be trained and supervised in safeguarding matters to raise awareness and ensure they have the necessary skills to identify abuse and respond.

GPs need to raise awareness of safeguarding in their communities and forge links with other services and stakeholders including local service user and carer groups (such as those offered through organisations like the Alzheimer's Society or National Autistic Society). Interventions should be aimed at making life easier, such as providing mobility aids or treating physical and mental illness to help individuals maintain independence. Such actions reduce barriers to patients making their own

choices and reduce their reliance on others. Even when a person requires a high level of personal care, it is important to ensure that services are organised around the individual. The person's choices need to be heard and where possible form part of the plan. Compassion, dignity, and respect are fundamental to all aspects of care. The introduction of personal budgets for social care[17] is one key way that individuals are being helped to take control of the care that they receive. Personal health budgets are to be rolled out in 2013.[18]

In England and Wales, statutory requirements for safeguarding adults are set out in the Department of Health document *No Secrets*,[1] and they continue to inform safeguarding practice. This establishes the principles of multiagency working and sets out how this should be achieved locally. In Scotland, the Adult Support and Protection (Scotland) Act 2007[19] describes the function of adult protection committees and sets out the requirements for multiagency working. For Northern Ireland, procedures are described by the Department of Health, Social Services, and Public Safety.[20]

The Care Quality Commission has a central role in overseeing safeguarding practice for England and Wales through its role in eliminating poor quality care and protecting the rights of individuals.[21] It emphasises that a central pillar in safeguarding practice is the principle of safe and proportionate information sharing to protect people at risk, to work in partnership with other agencies, and to promote adherence to standards. This can present particular challenges for clinicians, who are used to protecting confidentiality.

Serious case reviews often identify lack of information sharing between agencies as an issue. Doctors must therefore ensure that they share information about their concerns while respecting individuals' right to confidentiality. Patients and carers need to be informed that their right to confidentiality is not absolute and that information may be shared in some circumstances where there is a significant risk of harm to others and in cases where it is in the public interest.[22] An example might be that a patient tells their doctor that their mother has been physically abused by a nurse in hospital, but says she does not want to report it. The doctor should explain that this is a serious allegation and that patients other than their relative may be at risk of harm, therefore further inquiries are needed.

When should I refer?

Doctors and health professionals need to familiarise themselves with the policies and procedures concerning safeguarding in their region. There is international variation depending on the law of the country. The United Nations Declaration on Human Rights informs the development of law for the protection of individuals throughout the world (www.un.org/en/documents/udhr/index.shtml).

All concerns regarding significant risk of abuse should be reported to the local services responsible for safeguarding. In England and Wales this would be the local safeguarding investigating team, the lead agency for safeguarding being the local authority.[1] Under section 75 of the Health and Social Care Act 2012,[23] the local authority is able to delegate this authority to other statutory organisations such as NHS partnerships. Doctors need to be aware of how and where to report in their local area. Most safeguarding boards have contact details and information on their websites.

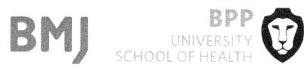

In the UK there is a well established network of named professionals with experience in safeguarding for children and young people, as laid out in an intercollegiate document on safeguarding children and young adults.[24] Similar roles for safeguarding adults are currently not statutory requirements but are being introduced across the country and becoming part of provider contracts. These can be a valuable source of support and expertise where available. If unsure, doctors should always make a referral for investigation. There is no predetermined threshold for intervention where there are safeguarding concerns. All responses are bespoke and depend on the circumstances of the case.

Contributors: All authors contributed to the design and writing of this article.

Competing interests: We have read and understood the BMJ Group policy on declaration of interests and have no relevant interests to declare.

Provenance and peer review: Not commissioned; externally peer reviewed.

1   Department of Health. *No secrets: Guidance on developing and implementing multi-agency policies and procedures to protect vulnerable adults from abuse* . DoH, 2000.
2   Flynn M. South Gloucestershire Safeguarding Adults Board. *Winterbourne View Hospital. A serious case review* . South Gloucestershire Council, 2012.
3   Francis R. Report of the Mid Staffordshire NHS Foundation Trust public inquiry. Mid Staffordshire NHS Foundation Trust Public Inquiry, 2013.
4   Law Commission. *Adult social care* . Stationary Office, 2011.
5   Department of Health. *Report on the consultation of the review of "No Secrets."* DoH, 2009.
6   Morgan A. *Clinical governance and adult safeguarding—an integrated process* . Department of Health, 2010.
7   NHS Information Centre, Social Care Team. Abuse of vulnerable adults in England 2010-11: Experimental statistics final report. 2012.
8   Cooper C, Selwood A, Livingston G. The prevalence of elder abuse and neglect: a systematic review. *Age Ageing* 2008;37:151-60.
9   Yan E, Tang CSK. Elder abuse by caregivers: a study of prevalence and risk factors in Hong Kong Chinese families. *J Fam Violence* 2004;19:269-77.
10   Martin SL, Ray N, Sotres-Alvarez D, Kupper LL, Morracco KE, Dickens PA, et al. Physical and sexual assault of women with disabilities. *Violence Against Women* 2006;12:823-37.
11   Cooper C, Selwood A, Blanchard M, Walker Z, Blizard R, Livingston G. Abuse of people with dementia by family carers: representative cross sectional survey. *BMJ* 2009;338:b155.
12   Sasaki M, Arai Y, Kumamoto K, Abe K, Arai A, Mizuno Y. Factors relating to potentially harmful behaviours towards disabled older people by family caregivers in Japan. *Int J Geriatr Psychiatry* 2007;22:250-7.
13   Manthorpe J, Martineau S. Serious case reviews in adult safeguarding in England: an analysis of a sample of reports. *Br J Soc Work* 2010;41:224-41.
14   General Medical Council. Raising and acting on concerns about patient safety (2012). www.gmc-uk.org/guidance/ethical_guidance/ raising_concerns.asp.
15   Department of Health. Statement of government policy on adult safeguarding. 2011. https://www.gov.uk/government/uploads/system/ uploads/attachment_data/file/147310/dh_126770.pdf.pdf.
16   Department for Constitutional Affairs. *Mental Capacity Act 2005: Code of practice* . Stationery Office, 2007.
17   Community Care, Services for Carers and Children's Services (Direct Payments) (England) Regulations 2009 (SI 2009/1887). www. legislation.gov.uk/uksi/2009/1887/contents/made.
18   Forder J, Jones K, Glendinning C, Caiels J, Welch E, Baxter K, et al. Evaluation of the personal health budget pilot programme. Department of Health, 2012. https://www.phbe.org.uk/index. php?action=frDownload
19   Scottish Government. The Adult Support and Protection (Scotland) Act 2007. Part 1: Draft guidance for adult protection committees. Scottish Government, 2008. www.scotland.gov.uk/ Publications/2008/05/21163507/0.
20   Department of Health, Social Services and Public Safety. *Adult safeguarding in Northern Ireland—regional and local partnership arrangements* . Department of Health, Social Services and Public Safety, 2010.
21   Care Quality Commission. *Our safeguarding protocol. The Care Quality Commission's responsibility and commitment to safeguarding* . Care Quality Commission, 2013.
22   General Medical Council. Confidentiality. 2009. www.gmc-uk.org/ guidance/ethical_guidance/confidentiality.asp.
23   UK Government. Health and Social Care Act 2012. www.legislation.gov. uk/ukpga/2012/7/contents/enacted.
24   Safeguarding children and young people: roles and competences for health care staff. Intercollegiate document September 2010. Royal College of Paediatrics and Child Health, 2010. www.rcpch.ac.uk/ system/files/protected/page/Safeguarding%20Children%20and%20 Young%20people%202010.pdf.

More titles in
The BMJ Series

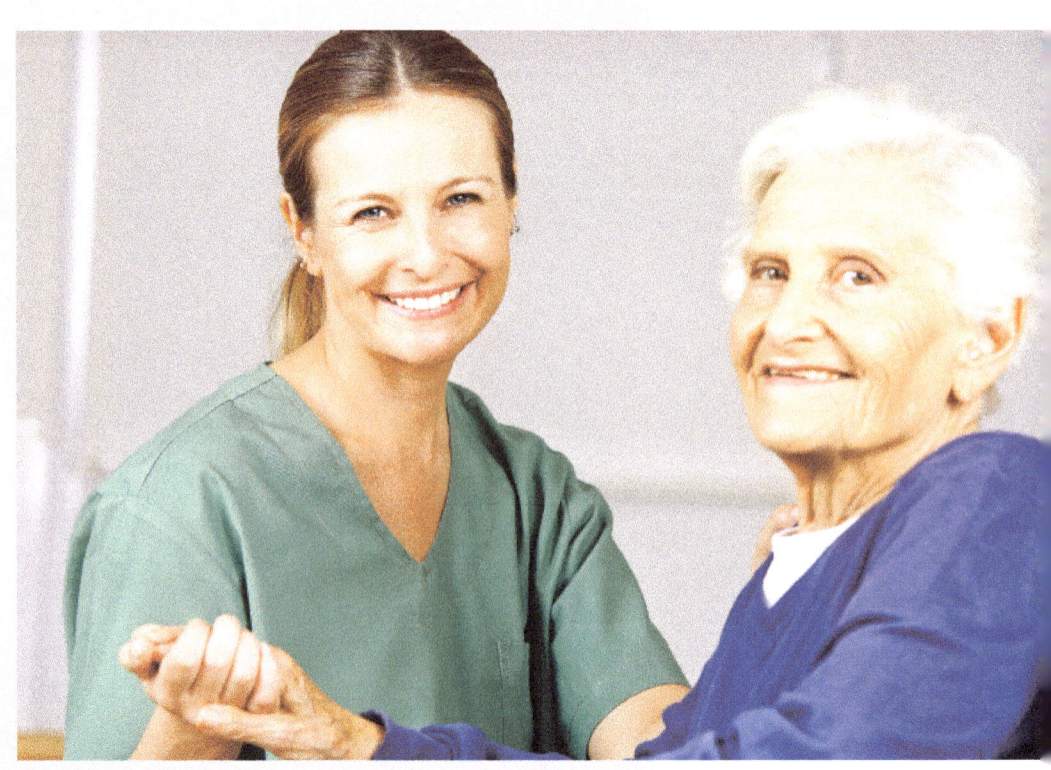

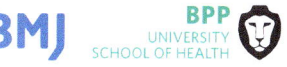
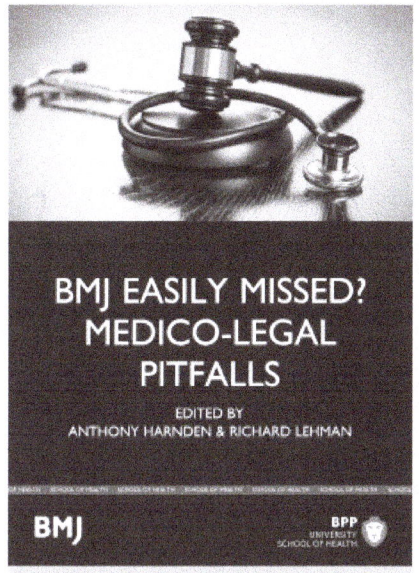
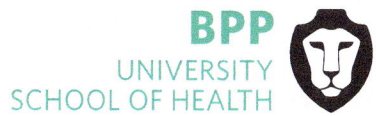

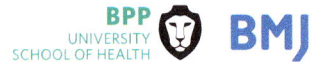

More titles in
The BMJ Easily Missed? Series

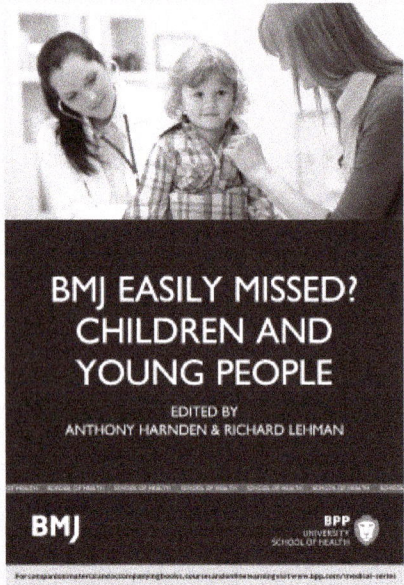

**BMJ EASILY MISSED?
CHILDREN AND
YOUNG PEOPLE**

EDITED BY
ANTHONY HARNDEN & RICHARD LEHMAN

BMJ

£29.99

January 2016

Paperback

978-1-472739-13-1

This book brings together a series of useful articles on a range of important diagnoses in children and young people that may be easily missed at first presentation in primary care. The spectrum of conditions ranges from coarctation of the aorta, biliary atresia and congenital cataract in neonates, orthopaedic presentations such as Perthes disease and slipped femoral epiphysis and infections such as septic arthritis and malaria. All articles describe data to support the assertion that the conditions are often overlooked in primary care and that failure to recognise the diagnosis may have serious implications for the child or young person.

This book provides the reader with:

- Diagnoses in children and young people that are important not to miss

- Evidence that the diagnoses are easily missed in primary care

- Succinct articles with specific learning points and take home messages

- Spectrum of ages from neonates to adolescents

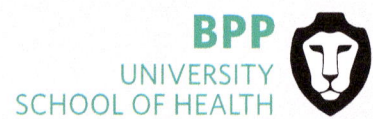

www.bpp.com/medical-series

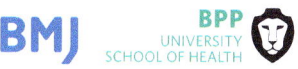

More titles in The BMJ Research Methods and Reporting Series

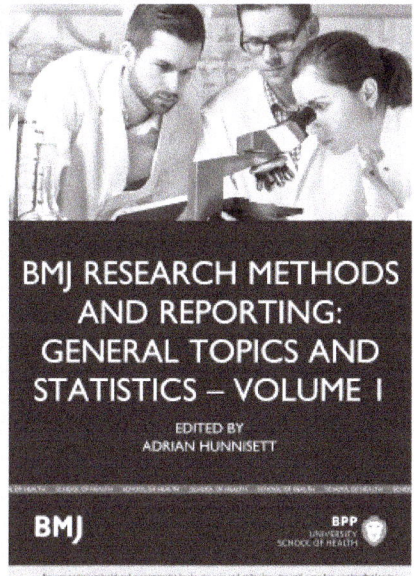

This book is the first of two volumes drawing together a collection of articles previously published in The BMJ covering contemporary issues in research. The articles give key messages about the 'nuts and bolts' of doing research, particularly with reference to statistical approaches, methods and interpretation. Each article also provides linked information and explicit evidence to support the statements made. The topics covered answer key questions asked by researchers on subjects such as confidence intervals, p values, same size calculations, use of patient reported outcome measures, conundrums in the application of RCT and more complex statistical analysis. It also highlights implementation research and prognostic research. Each article is written by an expert in the field and the volume brings together a masterclass in research topics.

£29.99

February 2016

Paperback

978-1-472745-56-9

BPP
UNIVERSITY
SCHOOL OF HEALTH

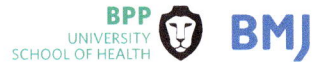

More titles in The BMJ Research Methods and Reporting Series

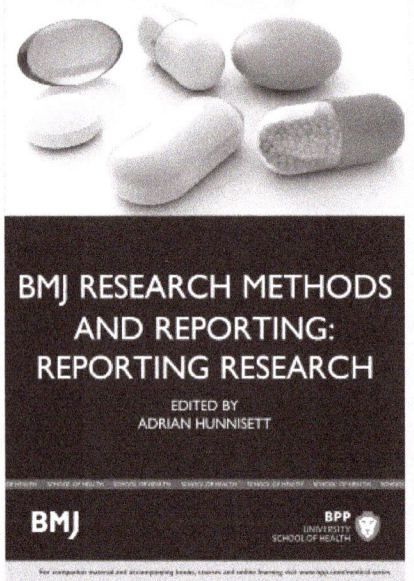

This book is the third of three volumes drawing together a collection of articles previously published in The BMJ covering contemporary issues in research. In this volume, the articles give key messages about the 'nuts and bolts' of doing research, particularly with reference to how research findings should be reported. Each article also provides linked information and explicit evidence to support the statements made. The topics covered take a look at guidelines such as CONSORT, SPIRIT, GPP2, PRISMA and the IDEAL framework for surgical innovation. It also gives some guidance on economic evaluations, policy and service interventions and publication guidelines, as well as providing useful tips on preparing data for publication. Each article is written by an expert in the field and the volume brings together a masterclass in research reporting.

£29.99

February 2016

Paperback

978-1-472745-57-6

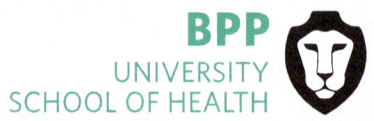

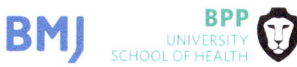
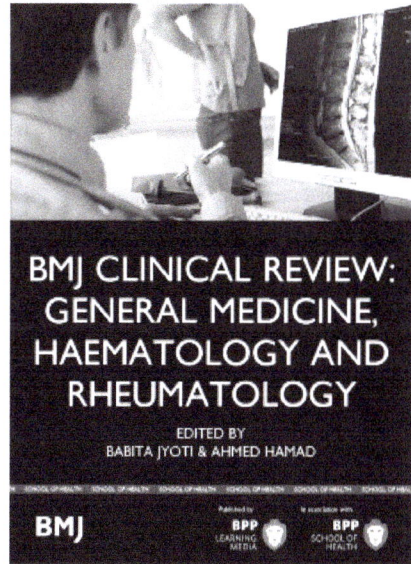
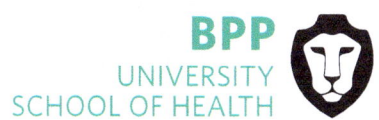

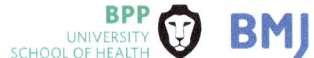

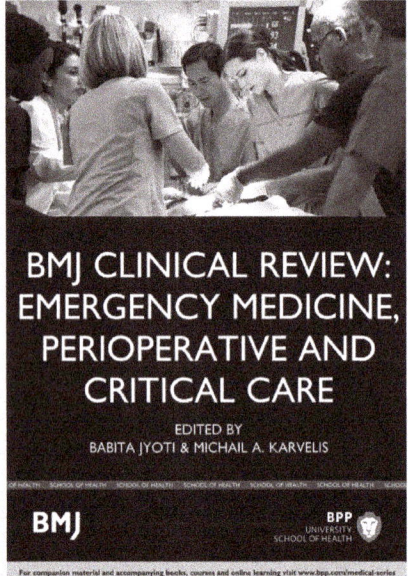
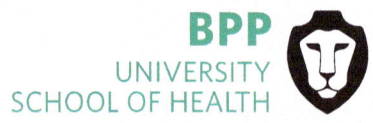

More titles from BPP School of Health

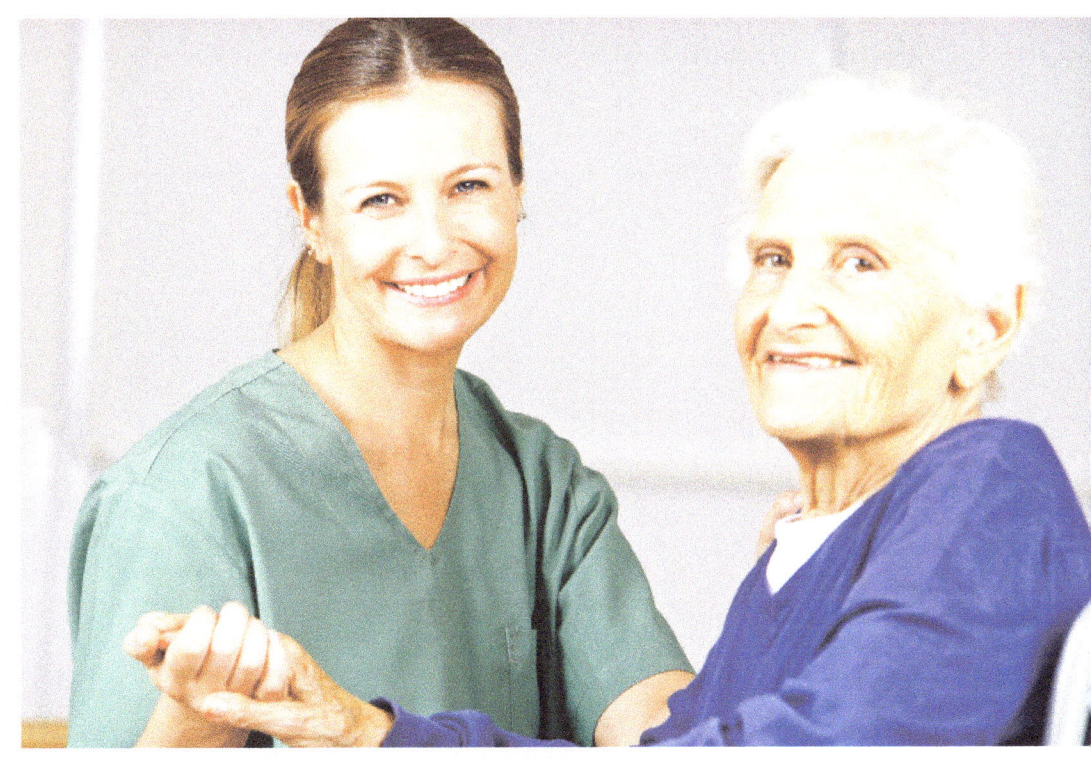

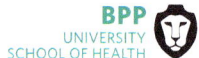

More titles in The Progressing Your Medical Career Series

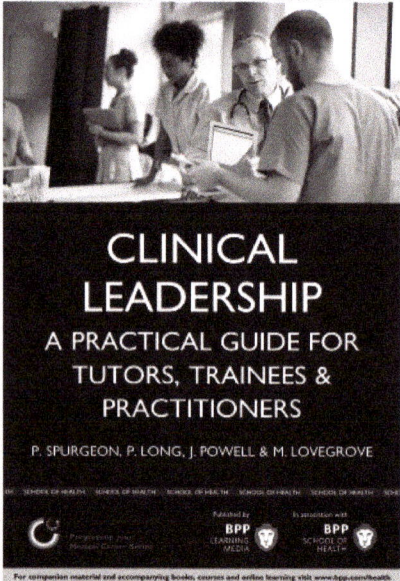

CLINICAL LEADERSHIP

A PRACTICAL GUIDE FOR TUTORS, TRAINEES & PRACTITIONERS

P. SPURGEON, P. LONG, J. POWELL & M. LOVEGROVE

£24.99

June 2015

Paperback

978-1-472727-83-1

Are you a healthcare professional or student who wishes to acquire and develop your leadership and management skills? Do you recognise the role and influence of strong leadership and management in modern healthcare?

Clinical leadership is something in which all healthcare professionals can participate in, in terms of driving forward high quality care for their patients. In this up-to-date guide, the authors take you through the latest leadership and management thinking, and how this links in with the Clinical Leadership Competency Framework. As well as influencing undergraduate curricula this framework forms the basis of the leadership component of the curricula for all healthcare specialties, so a practical knowledge of it is essential for all healthcare professionals in training.

Using case studies and practical exercises to provide a strong work-based emphasis, this practical guide will enable you to build on your existing experiences to develop your leadership and management skills, and to develop strategies and approaches to improving care for your patients.

This book addresses:

- Why strong leadership and management are crucial to delivering high quality care;
- The theory and evidence behind the Clinical Leadership Competency Framework;
- The practical aspects of leadership learning in a wide range of clinical environments
- How clinical professionals and trainers can best facilitate leadership learning for their trainees and students within the clinical work-place.

Whether you are a student just starting out on your career, or an established healthcare professional wishing to develop yourself as a clinical leader, this practical, easy-to-use guide will give you the techniques and knowledge you require to excel.

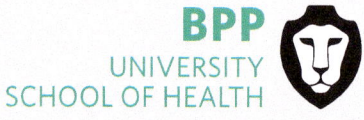

BPP
UNIVERSITY
SCHOOL OF HEALTH

www.bpp.com/medical-series

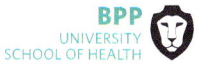

More titles in The Progressing Your Medical Career Series

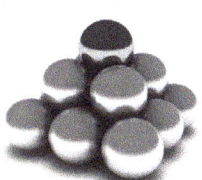

MEDICAL LEADERSHIP
A PRACTICAL GUIDE FOR TUTORS & TRAINEES

PROFESSOR PETER SPURGEON & DR BOB KLABER

Foreword by Professor Parveen Kumar CBE MD FRCP FRCP(E) FRCPath
Consultant Physician & Gastroenterologist
President of the Royal Society of Medicine
Co-author of Kumar & Clark's 'Clinical Medicine'

For companion material and accompanying books, courses and online learning visit www.bpp.com/health

£19.99
November 2011
Paperback
978-1-445379-57-9

Are you a doctor or medical student who wishes to acquire and develop your leadership and management skills? Do you recognise the role and influence of strong leadership and management in modern medicine?

Clinical leadership is something in which all doctors should have an important role in terms of driving forward high quality care for their patients. In this up-to-date guide Peter Spurgeon and Robert Klaber take you through the latest leadership and management thinking, and how this links in with the Medical Leadership Competency Framework. As well as influencing undergraduate curricula and some of the concepts underpinning revalidation, this framework forms the basis of the leadership component of the curricula for all medical specialties, so a practical knowledge of it is essential for all doctors in training.

Using case studies and practical exercises to provide a strong work-based emphasis, this practical guide will enable you to build on your existing experiences to develop your leadership and management skills, and to develop strategies and approaches to improving care for your patients.

This book addresses:

- Why strong leadership and management are crucial to delivering high quality care

- The theory and evidence behind the Medical Leadership Competency Framework

- The practical aspects of leadership learning in a wide range of clinical environments (eg handover, EM, ward etc)

- How Consultants and trainers can best facilitate leadership learning for their trainees and students within the clinical work-place

Whether you are a medical student just starting out on your career, or an established doctor wishing to develop yourself as a clinical leader, this practical, easy-to-use guide will give you the techniques and knowledge you require to excel.

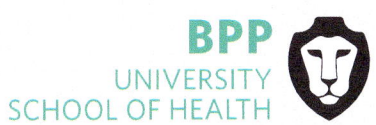

BPP
UNIVERSITY
SCHOOL OF HEALTH

www.bpp.com/medical-series

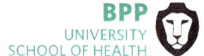

More titles in The Progressing Your Medical Career Series

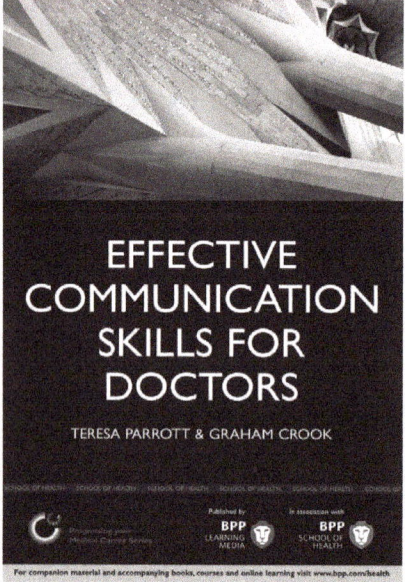

£19.99

September 2011

Paperback

978-1-445379-56-2

Would you like to know how to improve your communication skills? Are you looking for a clearly written book which explores all aspects of effective medical communication?

There is an urgent need to improve doctors' communication skills. Research has shown that poor communication can contribute to patient dissatisfaction, lack of compliance and increased medico-legal problems. Improved communication skills will impact positively on all of these areas.

The last fifteen years have seen unprecedented changes in medicine and the role of doctors. Effective communication skills are vital to these new roles. But communication is not just related to personality. Skills can be learned which can make your communication more effective, and help you to improve your relationships with patients, their families and fellow doctors.

This book shows how to learn those skills and outlines why we all need to communicate more effectively. Healthcare is increasingly a partnership. Change is happening at all levels, from government directives to patient expectations. Communication is a bridge between the wisdom of the past and the vision of the future.

Readers of this book can also gain free access to an online module which upon successful completion can download a certificate for their portfolio of learning/ Revalidation/CPD records.

This easy-to-read guide will help medical students and doctors at all stages of their careers improve their communication within a hospital environment.

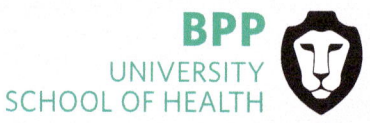

BPP
UNIVERSITY
SCHOOL OF HEALTH

www.bpp.com/medical-series

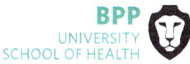

More Titles in The Progressing Your Medical Career Series

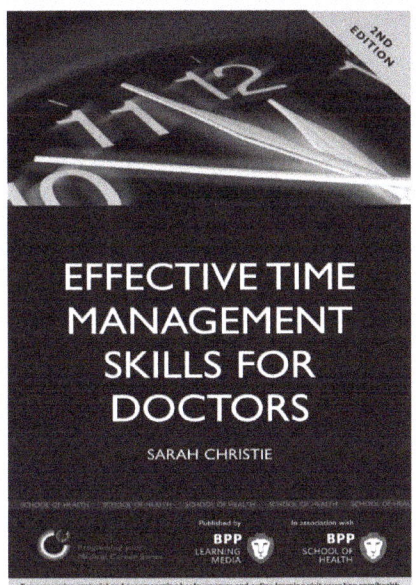

£19.99

October 2011

Paperback

978-1-906839-08-6

Do you find it difficult to achieve a work-life balance? Would you like to know how you can become more effective with the time you have?

With the introduction of the European Working Time Directive, which will severely limit the hours in the working week, it is more important than ever that doctors improve their personal effectiveness and time management skills. This interactive book will enable you to focus on what activities are needlessly taking up your time and what steps you can take to manage your time better.

By taking the time to read through, complete the exercises and follow the advice contained within this book you will begin to:

- Understand where your time is being needlessly wasted

- Discover how to be more assertive and learn how to say 'No'

- Set yourself priorities and stick to them

- Learn how to complete tasks more efficiently

- Plan better so you can spend more time doing the things you enjoy

In recent years, with the introduction of the NHS Plan and Lord Darzi's commitment to improve the quality of healthcare provision, there is a need for doctors to become more effective within their working environment. This book will offer you the chance to regain some clarity on how you actually spend your time and give you the impetus to ensure you achieve the tasks and goals which are important to you.

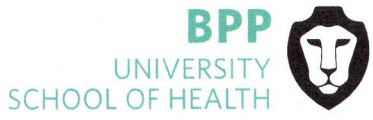

BPP
UNIVERSITY
SCHOOL OF HEALTH

www.bpp.com/medical-series

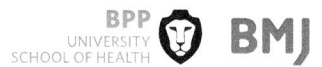